CC Chatterjee's

Manual of
Practical
Physiology

As per Medical Council of India: *Competency based Undergraduate Curriculum for the Indian Medical Graduate*

CC Chatterjee's

Manual of Practical **Physiology**

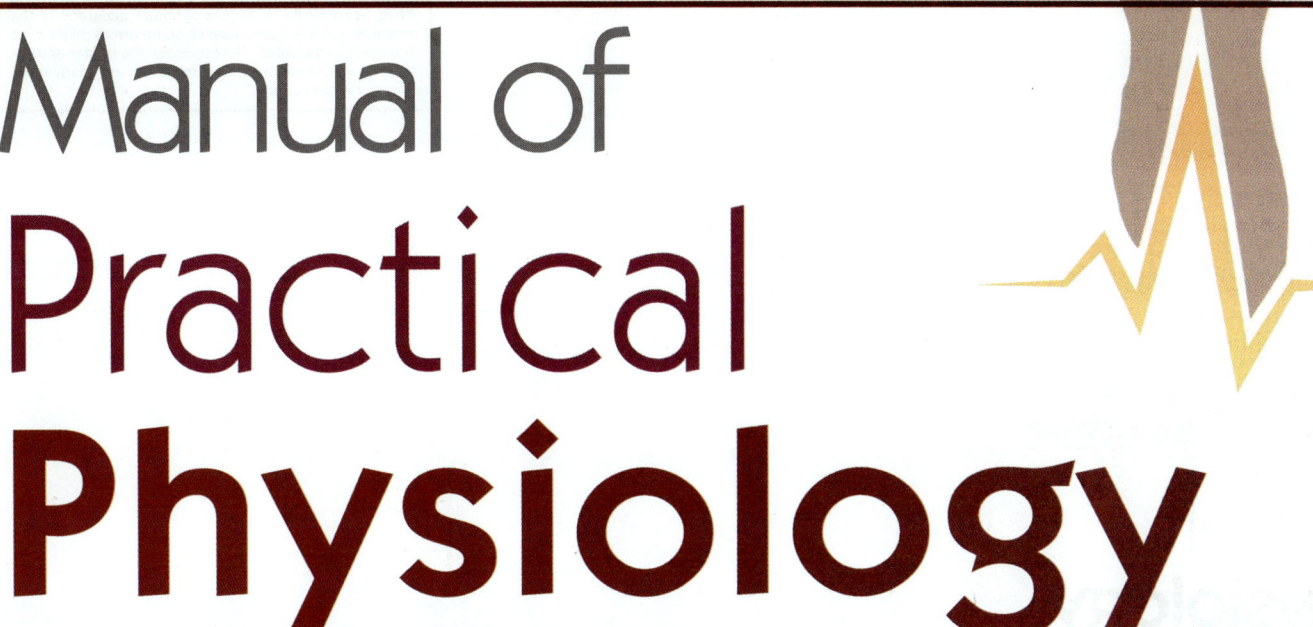

As per Medical Council of India: *Competency based Undergraduate Curriculum for the Indian Medical Graduate*

Nitin Ashok John MD, DIH, PGDMLE, PGDHA
Professor and Head
Department of Physiology
Dr. Ram Manohar Lohia Institute of Medical Sciences
Lucknow, UP

Surrinder H Singh MBBS, MD, FIMSA, MAMS, FIMA-MS
Ex-Professor of Physiology
Lady Hardinge Medical College
New Delhi
Visiting Faculty and Consultant
Pt Deendayal Upadhyaya Institute for
Physically Handicapped
New Delhi

Yuvraj Gharu MBBS, MD
Professor
Department of Physiology
Indira Gandhi Medical College
Shimla, HP

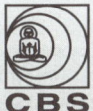

CBS

CBS Publishers & Distributors Pvt Ltd

New Delhi • Bengaluru • Chennai • Kochi • Kolkata • Mumbai
Hyderabad • Jharkhand • Nagpur • Patna • Pune • Uttarakhand

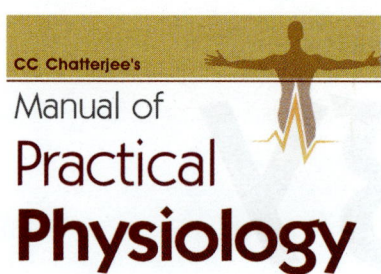

CC Chatterjee's
Manual of
Practical
Physiology

ISBN: 978-93-89017-64-9

Copyright © Authors and Publisher

First Edition: 2020

Reprint: 2021

Published by Satish Kumar Jain and produced by Varun Jain for

CBS Publishers & Distributors Pvt Ltd

4819/XI Prahlad Street, 24 Ansari Road, Daryaganj, New Delhi 110 002, India
Ph: 011-23289259, 23266861, 23266867   Website: www.cbspd.com
Fax: 011-23243014   e-mail: delhi@cbspd.com; cbspubs@airtelmail.in
Corporate Office: 204 FIE, Industrial Area, Patparganj, Delhi 110 092

Ph: 011-4934 4934   Fax: 011-4934 4935   e-mail: publishing@cbspd.com; publicity@cbspd.com

Branches

• **Bengaluru:** Seema House 2975, 17th Cross, K.R. Road, Banasankari 2nd Stage, Bengaluru 560 070, Karnataka
  Ph: +91-80-26771678/79   Fax: +91-80-26771680   e-mail: bangalore@cbspd.com
• **Chennai:** 7, Subbaraya Street, Shenoy Nagar, Chennai 600 030, Tamil Nadu
  Ph: +91-44-26680620, 26681266   Fax: +91-44-42032115   e-mail: chennai@cbspd.com
• **Kochi:** 42/1325, 1326, Power House Road, Opp. KSEB, Power House, Ernakulam 682018, Kochi, Kerala
  Ph: +91-484-4059061-65   Fax: +91-484-4059065   e-mail: kochi@cbspd.com
• **Kolkata:** No. 6/B, Ground Floor, Rameswar Shaw Road, Kolkata 700014 (West Bengal), India
  Ph: +91-33-2289-1126, 2289-1127, 2289-1128   e-mail: kolkata@cbspd.com
• **Mumbai:** PWD Shed, Gala No. 25/26, Ramchandra Bhatt Marg, Next to JJ Hospital, Gate No. 2 Opp. Union Bank of India, Noorbaug, Mumbai 400009, Maharashtra, India
  Ph: +91-22-66661880/89   e-mail: mumbai@cbspd.com

Representatives

• **Hyderabad** 0-9885175004   • **Jharkhand** 0-9811541605   • **Nagpur**   0-9421945513
• **Patna**   0-9334159340   • **Pune**   0-9623451994   • **Uttarakhand** 0-9716462459

Printed at Goyal Offset Works Pvt. Ltd. Haryana, India

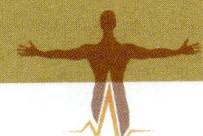

Preface

It gives us immense pleasure to author the *CC Chatterjee's Manual of Practical Physiology* as per PC, MCI BOG competency-based curriculum 2018. This practical manual is also immensely helpful for students of paramedical courses, Pharmacy, Nursing and AYUSH (Ayurvedic, Unani, Siddha and Homeopathy) as it has also been meticulously covering their prescribed practical physiology curriculum.

The salient features of the Manual are:

1. Simple and easy to understand format of practicals is supplemented with frequently asked viva voce questions and answers.
2. Spotters for haematology, clinical and amphibian experiments have been separately covered in detail.
3. Coloured photographs and diagrams especially of haematology shall give clear picture of morphological features of cells in health and diseased.
4. The new practicals as per MCI BOG competency-based curriculum has been introduced: Basic Life Support, Anthropometric Measurements, Interpretation of Growth Chart, Harvard Fitness Index, etc. have been covered in this edition.
5. This book also incorporates the practicals written by the legendary physiologist CC Chatterjee.

We especially thank:

a. Dr Jyoti John, Additional Professor, Department of Biochemistry, for writing a practical photometric colorimetry.
b. Dr Deepak Maluya, Professor and Head, Department of Anaesthesia, and Ex-Director, Dr. Ram Manohar Lohia Institute of Medical Sciences, Lucknow, for writing practical on basic life support.
c. Dr Abhishek Madhura, Assistant Professor, Pediatric Government Medical College, Nagpur, for writing practicals in interpretation of growth chart.

We are thankful to Mr SK Jain, CMD, CBS Publishers & Distributors, New Delhi.

In spite of our best efforts, errors if any, due to omission or commission, may be excused. Your valuable suggestions will help us to update the book further.

Nitin Ashok John
Surrinder H Singh
Yuvraj Gharu

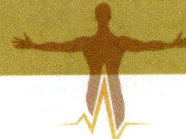

Contents

Preface   *v*

Unit 1
Haematology Practicals with Spotters

1. Introduction   3

2. Collection of Blood Samples   11

3. Haemocytometry   18

4. Estimation of Haemoglobin   26

5. Determination of Red Blood Cells Count   35

6. Determination of Red Blood Cell Indices   41

    Genesis of White Blood Cells and Red Blood Cells 45
    Genesis of Monocytes and Lymphocytes 46
    Structure of Platelet and its Genesis 47

7. Determination of Total Leucocyte Count   48

8. Preparation of Peripheral Blood Smear and Determination of   53
    Differential Leucocyte Count

9. Arneth Count   62

10. Determination of Absolute Eosinophil Count   67

11. Determination of Blood Groups (A, B, O and Rh System)   71

12. Determination of Bleeding Time (BT) and Clotting Time (CT)   77

13. Platelet Count   84

14. Reticulocyte Count　　　　　　　　　　　　　　　　　　89

15. Determination of Erythrocyte Sedimentation Rate (ESR) and　　92
Packed Cell Volume (PCV)

16. Determination of Osmotic Fragility of Red Blood Cells　　　97

Spotters　　　　　　　　　　　　　　　　　　　　　　103

Unit 2
Clinical Practicals with Spotters

1. General Clinical Examination　　　　　　　　　　　　　121

2. Examination of Arterial Pulse　　　　　　　　　　　　　126

3. Blood Pressure Recording　　　　　　　　　　　　　　131

4. Cardiorespiratory Response to Exercise　　　　　　　　140

5. Autonomic Function Test　　　　　　　　　　　　　　142

6. Clinical Examination of Cardiovascular System　　　　　147

7. Electrocardiography: Recording of Normal Electrocardiogram　153

8. Experiment to Record Blood Flow in the Arm　　　　　　164

9. Spirometry—Measurement of Lung Volume and Capacities and　167
Recording Peak Expiratory Flow

10. Clinical Examination of the Respiratory System　　　　　174

11. Stethography Recording of Respiratory Movements　　　　180

12. Determination of Physical Fitness of the Subject　　　　　184

13. Examination of Abdomen　　　　　　　　　　　　　189

14. Reproduction　　　　　　　　　　　　　　　　　194

15. Pregnancy Diagnostic Test ... 198

16. Examination of Central Nervous System ... 201

17. Examination of the Sensory System ... 204

18. Examination of the Motor System ... 211

19. Reflexes ... 216

20. Cranial Nerves ... 224

21. Cerebellar Function Tests ... 238

22. Perimetry ... 242

23. Electroencephalogram (EEG) ... 249

Clinical Spotters ... *257*

Unit 3
Amphibian Practicals with Spotters

1. Introduction to Amphibian Experiments ... 283

2. Apparatus for Amphibian Experiments ... 285

3. Nerve Muscle Preparation ... 293

4. Simple Muscle Twitch ... 295

5. Effect of Temperature on Simple Muscle Twitch ... 298

6. Velocity of Nerve Impulse ... 300

7. Effects of Two Successive Stimuli ... 303

8. Genesis of Fatigue in the Isolated Nerve Muscle Preparation ... 306

9. Effect of Increasing the Strength of Stimulus ... 309

10. Genesis of Tetanus ... 312

11. Effect of After Load and Free Load on Muscle Contraction and Calculation of Work Done ... 315

12. Recording of Normal Cardiogram   318

13. Effect of Temperature on Frog's Heart   321

14. Properties of Cardiac Muscle   323

15. Properties of Cardiac Muscle II   327

16. Effects of Various Drugs on the Frog Heart Muscle   330

Spotters   *333*

Appendices   *349*

     1. Photometry and Spectrophotometry   349
     2. Artificial Respiration or Resuscitation   352
     3. Anthropometric Measurement   356
     4. Interpretation of Growth Chart   360

Haematology Practicals with Spotters

PY 2.11*, PY 2.12*, PY 2.13*

1. Introduction
2. Collection of Blood Samples
3. Haemocytometry
4. Estimation of Haemoglobin
5. Determination of Red Blood Cells Count
6. Determination of Red Blood Cell Indices
7. Determination of Total Leucocyte Count
8. Preparation of Peripheral Blood Smear and Determination of Differential Leucocyte Count
9. Arneth Count
10. Determination of Absolute Eosinophil Count
11. Determination of Blood Groups (A, B, O and Rh System)
12. Determination of Bleeding Time (BT) and Clotting Time (CT)
13. Platelet Count
14. Reticulocyte Count
15. Determination of Erythrocyte Sedimentation Rate (ESR) and Packed Cell Volume (PCV)
16. Determination of Osmotic Fragility of Red Blood Cells
    Spotters

*Competency achievement as per competency based Undergraduate Curriculum for the Indian Medical Graduate, 2018, 1; Medical Council of India.

1

Introduction

I. THE STUDY OF COMPOUND MICROSCOPE

Learning Objectives

The student after completing the practical should be able to:
1. Identify and able to explain the uses of parts of a compound microscope.
2. Focus the given blood smear using low power, high power and oil immersion objective lenses.
3. Enlist precautions to be taken while using the microscope.
4. Discuss the care to be taken while transporting, handling, and cleaning and storage of the microscope.
5. Understand the importance of learning microscopy and its implication in clinical practice.

Aim of experiment: To study the compound microscope.

Instrument: Compound microscope.

Description of the instrument: Microscope is an instrument used to visualize objects which cannot be seen by the naked eye. Microscope may be simple or compound microscope. The compound microscope is commonly used by the students in haematology lab.
1. A simple microscope consists of a lens or set of lenses which produces an erect enlarged virtual image. Simple microscope does not produce high magnification.
2. The compound microscope is an instrument for magnifying small objects. It is consisting of an objective lens of short focal length for forming a real image of the object inside the microscope (Fig. 1.1) and is further magnified by a second lens (eyepiece) of longer focal length forming enlarged inverted virtual image of the object (Fig. 1.2). Refer to Fig. 1.1. The objective and eyepiece together allow much higher magnification and reduces chromatic aberration.

PRINCIPLE OF WORKING OF A COMPOUND MICROSCOPE

Principle: The objective lens focuses a real image (Fig. 1.1) of the object inside the microscope. That image is then magnified by a second lens or group of eyepiece lenses producing enlarged inverted virtual image (Fig. 1.2) of the object.

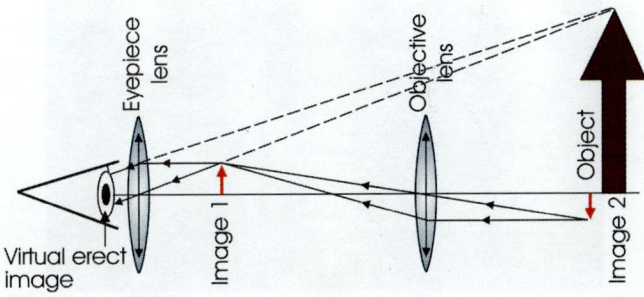

Fig. 1.1: Image formation under compound microscope

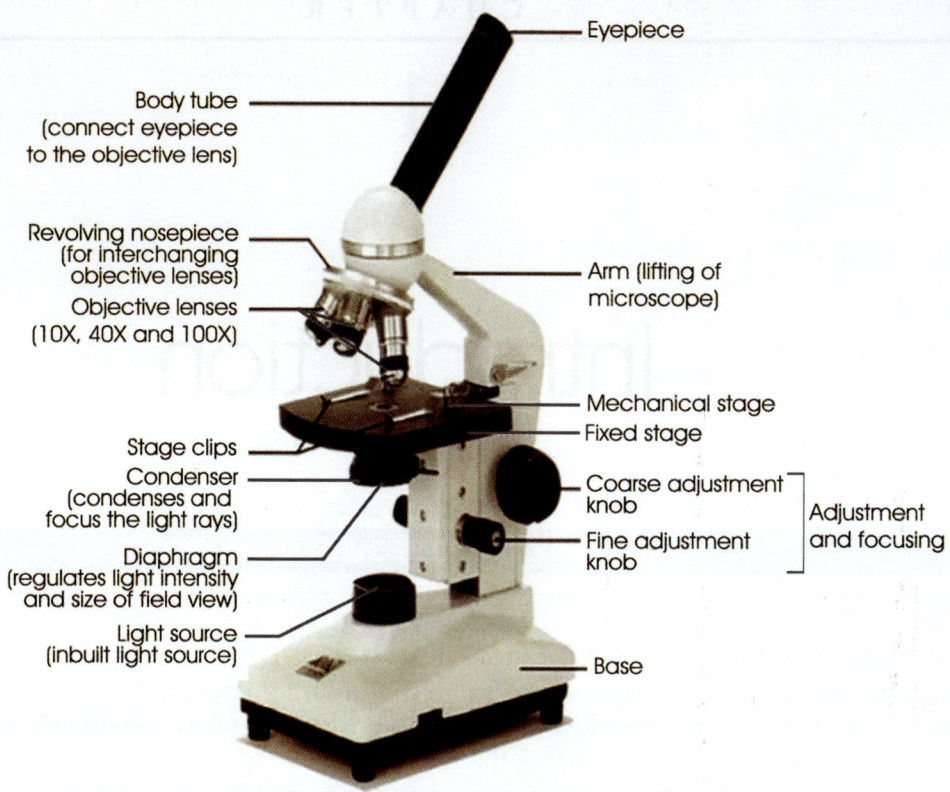

Eyepiece

Body tube
(connect eyepiece
to the objective lens)

Revolving nosepiece
(for interchanging
objective lenses)

Objective lenses
(10X, 40X and 100X)

Arm (lifting of
microscope)

Mechanical stage
Fixed stage

Stage clips

Condenser
(condenses and
focus the light rays)

Coarse adjustment
knob

Fine adjustment
knob

Adjustment
and focusing

Diaphragm
(regulates light intensity
and size of field view)

Light source
(inbuilt light source)

Base

Fig. 1.2: Compound microscope

PARTS OF THE MICROSCOPE

Eyepiece lens: These are the lens at the top through which we make our observations. They are usually of 10X power.

Tube: It connects the eyepiece to the objective lenses.

Revolving nosepiece: It holds two or more objective lenses and can be rotated to easily change power.

Objective lenses: The three objective lenses commonly present on a microscope are having 10X, 40X and 100X powers. Together with a 10X eyepiece lens the total magnifications produced will be of 100X (10X times 10X), 400X and 1000X.

> **Key Notes**
>
> The oil immersion lens the highest magnification and least working length. It is so called oil immersion lens because it is to be used with a drop of oil having the same refractive index as that of the glass slide so that the loss of light rays coming from the object can be minimized. Cedar wood oil is commonly used to minimize the loss of light rays coming from the object as its refractive index is 1.515 which is the same as that of glass.

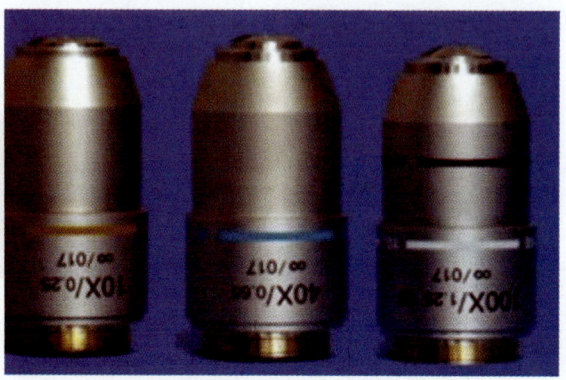

Fig. 1.3: Objective lenses of microscope

Arm: The handle supports the optical system of lenses and can be used for lifting the microscope.

Illumination: Light from an electric bulb or sunlight acts as the source of illumination. The light rays are reflected by a plane concave mirror provided at the base. Modern microscope has inbuilt light source of 110 volts in place of a mirror.

Stage: It consists of a horizontal platform on which the slide is mounted. The stage clips hold the slides in place and keeps it stable. It has a central aperture which allows the reflected light rays to fall on the object. A mechanical stage is fitted to the fixed stage so that the object can be moved from side to side or from front to back.

Substage: This is located below the stage and it consists of a condenser and an iris diaphragm. The condenser consists of lenses which condenses and focuses the light rays from the mirror on to the object. The condenser can be lowered or raised by moving of the knob which is located at the side. The iris **diaphragm** is used to control the amount of light reaching the object.

Diaphragm: The diaphragm consists of varied sized holes due to which various intensity of light can be projected upward into the slide. The setting of diaphragm is carried out by the observer depending on transparency of the specimen, the degree of contrast expected and the type of objective lens which is in use.

Focus adjustment knobs: There are two focus adjustment knobs present at the side of the microscope. The bigger knob is utilized for coarse adjustment and focusing while the smaller knob is utilized for fine focusing. The distance between the objective lens and object can be adjusted using these knobs so that the object lies at the focal length of the objective.

Base: The microscope has a solid base which provides stability.

II. MAGNIFICATION

The product of power of eyepiece and that of power of objective determines the total magnifying power of the microscope. The total magnification achieved when viewing an image under a compound microscope, under the low-power lens (10X), the high-power lens (40X), and the oil-immersion lens (100X) shall be the power of the eyepiece which is 10X multiplied with power of lenses, that is, 10X, 40X and 100X respectively. Thus, magnification achieved is 100X with the low-power lens, 400X with the high-power lens, and 1000X with the oil-immersion lens.

III. RESOLUTION

The **resolution** of the microscope refers to the ability to see two items as separate objects and with clarity under the microscope. The resolving power depends on the numerical aperture of the lens and the wavelength of the light used for visualization. Shorter the wavelength of light, better will be the resolution. The **numerical aperture (NA)** refers to the widest cone of light entering the lens.

IV. WORKING DISTANCE

At low magnification your working distance is more and so vice versa when magnification is increased. This objective has the least working distance when observed under oil immersion lenses.

V. FOCUSING PROCEDURE

Under Low Power (10X)

a. Keep the slide to be focused on the mechanical stage and ensure that the stage clips are approximated so that it does not get displaced.
b. Focus the light on the object by adjusting the concave mirror.
c. Lower the low power objective (10X).
d. Lower the condenser from the higher position till the object is properly illuminated;
e. Keep the iris diaphragm partially opened and adjust the focus with the fine adjustment for a sharper image.

For High Power Magnification (40X)

a. Place the slide to be focused on the mechanical stage and ensure that the stage clips are approximated so that it does not get displaced.

b. First focus under low power and carefully observe and select the required area.

c. Rotate the revolving nosepiece and focus the high-power objective lens into visualization position.

d. Keep the iris diaphragm half opened.

e. Use plane mirror to condense the light on the object.

f. Raise the condenser and keep it in high position

g. Use the fine focusing knob to focus the object and visualize and note your observations carefully.

Under Oil Immersion (100X)

a. Place the slide to be focused on the mechanical stage and ensure that the stage clips are approximated so that it does not get displaced.

b. Place a drop of cedar wood oil over the area which is to be visualized

c. Keep the condenser at the highest position

d. Keep the iris diaphragm fully opened

e. Adjust the plane mirror to focus the light on the object.

f. Adjust the objective lens as it touches the slide, ensure that the slide is not broken.

g. Visualize the object and note your observations

Note: In microscope having inbuilt light source; there is no mirror and hence no such mirror adjustment are required.

BENEFITS OF USING A COMPOUND MICROSCOPE

The compound microscope is simple and convenient to use; it has also inbuilt light source; they have multiple lenses with varied magnification power (for example, 10X, 40X and 100X) that reveals a greater amount of details; and being small in size it is convenient to store and handle easily.

Precautions

1. **Transporting the microscope:** Handle the microscope with care. Support the base of the microscope and hold it uprightly while lifting it. Do not swing the microscope.

2. **Handling and cleaning the microscope:** Clean the eyepiece and objective lens gently with xylene before using the microscope. Do not touch the lens with hand as this will leave a fingerprint marks on lens; which will smudge the images. Use sterile gauze piece for cleaning the lenses and the glass slide.

3. **Care while using:** Do not lower the optical tube when you are looking through the eyepiece. After using the oil immersion lens, it should be cleaned with cotton soaked in xylol. Prefer minimal use of fine adjustment while viewing through low power, high power or oil immersion lens.

4. **Cleaning:** The students should clean all slides, place materials in rack or assigned appropriate place, and finally clean the work area. Discard the cover slips in the bin.

Types of Microscopes

1. **Simple microscope:** Simple microscope has a single lens for magnification. It has lower magnification as compared to compound microscope.

2. **Compound microscope:** The common magnifications of a compound microscope are 10X, 40X and 100X. The compound microscopes have high magnification but a low resolution.

3. **Dissection microscope or stereoscope:** This microscope is binocular (two eyes) and provides a three-dimensional image of the specimen and is especially used for studies related to anatomical dissection.

4. **Confocal microscope:** This microscope uses laser light which scan across the specimen and image is focused on a digital computer screen for further studies and evaluation.

5. **Scanning electron microscope:** They use electrons (negatively charged electrical particles) to magnify objects up to two million times. The 3-dimensional image is formed. The magnification and resolution of scanning electron microscope is high.

6. **Transmission electron microscope:** They also use electrons for illumination, but instead of scanning the surface (as with Scanning Electron Microscope) electrons are made to pass through very thin specimens. This forms a 2-dimensional view. The magnification and resolution of transmission electron microscope is high.

7. **Fluorescence microscope:** This type of microscope utilizes fluorescence to create an image. The sample specimens are stained with a fluorescent dye which gets bounded to specific component of the specimen. The light of a specific wavelength (or wavelengths) is absorbed by the fluorophores. This cause them to emit light of longer wavelengths producing auto fluorescence image based on their chemical constitutional makeup.

8. **Bright field microscope:** The bright field microscopes use transmitted light to observe targets at high magnification. They are used to observe live or stained cells.

9. **Phase contrast microscope:** The phase contrast microscopes are used for viewing transparent, unstained, live cells. Phase-contrast microscopy converts phase shifts in light passing via the transparent specimen to bright outlook of the image, thereby making them visible and identifiable so that their characteristics can further be studied.

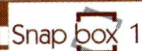
Snap box 1

Clinical Perspective

Microscope has been a diagnostic tool in clinical practice. Microscope has been in use for manual blood cell count of red blood cell, white blood cell, platelet, reticulocyte, Arneth, absolute eosinophil count, sperm count, etc. It is immensely helpful in histological and histopathological studies. Its application in diagnosis of anaemia, malaria, filaria, leukemia, diagnosis of cancerous conditions, parasitic disorders, cell culture studies, etc. has been boon to medical sciences.

EXERCISE FOR STUDENTS
OSPE Non-skilled

1. Label the parts of microscope in the figure below:

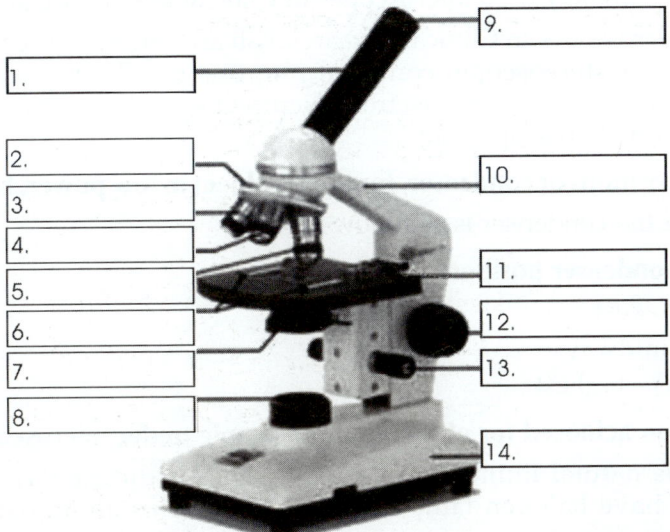

Fig. 1.4

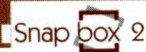
Snap box 2

Nobel Prize in Chemistry for the year 2014 was awarded to Eric Betzig, William Moerner and Stefan Hell 2014, for the development of super-resolved fluorescence microscopy. The newly developed technique brought optical microscopy into the Nano dimension.

Bibliography

Lippincott-Schwartz J. Profile of Eric Betzig, Stefan Hell, and W. E. Moerner, 2014 Nobel Laureates in Chemistry. ProcNatlAcadSci USA. 2015 Mar 3;112(9):2630–2.

VIVA VOCE QUESTIONS

Q1. What is the power of eyepiece lens?

Ans. The power of eyepiece lens usually 10X or 15X power.

Q2. What is the function of tube in compound microscope?

Ans. The tube connects the eyepiece to the objective lenses.

Q3. What is the function of arm in compound microscope?

Ans. The arm supports the tube and connects it to the base.

Q4. What is the function of base in compound microscope?

Ans. The base is the bottom of the microscope, used for support.

Q5. What is the source of illumination in your compound microscope?

Ans. The microscope has a mirror which reflect light from an external light source up via the bottom of the stage. In modern compound microscope a light source of 100 volts is inbuilt instead of mirror.

Q6. What is the function of stage in compound microscope?

Ans. The stage is flat platform where slides are placed. The stage clips keep the slide approximated in place. A mechanical stage is fitted to the fixed stage so that the object can be moved from side to side or from front to back.

Q7. What is the function of nosepiece in compound microscope?

Ans. The nosepiece is the part that holds two or more objective lenses which can be rotated to change power.

Q8. What are the power of objective lenses of compound microscope?

Ans. The power of objective lenses of compound microscope commonly used are of power 10X, 40X and 100X.

Q9. What are the types of commonly used microscopes in Clinical Research Lab?

Ans. The commonly used microscopes in Clinical Research Lab are simple microscope, compound microscope, dissection microscope or stereoscope, confacial microscope, fluorescence microscope, bright field microscope, phase contrast microscope, electron microscope (includes transmission electron microscope and the scanning electron microscope), etc.

Q10. Which are the desired positions of condenser, for seeing object in low power, high power and oil immersion?

Ans. The desired position of the condenser is as follows:

Objective lens power condenser position
  i. Low power (10X)—lowest
  ii. High power (40X)—midway
  iii. Oil immersion (100X)—highest

Q11. How are the illumination achieved for observation of sample under microscope?

Ans. The normal daylight is natural illuminating source which is directed via a mirror on to the sample. Modern microscopes have halogen lamp, LEDs and lasers as an adjustable and controllable light source.

Q12. What is the role of condenser in the microscope?

Ans. The condenser is a lens designed to focus light from the illumination source onto the sample. The condenser consists a diaphragm to control the quality and intensity of the illumination.

Q13. What do you understand by magnification of a compound optical microscope?

Ans. The magnification of a compound optical microscope is the product of the powers of the ocular (eyepiece) lens and the objective lens.

Q14. How much is the total magnification achieved when viewing an image under a compound microscope, under the low-power lens (10X), the high-power lens (40X), or the oil-immersion lens (100X)?

Ans. The total magnification achieved when viewing an image under a compound microscope, under the low-power lens (10X), the high-power lens (40X), or the oil-immersion lens (100X) is obtained by multiplying the power of the eyepiece which is 10X with power of the lens, thus the total magnifications of the low-power lens will be 100X, 400X of the high-power lens, and 1000X of the oil-immersion lens.

Q15. What is the principle advantage of an oil immersion objective?

Ans. The oil-immersion objectives offer greater resolution at high magnification.

Q16. Which oil is used for magnification under oil immersion objective? What is its advantage?

Ans. Cedar wood oil is used as index-matching material. The refractive index of the cedar wood oil is higher than air; due to which the objective lens achieve a larger numerical aperture (greater than 1). The larger numerical aperture allows minimal refraction enabling more light to be transmitted and object can be observed with clarity.

Q17. Define numerical aperture, working distance and resolving power of the lens.

Ans. The numerical aperture is a measure of the amount of light entering the objective lens. The working distance is approximately equal to the focal length. The resolving power of an objective lens is measured by its ability to differentiate two lines or points in an object:

$$\text{Minimum separable difference} = \frac{0.61 \times \text{wavelength of light}}{\text{Numerical aperture}}$$

Q18. What will happen to image under focus, if the aperture of oil immersion objective lens is more than a pin-hole aperture?

Ans. In case the aperture of oil immersion lens is more than a pin-hole; spherical and chromatic aberration would distort the image.

Q19. What is phase contrast microscopy?

Ans. The phase contrast microscopy is an optical microscopy illumination technique; in which small phase shifts in the light passing through a transparent specimen are converted into amplitude for contrast changes in the image. This microscope technique made it possible to study the cell cycle in live cells.

Q20. Name the variants of the electron microscopes.

Ans. The major variants of electron microscopes are scanning electron microscope (SEM) and the transmission electron microscope (TEM).

Q21. What is fluorescence microscopy?

Ans. The sample is illuminated through the objective lens by narrow set of wavelengths of light. The light interacts with fluorophores in the sample eventually emitting light of a longer wavelength. The emitted light which forms up the image. This illuminating technique with the aid of fluorophores is called fluorescence microscopy.

Q22. Enlist the applications of optical microscopy.

Ans. Optical microscopy is used in histopathological studies for medical diagnosis and so also in nanotechnology, biotechnology, pharmaceutical research, microbiology, microelectronics and mineralogy.

Q23. How does digital microscope work?

Ans. The digital microscope uses optics and a digital camera to output an image to a monitor. A digital microscope often has its own in-built LED light source. The image is focused on the monitor.

Q24. What are the monocular, binocular and trinocular microscope?

Ans. A. Monocular microscope has provision for one eyepiece for viewing the specimen.
B. Binocular microscope has provision for two eyepieces; and is comfortable and easy to use.
C. Trinocular microscope has provision for third eyepiece tube that can be used by the third individual, for example, a learner student simultaneously or by a CCD camera.

Q25. What is the basic precaution to be taken in use of a microscope after its use?

Ans. The basic precaution to be taken in use of a microscope after its use is: Switch off the microscope when not in use. Place it in rack. Support the base of the microscope and hold it uprightly while lifting it. Do not swing the microscope.

Q26. Who received the Nobel Prize in Physics in 1986 for his work in scanning tunneling microscopy?

Ans. Gerd Binnig along with his colleague Heinrich Rohrer was awarded the Nobel Prize in Physics in 1986 for his work in scanning tunneling microscopy. Binnig and Rohrer developed the powerful microscopy technique that could form an image of individual atoms on a semiconductor surface or metal by scanning the tip of a needle over the surface at a height of only a few atomic diameters.

Q27. What are the advantages of binocular microscope?

Ans. The advantages of binocular microscope are the true depth perception of an image and moreover the use of dual eyepieces reduces strain on eyes especially when work on microscope is to be carried for long hours.

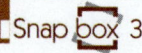 Snap box 3

HISTORICAL ASPECTS—INVENTION OF MICROSCOPE

Zacharias Jansen (1580–1638): He was a Dutch spectacle-maker from Middelburg and credited with inventing the first microscope. Although Zacharias Jansen (often written as Zacharias Janssen or Zacharias Jansen) is generally believed to be the first creator of a compound microscope, the accomplishment is dated around the 1590's, and many scholars believe that his father Hans must have played an important role in the creation of the instrument.

Anton van Leeuwenhoek (1632–1723): The father of microscopy Anton van Leeuwenhoek of Holland made several biological discoveries. He was the first to see and describe bacteria, yeast plants, the teeming life in a drop of water and the circulation of blood corpuscles in capillaries.

Robert Hooke (1635–1703): He was the English father of microscopy and he re-confirmed Anton van Leeuwenhoek's discoveries of the existence of tiny living organisms in a drop of water. Hooke made a copy of Leeuwenhoek's light microscope and then improved upon his design.

James Hillier (1915–January 15, 2007): Physicist James Hillier is recognized for his contributions to the development of the electron microscope. Hillier's work on the electron microscope began in college. He and a fellow graduate student built a model that magnified 7,000 times in the year 1937.

Bibliography

1. Ball, Vicent and Bauslaugh, Cheryl (January 18, 2007). "James Hillier". Brantford Expositor.pp. A1-A2, A8, A10-A11.

2. Frank N. Egerton (2006). "A History of the Ecological Sciences, Part 19: Leeuwenhoek's Microscopic Natural History". *Bulletin of the Ecological Society of America.* 87: 47

3. Franz Josef Giessibi, Christoph Gerber and G. Binnig, "A low-temperature atomic force/scanning tunneling microscope for ultrahigh vacuum", J. Vac. Sci. Technol. B9, 984–988 (1991).

4. Hall, AR (1951). "Robert Hooke and Horology". Notes and Records of the Royal Society of London. 8 (2): 167–177.

5. JD North, JJ Roche (2012). The Light of Nature: Essays in the History and Philosophy of Science presented to AC Crombie, Springer Science and Business Media. page 202.

OBSERVATIONS: EXERCISE FOR STUDENTS

1. Draw a well-labelled diagram of microscope. Describe its parts and their functions.

....

....

....

....

....

....

....

....

....

....

2

Collection of Blood Samples

Learning Objectives

The student after completing the practical should be able to:
1. Discuss the various methods of collection of blood sample.
2. Describe the common anticoagulants used *in vitro* and *in vivo*.
3. Draw capillary and venous blood.
4. Describe the precautions to be taken while withdrawing capillary and venous blood.
5. Discuss the significance and drawback of storage of blood.

Aim of experiment: To study the methods of collection of blood sample.

Materials: Disposable sterile lancet, 5 ml syringe, 22/23 gauze needle, cotton and spirit.

BASIC GUIDELINES FOR BLOOD COLLECTION

1. The use of sterile lancet with around 4 mm penetrating sharp points is recommended for purpose of pricking.
2. The cotton, gauze, needle and lancet should be sterile and autoclaved.
3. Disposable gloves should be worn prior to collection of blood sample.
4. The area from where blood sample is to be obtained is cleaned with methylated spirit. The area is made to dry before pricking is initiated.
5. Necessary instruction regarding the procedure should be given to subject prior to starting the procedure.

SOURCES FOR BLOOD COLLECTION

1. Capillary blood
2. Venous blood

Methods of Collection of Blood Sample

Principle: The two types of collection methods of blood samples are commonly employed in hematology and these are: **Capillary (peripheral) blood sampling** in which blood is collected by skin puncture and **venous blood sampling** via veins. The capillary blood is preferred when a little amount of blood is required for hematological investigations while venous blood sampling is done if large amount of blood is required.

Materials: Disposable sterile lancet, 5 ml syringe, 22/23 gauze needle, cotton and spirit.

- **Collection of capillary blood sample:** The site for collecting capillary blood is from fingertip and ear lobe in an adult and from the ball of the heel in infants.

Finger Prick Method (Fig. 2.1)

1. Clean the ring or middle finger with a spirit swab. Allow the area to dry.
2. Prick the fingertip using aseptic precaution using a sterile lancet. The prick should be deep enough to ensure a free flow of blood. The given prick should not be more than 3–4 mm deep.

3. Do not squeeze the finger to obtain blood, first drop of blood and it is to be wiped with sterile cotton. As first drop of blood is admixed with tissue fluids, it may interfere with the proper reporting of results. Always allow the blood to free flow.

4. The subsequent drop is collected and utilized to conduct various estimation. (For example, the blood is drawn into WBC/RBC pipette for carrying white blood cell count/red blood cell count or utilize for other practicals such as blood grouping, bleeding time and clotting time, etc.)

5. Apply firm pressure over the bleeding site by using cotton gauze and instruct the patient to hold it till the process of bleeding is stopped.

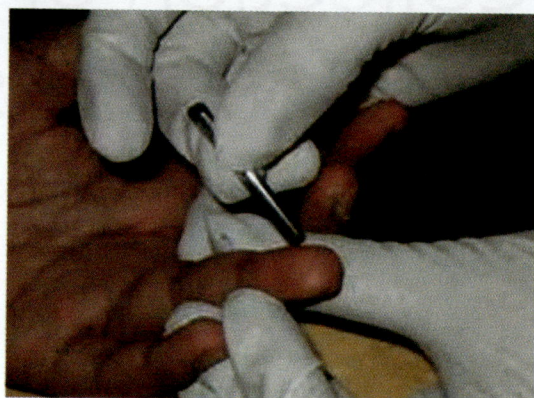

Fig. 2.1: Method of finger pricking

Precautions

1. Clean and scrub hand with soap and antiseptic solution. Dry your hand and always wear gloves for withdrawing any blood sample. Clean the fingertip area with spirit and allow it to dry.
2. The sterile disposable lancet must be used for pricking.
3. Ensure that you do not squeeze the finger in attempt to draw the blood as this dilutes the blood with tissue fluid.
4. Discard the first drop of blood as it gets admixed with tissue fluid.
5. Collect the blood from any one of the middle fingers; as palmar fascia of middle fingers is limited to hand itself while palmar fascia of thumb and little finger are in continuity with the limb.

Pricking the Ear Lobe (Fig. 2.2)

Method

1. Gently rub the ear lobe to make it warm. Clean the ear lobe area with methylated spirit and allow it to dry.
2. Make a single firm prick to a depth of 2–3 mm with a sterile needle of 22/23 gauze.
3. Wipe away the first few drops and collect the sample as the blood spontaneously flows thereafter.
4. Apply gentle pressure by cotton/gauze piece to ensure stoppage of bleeding.

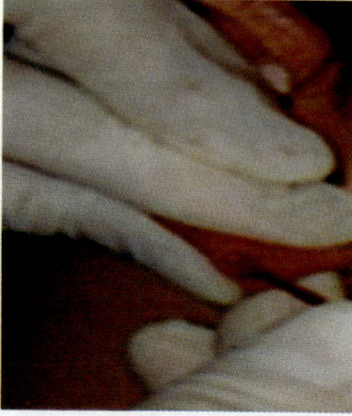

Fig. 2.2: Collection of capillary blood: Pricking of ear lobe

Pricking the Heel *(Fig. 2.3)*

Method

This method is used to obtain sample of blood in infants.

1. Warm the heel by gently rubbing it.
2. Clean the selected punctured site with methylated spirit and allow to dry it.
3. Give a deep prick on the lateral or medial parts of the plantar surface of the heel.
4. Ensure that you do not puncture posterior curvature and central plantar area as this may injure the tarsal bone.

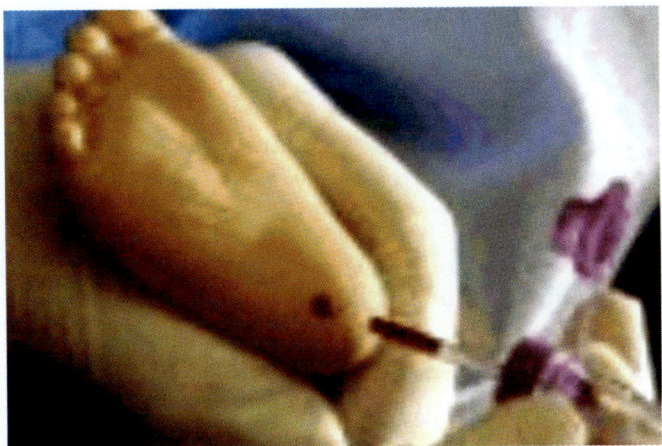

Fig. 2.3: Pricking of heel in infant to collect capillary blood

Collection of Venous Blood *(Fig. 2.4)*

Venous blood for hematological examinations can be obtained from the ante-cubital vein.

1. The subject is to be instructed to sit comfortably with his arm resting on the table.
2. Identify and locate a vein in the ante-cubital-fossa.
3. Apply a tourniquet around the upper arm and ask the subject to close his fist firmly in order to make the vein prominent.
4. Clean the skin over the selected area with spirit and allow it to dry.
5. Take a sterile dry 5 ml syringe with a 22 or 23 gauze needle and introduce the tip of the needle under the skin near the vein; and puncture the vein from the side; taking care to avoid a counter puncture. Ensure to keep the level of the needle up.
6. When blood flows into the syringe release the tourniquet and draw the required amount of blood.
7. As blood appears in the barrel pull the piston gently so that blood is further drawn in.
8. The needle should be withdrawn gently. Using a sterile cotton swab apply pressure and then instruct the subject to press the site firmly with aid of cotton swab for 2–3 minutes or till the bleeding stops.
9. Remove the needle from the syringe and deliver the blood into a sterile container containing anticoagulant.
10. Mix the blood with the anticoagulant by shaking the closed bottle gently over the table.
11. Rinse the needle and syringe with water and arrange for disposal.

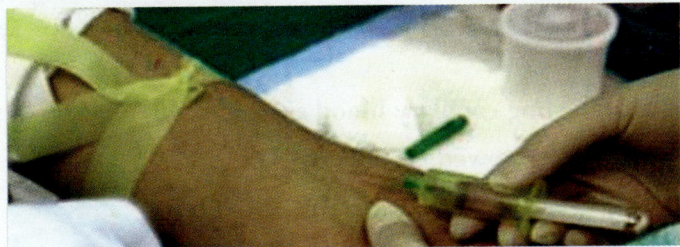

Fig. 2.4: Collecting venous blood sample

Precautions

1. Clean and scrub hand with soap and antiseptic solution.
2. Wear gloves prior to withdrawing the blood.
3. Always use sterile disposable needle and syringe for drawing the blood.
4. The area selected for puncture should be cleaned with methylated spirit and dry it.
5. The needle should be placed obliquely between 20–40%. This will prevent damaging the veins. Ensure needle is pierced gently, slowly and steadily. Feel the loss of resistance after needle passes 1–1.5 cm beneath.
6. Remove the tourniquet before drawing back the piston for collecting blood.
7. Ask the subject to press over the punctured area with cotton gauze piece for 3–5 minutes.
8. The blood should be emptied into appropriate bottle depending on the investigation for which the sample has been collected.

Anticoagulants

Anticoagulants prevent blood coagulation and allow separation of the blood into liquid (plasma) and cellular components. The plasma contains coagulation factors.

Anticoagulants

The common anticoagulants used are 3.8% trisodium citrate, potassium oxalate, ethylenediaminetetraacetic acid (EDTA), heparin, potassium ammonium oxalate and dicoumerol.

1. **Trisodium citrate:** 3.8% of trisodium citrate dissolved in distilled water is used as anticoagulant as it is isotonic with plasma. It prevents clotting of blood as it causes Ca^{++} to precipitate out as calcium sodium citrate. It is the anticoagulant of choice for prothrombin time, coagulation studies, and erythrocyte sedimentation rate (ESR).

2. **Double oxalate: Potassium ammonium oxalate:** In the double oxalate mixture, potassium oxalate and ammonium oxalate are mixed in ratio of 2:3. The solution of double oxalate contains 1.2% of ammonium oxalate and 0.8% potassium oxalate. It acts as anticoagulants and produces chelation of calcium.

   Action of double oxalate: The potassium oxalate causes shrinking of RBC while ammonium oxalate causes swelling of RBC. This opposing effect of the two salts maintains the volume of the red blood cells. Hence it is used as an anticoagulant for the determination of packed cell volume (PCV), WBC count, RBC.

3. **EDTA:** Ethylenediaminetetraacetic acid is a chelating agent which sequesters calcium, thereby rendering its unavailability for clotting. The chelating effect is achieved with a sample of 1.2 mg of EDTA/ml of blood. The EDTA is used for all hematological examination except coagulation studies. It inhibits aggregation of platelets and hence used in platelet count estimation.

4. **Acid citrate dextrose and citrate phosphate dextrose adenine** are used as an anticoagulant in blood bank for storage of blood, preserving blood specimens for tissue typing and for plasmapheresis.

5. **Sodium flouride:** 1 mg thymol along with 10 mg of sodium flouride exhibits an anticoagulant effect. It is used as anticoagulant for blood sugar estimation.

6. **Heparin:** It is a naturally occurring anticoagulant. It can be used both *in vivo* and *in vitro*. It facilitates the action of anti-thrombin III and inactivates clotting factors IX, X, XI and XII. Hence they are not available for the formation of prothrombin activator and thrombin, therefore, fibrinogen cannot be converted to fibrin. The sodium or lithium salt of heparin at a concentration of 10–20 IU/ml of blood is used for evaluating osmotic fragility of red blood cell and glucose-6-phosphate dehydrogenase enzymatic assay. Heparin is used as anticoagulants for estimation of electrolyte levels and in blood gas analysis.

EXERCISE FOR STUDENTS

OSPE Skilled

Q1. Perform the procedure of collecting capillary blood sample from fingertip in provided WBC / RBC pipette.

Finger prick method: Steps to be followed by student

1. Cleans the ring or middle finger with a spirit swab. (Yes/No)
2. Allows the wiped area to dry. (Yes/No)
3. Pricks the fingertip using a sterile lancet. The prick is deep enough to ensure a free flow of blood. (Yes/No)

4. Does not squeeze the finger to obtain blood; first drop of blood is wiped with sterile cotton. (Yes/No)

5. Wipes the drop of blood with cotton swab and presses it. The subsequent drop is collected and utilized for collection. (Yes/No)

6. Draws the blood into WBC/RBC pipette up to 0.5 mark. (Yes/No)

Q2. Perform the procedure of collecting venous blood sample from the antecubital vein.

Venous Blood Sampling

Steps to be followed by student:

1. Asks the subject to sit comfortably; with his arm resting on the table. (Yes/No)

2. Identify a vein in the antecubital fossa. (Yes/No)

3. Applies a tourniquet around the upper arm and ask the subject to close his fist firmly in order to make the vein prominent. (Yes/No)

4. Cleans the skin over the selected area with spirit and allow it to dry. (Yes/No)

5. Takes a sterile dry 5 ml syringe with a 23 gauze needle and introduce the tip of the needle under the skin near the vein; and puncture the vein from the side; taking care not to counter puncture. (Yes/No)

6. When blood flows into the syringe; releases the tourniquet and draw the required amount of blood. (Yes/No)

7. As blood appears in the barrel pulls the piston gently so that blood is further drawn in. (Yes/No)

8. The needle is withdrawn gently. Using a sterile cotton swab instruct subject to apply pressure for 2–3 minutes at the site of puncture to prevent blood loss. (Yes/No)

9. Remove the needle from the syringe and deliver the blood into a sterile container containing anticoagulant. (Yes/No)

10. Mix the blood with the anticoagulant by shaking the closed bottle gently over the table. (Yes/No)

11. Rinse the needle and syringe with water and arrange for disposal. (Yes/No)

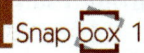 Snap box 1

Blood collection tubes: The blood collection tubes are drawn in a specific recommended order and specific tubes (blood collection tube top colors) to avoid cross-contamination of additives between the tubes; for example, blood culture bottle or tube (yellow/yellow-black top), EDTA (lavender top), coagulation tube (light blue top), lithium heparin anticoagulant and a gel separator (light green top), oxalate/fluoride (light gray top), acid citrate dextrose (pale yellow top), etc.

VIVA VOCE QUESTIONS

Q1. Describe the types of samples collected for haematological investigations.

Ans. *The types of samples collected for haematological investigations are:*

1. **Whole blood:** It is utilized for conducting complete blood counts, reticulocytes count and preparation of peripheral blood smear.

2. **Serum:** The blood when collected in a test tube clot at room temperature and a straw colour clear fluid which appears is the serum. Serum is clear fluid which separates from the clotted blood. The serum is devoid of white blood cells, red blood cells, platelets and fibrinogen. It is used for conducting various biochemical parameters and serum protein electrophoresis. They do not contain coagulation factors.

3. **Plasma:** This centrifugation of anti-coagulated blood forms plasma which is used for coagulation studies. It is pale yellow liquid which contains white blood cells, red blood cells, platelets and fibrinogen.

Q2. Describe the complications due to faulty method of capillary blood sampling.

Ans. *The complications due to faulty method of capillary blood sampling are:*

1. Laceration of tibial artery while puncturing the medial aspect of the heel leads to collapse of veins.

2. Osteomyelitis of the calcaneus.

3. Hematoma formation at site of puncture.

4. Nerve damage at the site of puncture.

5. **Long-term effects:** Localized or generalized necrosis

Q3. What are the advantages of capillary blood sampling over venous blood sampling?

Ans. *The advantages of capillary blood sampling over venous blood sampling are:*

1. Capillary blood collection is simple and easy to obtain; while during venous blood collection it might be difficult to obtain blood especially in obese individual (more fat mass) and in infants.

2. The capillary blood can be collected from different available locations (fingertip, ear lobules, heel area in infants, etc.).

3. A person can self-perform the test. Especially advantageous in patients of diabetes mellitus for testing their blood sugar level at home.

Q4. Enlist the causes of collection artifacts in blood sampling for haematological investigations.

Ans. *The causes for artifacts in blood samples for haematological investigations are:*

1. **Inappropriate procedure employed for venipuncture:** Slow or traumatic venipuncture precipitate platelet clump and form clot which will decrease all blood cell counts and give error in result. Venipuncture with small gauge needle may cause shearing of red blood cells, thereby altering cell counts.

2. **Obtaining less blood sample in volume:** When small amount of blood (e.g. 0.5–1 mL) is poured into a standard 5 mL EDTA bottle; the red blood cells, will shrink as EDTA is hypertonic. This will decrease the mean cell volume (MCV) and increase mean cell haemoglobin concentration (MCHC) and affect cell counts and blood indices value. The crenation of red blood cells can be observed in the blood smear.

3. **Inadequate mixing of anticoagulant:** Inadequate mixing will produce clotting of blood.

4. **Dilution with fluids:** The blood collected for haematologic testing through an in-dwelling catheter in critically ill patients may be admixed with fluids as IV line of fluids and antibiotic is given through same line. Discard first 3 mL of blood to avoid dilutional effects.

Q5. How should the needle, syringe and blood sample be disposed?

Ans. The needle and syringe must be disposed of in approved sharps disposal containers. Other contaminated waste must be discarded in an appropriate bio-hazard bag.

Q6. Which toxic symptoms may occur because of sodium oxalate ingestion?

Ans. It can cause burning pain in the mouth, throat and stomach, bloody vomiting, headache, muscle cramps, convulsions, hypotension, heart failure, shock, coma, and possible death. Mean lethal dose by ingestion of oxalates is 10–15 grams (per MSDS).

Q7. What is the role of EDTA in chelation therapy?

Ans. EDTA is used to bind metal ions in the practice of chelation therapy, e.g. for treating mercury and lead poisoning. It is also used to remove excess iron from the body.

Q8. Which of the market products have EDTA as a component?

Ans. Shampoos, cleaners and other personal care products have EDTA salts as component and are used as a sequestering agent to improve their stability in air.

Q9. When was sodium citrate first used as anticoagulant in blood transfusion?

Ans. Belgiuin doctor Albert Hustin and Argentine Physician Luis Agote successfully used sodium citrate as anticoagulant in blood transfusions in 1914.

Q10. What is the role of sodium citrate in coagulation?

Ans. The citrate ion chelates calcium ions in the blood by forming calcium citrate complexes, disrupting the blood clotting mechanism.

Q11. Where from is heparin produced in the human body?

Ans. Yes, heparin is a naturally occurring anticoagulant produced by basophils and mast cells.

Q12. Explain the mechanism of anticoagulant effect of heparin.

Ans. It facilitates the action of anti-thrombin III and inactivates clotting factors IX, X, XI and XII. Hence these clotting factors are unavailable for the formation of prothrombin activator and thrombin, thereby fibrinogen cannot be converted to fibrin.

Q13. Why blood sample is collected for?

Ans. Blood samples are collected for the purpose of clinical investigation for evaluating the underlying cause of the disease which is reflected by the altered levels of hematological parameters which include cell count, electrolyte levels, glucose, lipids and protein levels.

Q14. How knowledge of anticoagulants and collection of blood sample useful for students?

Ans. The knowledge of anticoagulants and collection of blood sample will help students to gain expertise so that they can confidently draw blood sample while performing experiments and while conducting research.

Q15. Discuss the role of blood analysis and use of anticoagulants in research.

Ans. Blood analysis is one of the most important diagnostic tools while exploring therapeutic effects in clinical trial. Anticoagulants are commonly being used in pharmacological *in vitro* experiments (e.g. heparin, sodium citrate, etc.) and *in vivo* experiments (heparin, warfarin, streptokinase, etc.) while some are used for both *in vitro* and *in vivo* experiments.

Q16. Discuss the indications for anticoagulants in clinical practice.

Ans. The anticoagulants are recommended in clinical conditions like myocardial infarction, venous thrombosis, pulmonary emboli, etc. and also to prevent transient ischemic attacks and risk of recurrent myocardial infarction.

Q17. Which is the most commonly used vein for venepuncture for collection of blood sample?

Ans. The median cubital vein which is a superficial vein is the most commonly used vein for venipuncture for collection of blood sample.

Q18. What are the advantages of low molecular weight heparin over heparin?

Ans. The molecular weight of heparin is 15,000 while that of low molecular weight heparin is 4000–5000. The low molecular weight heparin is easy to administer, dosage and its anticoagulant effect easily predictable; dose is calculated based on body weight, lab monitoring not essential in all patients and there is less chance of occurrence of immune-mediated thrombocytopenia.

OBSERVATIONS: EXERCISE FOR STUDENTS

1. Discuss the various methods of blood collection.
2. Discuss the precaution to be taken while drawing blood by capillary method and venous method.
3. What are the advantages of capillary blood sampling over venous blood sampling?
4. Describe the types of samples collected for hematological investigations.
5. Describe and discuss the role and nature of various anticoagulants used in for collecting blood sample.

....

....

....

....

....

....

....

Haemocytometry

Learning Objectives

After learning this practical the student should be able to:

1. Describe the components and the uses of haemocytometer.
2. Identify the squares used for white blood cell and red blood cell count.
3. Draw and dilute the blood sample for red and white blood cell counts in respective pipettes.
4. Discuss the precautions to be taken while diluting the blood.
5. Charge the Neubauer cell counting chamber.
6. Enlist the precautions to be taken during charging of Neubauer chamber.
7. To calculate the volume and area of squares used for WBC and RBC count.

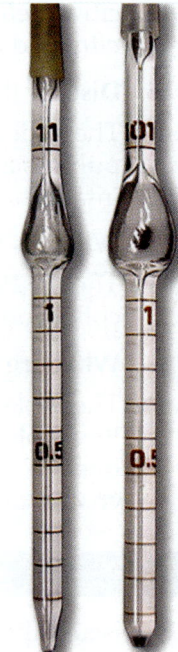

Aim of experiment: To study the details of Neubauer's cell counting chamber, its use and procedure of charging the Neubauer's chamber.

Instruments: Materials and chemicals: Lancet for making a sterile finger prick, haemocytometer with coverslip (improved Neubauer chamber), white blood cell and red blood cell pipettes, white blood cell and red blood cell diluting fluids and microscope.

- **RBC pipette:** The part of RBC pipette is a narrrow stem which widens into a bulb. The stem is graduated and has two markings 0.5 and 1.0 mark. Stem extends as bulb which carries the red bead, and the bulb narrows above and has 101 as mark on it. This end is connected to a rubber tube which ends as mouthpiece. The red bead presence in the bulb along with markings helps in identifying the red blood cell pipette. The function of the red bead is to facilitate mixing in the bulb.

Fig. 3.1: WBC and RBC pipette

- **WBC pipette:** The structural feature of WBC pipette is same as the RBC pipette except that it has a smaller bulb capacity and it contains white coloured bead. The marking over the pipette are 0.5 and 1 over the stem and 11 above the bulb portion. The rubber tubing from the bulb ends in a white mouthpiece.

- **Haemocytometer:** It consists of a thick glass slide. There are three platform separated with each other by trenches and are also called gutters. The central platform is slightly lower than the side platforms. The central

Table 3.1: Difference between RBC and WBC pipette		
	WBC pipette	*RBC pipette*
Graduation on pipette	Stem: 0.5 and 1	Stem: 0.5
	Above bulb: 11	Above bulb: 101
Bulb size	Smaller	Larger
Bead of the bulb	White coloured bead	Red coloured bead
Mouthpiece	White in colour	Red in colour
Size of lumen of pipette	Larger	Smaller

platform is divided into two mirror coated floor pieces by an H-shaped groove. Thus, it the H-shaped trench or gutter enclosing the two floor pieces. The coverslip is placed on the side platforms and covers the central platform. The central platform is 0.1 mm lower than the two-side platforms. The distance between the coverslip and the central platform is 1/10 mm.

The central platform has lines engraved on both sides to form squares of different dimensions which are used for different cell counts especially red blood cell count and white blood cell count.

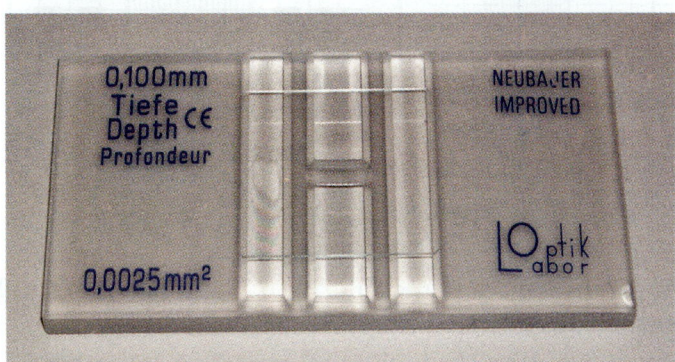

Fig. 3.2: Improved Neubauer chamber

A. Older Neubauer Chamber

The total engraved ruled area consists of a square having a dimension of 3 mm × 3 mm, which is divided into nine 1 mm squares. The nine squares consist of four corner squares which are used for the WBC count; and the central square for the RBC count. The WBC square is further divided into 16 squares of 1/16 sq.mm. The central large RBC square is of size of 1 mm square and has 16 groups of 16 small squares each **(while there are 25 groups of 16 small squares in modified improved Neubauer chamber).**

B. Improved Neubauer Chamber

The total engraved ruled area is of dimension of 3 × 3 mm, which is divided into nine 1 sq mm each. The nine squares comprise four corner squares for the WBC count; and the central square is used for the RBC count.
1. The central large RBC square is divided into 25 medium size square each having an area of 1/5 × 1/5 mm, thus total area of each medium size RBS square is 1/25 sq.mm. The central medium sized square and four corner medium sized squares are used for the RBC count. The area of the 5 medium sized square used in RBC count is 1/25 × 5 = 1/5 sq.mm. Moreover, the depth under the coverslip is 1/10 mm, the volume of five of the medium sized squares is 1/5 × 1/10 = 1/50 cu.mm.

🖋 Key Notes

The five medium square in which RBC are counted is 1/50 sq mm. This calculation is further confirmed by counting the area of even the smallest 16 squares of the five medium squares in which RBC count is conducted.

- The medium-sized square consists of 16 small squares thus 25 medium size RBC squares consist of—25 × 16 = 400 small squares. The smallest RBC square is 1/20 × 1/20 mm in size. Thus, the area of the smallest RBC square is 1/20 × 1/20 mm = 1/400 sq.mm. The depth under the coverslip is 1/10 mm, therefore the volume of the smallest RBC square will be 1/400 × 1/10 mm = 1/4000 cu.mm. Since
- Red blood cells are counted in 80 small squares.
- Therefore, the volume of 80 small size RBC squares is 1/4000 × 80 mm = 1/50 cu.mm.

---

2. Each WBC square is further divided into 16 squares of 1/16 sq.mm.

🖋 Key Notes

In improve Neubauer chamber, the each of the 25 RBC medium squares are demarcated from other by double or triple lines. While 16 medium size WBC squares are demarcated by single line.

Diluting fluids: The commonly used diluting fluids are:
1. **WBC diluting fluid (Türk's fluid):** It contains gentian violet (1%) 1 ml, glacial acetic acid (3%) 3 ml and 100 ml distilled water.

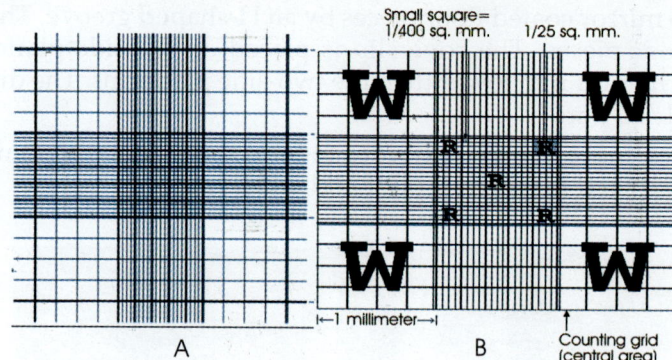

Fig. 3.3: A: Improved Neubauer chamber. B: Improved Neubauer chamber showing RBC and WBC squares utilized for cell counting

2. **RBC diluting fluid (Hayem's fluids):** Mercuric chloride 0.25 gm; Sodium sulphate 2.5 gm; Sodium chloride 0.5 gm and distilled water 100 ml

The functions of each constituent are explained with the concerned cell count.

Method

A. Study the Neubauer chamber and identify the squares for the RBC and WBC counts under the compound microscope. Study the squares under low power and then under high power. Identify the WBC and RBC pipette. Practice drawing the fluid in the pipette. Practice charging the Neubauer chamber.

B. The students should learn method of drawing sample in RBC/WBC pipette before proceeding for charging Neubauer chamber.

- *Drawing sample in RBC pipette—dilution for RBC count*:
  1. Take a clean and dry pipette.
  2. Pour the RBC diluting fluid (Hayem's fluid) in a watch glass.
  3. Clean the middle or the index finger with spirit. Give a finger prick using lancet, discard first drop, allow free flow and then suck blood up to 0.5 mark. No air bubbles should accumulate during the process.
  4. Wipe the tip of the pipette using sterile gauze, and then suck Hayem's fluid up to the 101 mark.
  5. Keep the pipette initially at an acute angle while sucking in the Hayem's fluid and then gradually make it vertical as the fluid reaches the 101 mark.
  6. Place the pipette in a horizontal position and firmly hold it between the palms.
  7. Mix the contents of the bulb between the palms of the two hands gently.
  8. Discard the fluid in the stem as it contains only diluting fluid.

- *Drawing sample in WBC pipette—Dilution for WBC count*:
  1. Draw the blood up to 0.5 marks in the WBC pipette.
  2. Holding the pipette almost vertical place it into the fluid. Draw the diluting fluid into the pipette slowly until the mixture reaches the 11 mark.
  3. Place the pipette in a horizontal position and firmly hold it between the palms.
  4. Mix the contents of the bulb between the palms of the two hands gently for at least 3 minutes to facilitate hemolysis of RBCs.
  5. Discard the fluid in the stem as it contains only diluting fluid.

C. **Charging the improved Neubauer chamber**
  1. Clean the haemocytometer and its coverslip with a sterile gauze piece and wait for 2 minutes to make it dry.
  2. Discard first two drops from the RBC/WBC pipette in order to expel the diluents from the stem.
  3. The drop of blood is formed at the tip of the pipette; thereafter the tip of the pipette is placed on the central platform near the edge of the coverslip. The fluid is drawn under coverslip by capillary action.

4. Ensure that no air bubbles are present and there is no overflow of fluid into the grooves.
5. After charging allow the cells to settle and then focus the cells under low power to ensure uniform distribution.
6. Conduct WBC count under four corner WBC squares under low power objective. Conduct RBC count in the central square of the Neubauer chamber under high power objective in the four medium sized corner square and one medium sized central square.

Precautions

1. The pipette and lancet should be clean and dry.
2. The finger should be cleaned with methylated spirit and allowed to dry.
3. The prick should be firm and bold so that after a single prick the blood flows freely.
4. The finger should never be squeezed to obtain blood.
5. The tip of the pipette should place over the drop and then sucked.
6. Ensure no air bubble is drawn into pipette.
7. Do not suck blood over 0.5 mark of the pipette.
8. Dilute the blood immediately with diluents up to 101 mark of RBC pipette or up to 11 mark of WBC pipette.
9. Ensure that tip of pipette is dipped into diluting fluid when sucking; so that air bubble do not enter in.
10. Hold the pipette gently horizontally between palms and rotate for 2–3 minutes for uniform mixing and then place it horizontally in the tray that you can charge after uniform mixing is achieved.

Rule for Cell Counting

Counting the Cells

1. **Counting cells that are on a line:** Cells that are on the line of a grid require special attention. Note that cells touching the left and lower borders are to be considered for counting while those at right and upper borders are omitted.

Precautions

1. Ensure that the Neubauer chamber, pipette, fingertip, lancet and coverslip is clean and dry.
2. The diluted blood sample after pipetting should be thoroughly mixed.
3. The air bubble should not be present in charging pipette or under coverslip of the counting chamber.
4. The chamber should be uniformly charged and ensure that there is no overflowing in the chamber
5. Note that cells touching the left and lower borders are to be considered for counting while those at right and upper borders are omitted.
6. Cell count should be started after they get equally distributed.

Sources of Error

1. Improper collection of blood sample: Blood collected less than that required for counting may give error in results.
2. Wet or contaminated pipettes: This may result in improper results.
3. Poor pipetting technique; for example, under collection below desired line with blood or diluting fluid; or over collection above desired line with blood or diluting fluid; or presence of air bubble in the pipette, etc.
4. Failure to discard 2 drops from the pipette tips before charging the haemocytometer.
5. Overcharging or undercharging the haemocytometer
6. Wet or contaminated coverslip and haemocytometers.
7. The cells in the counting chamber are unevenly distributed.
8. Error while counting cell.

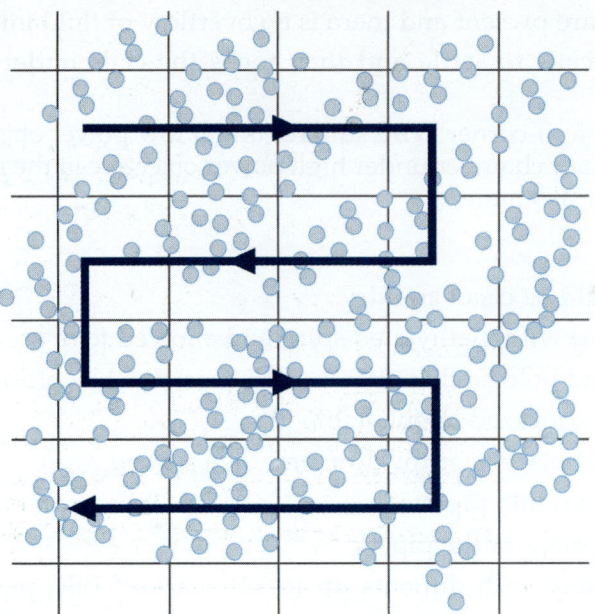

Fig. 3.4: Cell counting method: Count the cells in the first square and go in Z pattern for further counting

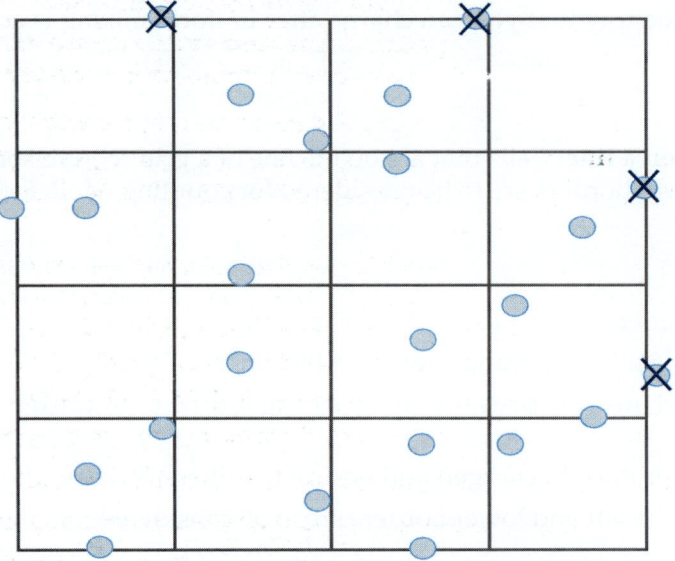

Fig. 3.5: Do not count cells on the top and right lines

OSPE SKILLED 1

Q1. Charge the Neubauer chamber with the provided RBC/WBC pipette having diluted blood after addition of respective diluting fluid and the wait period.

Choose any one of the pipette.

Ans. *Steps to be followed by student:*

1. Ensure that the haemocytometer and its coverslip are clean and dry. (Yes/No)

2. Discards the first two drops from the RBC/WBC pipette in order to expel the diluents from the stem. (Yes/No)

3. Gently applying pressure along the rubber tubing of pipette allows the drop of blood to be formed at the tip of the pipette; thereafter places the tip of the pipette on the central platform near the edge of the coverslip. The fluid is drawn under coverslip by capillary action. (Yes/No)

4. Ensure that no air bubbles are present and there is no overflow of fluid into the grooves. (Yes/No)

5. After charging allow the cells to settle and then focus the cells under low power to ensure uniform distribution. (Yes/No)

ADDITIONAL OSPE QUESTIONS FOR PRACTICE

- Focus an RBC counting square in the Neubauer chamber under 40X
- Dilute the given sample of blood for total WBC count
- Dilute the given sample of blood for RBC count
- Focus a WBC counting square under high power

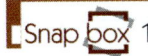 Snap box 1

Louis-Charles Malassez (1842–1909) was born on September 21 1842. He was a French anatomist. Malassez is known for his studies of microscopic anatomy, histology of blood cells, as well as for inventing the haemocytometer. In dentistry, he studied some ligament cells which are now named after him, called the epithelial cell rests of Malassez (ERM). A genus of fungi, Malassezia is also named after him, and includes species that can cause skin irritation.

VIVA VOCE QUESTIONS

Q1. What is haemocytometry? Who invented the haemocytometer?

Ans. The counting of blood cells after methodical dilution is termed haemocytometry and the instrument used to count the blood cells is called haemocytometer. Louis-Charles Malassez invented the haemocytometer.

Q2. Describe the gridded area of haemocytometer (improved Neubauer chamber).

Ans. The total ruled area is of dimension of 3 mm × 3 mm, which is divided into nine 1 mm squares areas. The nine squares comprise four corner squares for the WBC count; and the central square is used for the RBC count.

- The central large RBC square is divided into 25 medium size square each having an area of 1/5 × 1/5 mm, thus total area of each medium size RBS square is 1/25 sq. mm. The central medium-sized square and four corner medium-sized squares are used for the RBC count. The area of the 5 medium-sized square used in RBC count is 1/25 × 5 = 1/5 sq.mm. Moreover, the depth under the coverslip is 1/10 mm, the volume of five of the medium-sized squares is 1/5 × 1/10 = 1/50 cu.mm.
- Each WBC square is further divided into 16 squares of 1/16 sq.mm

Q3. Name the two common applications of haemocytometer.

Ans. The two common applications of haemocytometer include its use for blood count and sperm count.

Q4. Why do we discard the first two drops from the RBC or WBC pipette before charging the Neubauer chamber?

Ans. The first two drops from the RBC or WBC pipette are discarded before charging the Neubauer chamber as they contain only the diluting fluid.

Q5. What are the features of RBC diluting pipette?

Ans. *The features of RBC diluting pipette are*:
- The markings on the pipette include 0.5, 1 and 101
- The luminal diameter of the stem of RBC pipette is smaller when compared to that of WBC pipette.
- The bulb contains a red bead
- The volume of the bulb of the RBC pipette is larger than that of the WBC pipette.

Q6. How does the old Neubauer chamber differ from the improved Neubauer chamber?

Ans. The central (1 mm²) RBC large square in the old Neubauer chamber consisted of 16 medium size squares containing 16 small squares each while improved Neubauer chamber are having 25 medium size squares having 16 small squares each. The medium-sized 25 squares are demarcated among each other by triple lines.

Q7. Why should the tip of the pipette be wiped off before sucking the diluting fluid?

Ans. The tip of the pipette should be wiped off before sucking the diluting fluid to prevent the entry of the extra drop blood into the pipette which may give rise to false high cell counts and to avoid contamination of the diluting fluid.

Q8. Enlist the common causes of error while conducting haemocytometer counts.

Ans. *The common causes of error while conducting haemocytometer counts are*:
1. Improper collection of blood sample.
2. Wet or contaminated pipettes.
3. Poor pipetting technique.
4. Failure to discard two drops from the pipette tips before charging the haemocytometer.
5. Overcharging or undercharging the haemocytometer.
6. Wet or contaminated coverslip and haemocytometer.
7. The cells in the counting chamber are unevenly distributed.
8. Error while counting cell.

Q9. Enlist the applicability and use of a haemocytometer.

Ans. *The applicability and use of a haemocytometer are*:
1. Conduct blood counts for estimating red blood cell, white blood cell and platelet count.
2. Sperm counts
3. Recording cell growth over time in cell culture.
4. Haemocytometer is used in cell processing for downstream analysis: Investigations such as PCR and flow cytometry require accurate cell numbers.
5. Measurement of cell size: The real cell size can be ascertain by scaling cell to the width of a haemocytometer square.

Q10. Which studies in research can be carried using haemocytometer?

Ans. Haemocytometer is used in research for cell culture studies (subculturing cell growth over time) and cell processing for downstream analysis and for measurement of cell size in a micrograph.

Q11. Discuss examples of haemocytometry-based diagnosis.

Ans. Haemocytometry in clinical practice is an important tool for diagnosis. Some of the haemocytometry-based diagnosis are: Diagnosis of anaemia (if red blood cell count is decreased or polycythemia if it increased over and above the physiological limits), similarly increased WBC count indicates presence of bacterial infections, significant and progressive increased abnormal WBC count indicates leukaemia; increased platelet count indicates primary or secondary thrombocytosis (secondary to anaemia, inflammation, infection, carcinoma, etc.), decreased sperm count indicating sterility in males, etc.

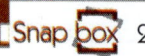 Snap box 2

The disposable plastic counting chamber with a grid pattern exactly the same as the improved Neubauer chamber are preferred today for cell count because they have
1. Precise fixed depth counting chamber having superior accuracy and reproducibility.
2. Reduces the risk of exposure to potentially infectious material.
3. Increases productivity as cleaning work interruptions eliminated.
4. These are light and non-breakable.

Bibliography

Absher, Marlene (1973). "Hemocytometer Counting": 395–397.

OBSERVATIONS: EXERCISE FOR STUDENTS

1. What is haemocytometry? Who invented the haemocytometer?
2. Describe the gridded area of haemocytometer.
3. Name the two common applications of haemocytometer.
4. Why do we discard the first two drops from the RBC or WBC pipette before charging the Neubauer chamber?

5. What are the features of RBC diluting pipette?
6. How does the old Neubauer chamber differ from the improved Neubauer chamber?
7. Why should the tip of the pipette be wiped off before sucking the diluting fluid?
8. Enlist the common causes of error while conducting haemocytometer counts.
9. Enlist the applicability and use of a haemocytometer.
10. Which studies in research can be carried using haemocytometer?
11. Discuss examples of haemocytometry-based diagnosis.

Estimation of Haemoglobin

Learning Objectives

After completion of practical the student should be able to:

1. Estimate the haemoglobin using Sahli's method.
2. Discuss the advantages and disadvantages of Sahli's method.
3. Enlist the precaution while estimating haemoglobin by Sahli's method.
4. Discuss the other methods for estimation of haemoglobin.
5. State the normal haemoglobin levels in males and females
6. Enlist various clinical conditions in which the haemoglobin levels are altered?
7. Able to classify anaemia on the basis of haemoglobin levels.
8. Describe the method of estimation of haemoglobin by internationally accepted cyanmethaemoglobin method.
9. Estimate oxygen carrying capacity of blood and iron content of haemoglobin.

Aim: Estimation of the haemoglobin concentration.

SAHLI'S ACID HAEMATIN METHOD

Material, apparatus and chemicals: Sahli's haemoglobinometer: It is a box containing comparator, haemoglobin tube, haemoglobin pipette, and stirrer.

Haemoglobin tube: It is graduated and calibrated on one side as gram per cent (gm%), from 2–22, and on in percentage (%), from 10 to 140 on other side. This tube is also known as Sahli-Adams tube.

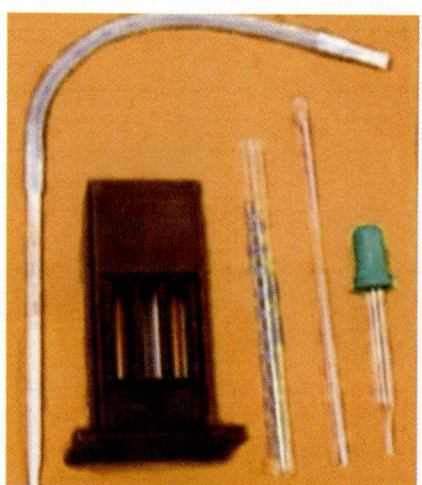

R-L dropper, stirring rod, haemoglobinometer tube, comparator box and haemoglobin pipette

Fig. 4.1: Haemocytometer

Comparator: It is a rectangular box of processed plastic polymer material having a centre slot for haemoglobin tube and two-colour standards for matching on either side. These standard brown tinted glass frame slots are provided on either side of the centre slot for the colour matching.

Haemoglobin pipette: The pipette bears a mark indicating 20 µL. It consists of tubing of rubber with mouth piece attach to it. The pipette is devoid of any bulb.

Stirrer: It is a thin glass rod which is used for stirring the solution.

Chemical solution: N/10 HCl bottle and distilled water.

Other Materials

Dropper: Ordinary glass dropper or Pasteur pipette which is an 8–10 inches glass tube with a long thin nozzle having a rubber teat is used as dropper.

Materials for a sterile finger prick: Sterile lancet, sterile gauze, cotton swabs and methylated spirit.

Principle: The Hb present in blood is converted to acid haematin on addition of N/10 HCl (hydrochloric acid). The observed golden brown colour depends on the concentration of Hb. The colour of the solution is matched against golden brown tinted glass colour of the comparator. The formed acid haematin appears golden brown in colour and this solution is diluted with distilled water till the colour matches with the standard colour. The Hb concentration is noted in gm% at the level where the colour of solution matches with that of comparator.

Procedure

1. Ensure that haemoglobinometer tube and pipette are clean and dry.
2. Add N/10 HCl in the haemoglobinometer tube up to its lowest mark (2 gm/dl or 10%) with the help of a dropper.
3. Clean the finger with methylated spirit using the cotton gauze and prick the finger under all aseptic precautions. Discard the first drop of blood.
4. Allow a large drop of blood to form on the fingertip, and then suck the blood up to 20 µL of the pipette.
5. Wipe the tip of the pipette to remove any blood which may remain on outside of the tube.
6. Transfer the blood from the haemoglobin pipette into the haemoglobinometer tube containing N/10 HCl by immersing tip of the pipette in N/10 HCl solution by blowing out blood from the pipette. Rinse the pipette by drawing N/10 HCl and blowing it for couple of time for uniform mixing. Ensure uniform mixing of content by using a stirrer.
7. Leave the solution in the haemoglobinometer tube for about ten minutes (for conversion of haemoglobin to acid haematin which occurs in the first ten minutes).
8. Dilute the acid haematin by adding distilled water drop by drop. Mix it with the stirrer. Match the colour of the solution in the haemoglobinometer tube with the standards of the comparator. After addition of every drop of distilled water, the solution should be mixed and the colour of the solution and should be compared with the standard of the comparator till it matches with that of the standard. Take care to hold the stirrer above the level of the solution while reading is being matched, otherwise at no stage should the stirrer should be taken out of the tube.
9. Note the reading when the colour of the solution exactly matches with the standard and express the haemoglobin content as gm per 100 ml of blood.

Precautions

1. All aseptic precautions should be used during pricking.
2. The first drop of blood should be discarded and do not squeeze the finger because tissue fluids which comes out gives lower values of haemoglobin.
3. Wait for at least ten minutes for the formation of acid haematin by the action of hydrochloric acid on Hb.
4. Avoid over dilution as later the solution cannot be concentrated to match with comparator colour.
5. Golden brown colour of the solution should be compared with the standard of the comparator till it matches with that of the standard of the comparator.
6. Match the colour in the comparator box in natural source of daylight.
7. Take care to hold the stirrer above the level of the solution. At no stage should the stirrer be taken out of the tube.

Advantages of Sahli's Acid Haematin Method

1. Shali's haemoglobin meter is portable, easy to carry anywhere (bed side in case of critical patient, outpatient department in hospital, at field visit during clinical studies, etc.) and hence test can be conducted as per convenience.
2. It is easy to perform and handle.
3. It is quick procedure and result can be noted immediately.
4. It is inexpensive test.
5. No technical expertise is required to conduct this test.

Disadvantages of Shali's Acid Haematin Method

1. The standard colouration on the haemoglobinometer fades away over the year and this will give wrong results.
2. It gives results in approximation only and not accurately and cannot be fully relied upon.
3. All types of haemoglobin's (oxyhaemoglobin, sulphaemoglobin) do not get converted to acid haematin and hence the value of Hb may be determined lesser than the actual value.
4. Individual variation in matching of colour is seen

Oxygen Carrying Capacity

1 gm of haemoglobin carries 1.34 ml of oxygen. Hence the oxygen carrying capacity is haemoglobin level × 1.34 ml

RESULTS

Hb concentration in the volunteer subject is .... by Sahli's method.

1 gm of haemoglobin carries 1.34 ml of oxygen, hence the oxygen carrying capacity in the subject is ....

NORMAL VALUES

Adult males: 14–18 gm/dl of blood (average is 15.5 gm/dl)
Adult females: 12–16 gm/dl of blood (average is 14 gm/dl)

OSPE I—SKILLED

Question: Draw the blood into haemoglobin tube for estimation of haemoglobin.

Steps to be followed by student

1. Sucks the blood into haemoglobin pipette and empty it into haemoglobinometer tube containing N/10 HCl. (Yes/No)
2. Ensures haemoglobinometer tube and pipette is clean and dry. (Yes/No)
3. Adds N/10 HCl in the haemoglobinometer tube up to its lowest mark (10 per cent or 2 gm %) with the help of a dropper. (Yes/No)
4. Draws blood up to 20 µL mark of the pipette from the given sample. (Yes/No)
5. Wipes the tip of the pipette and transfer the 20 µL of blood from the pipette into the haemoglobinometer tube containing N/10 HCl by immersing tip of the pipette in the acid solution and blowing out blood from the pipette. (Yes/No)
6. Leaves the solution in the haemoglobinometer tube for about ten minutes (for conversion of haemoglobin to acid haematin which occurs in the first ten minutes). (Yes/No)

The student should leave the tube in the comparator for acid haematin formation. The technician will take care of further step.

OSPE II—ANOTHER STUDENT

Note: A technician after waiting for 10 minutes has kept the haemoglobinometer tube ready. Golden brown colour of acid haematin is visible.

Question: Dilute the blood from given sample for estimation of haemoglobin.

Steps to be followed by student:

1. Dilutes the acid heamatin formed blood by adding distilled water drop by drop. Mixes it with the stirrer. Matches the colour of the solution in the haemoglobinometer tube with the standards of the comparator. Takes care to hold the stirrer above the level of the solution. (Yes/No)

2. After addition of every drop of distilled water, the student mixes the solution and compares the colour of the solution with the standard of the comparator till it matches with that of the standard. Takes care to hold the stirrer above the level of the solution. (Yes/No)

3. Throughout matching procedure takes care to hold the stirrer above the level of the solution. At no stage should the stirrer is taken out of the tube. (Yes/No)

4. Notes the reading when the colour of the solution exactly matches with the standard and expresses the haemoglobin content in gm%. (Yes/No)

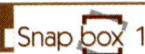 Snap box 1

Key Information

WHO Haemoglobin Colour Scale: The colour of a drop of blood is absorbed on a chromatography paper and the colour of the drop of blood is matched against a printed scale of colour corresponding to varied levels of haemoglobin ranging from 4 to 14 gram/dl.

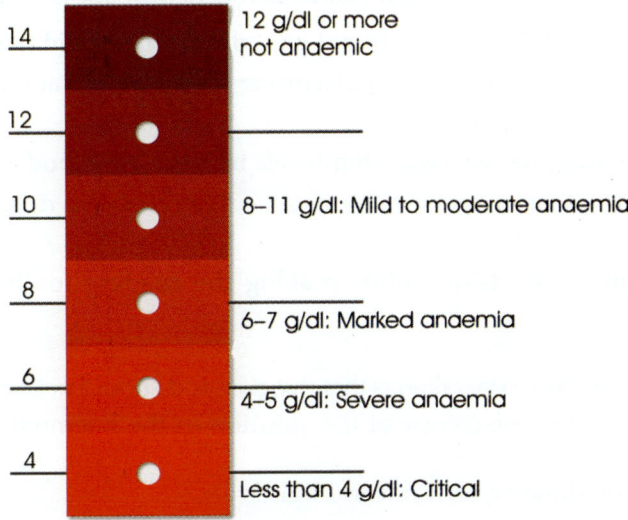

14		12 g/dl or more not anaemic
12		
10		8–11 g/dl: Mild to moderate anaemia
8		6–7 g/dl: Marked anaemia
6		4–5 g/dl: Severe anaemia
4		Less than 4 g/dl: Critical

Fig. 4.2: WHO haemoglobin colour scale

Bibliography

Cherian M, Emmanuel JC, Lewis SM et al. Evaluation of the haemoglobin colour scale. *Bull World Health Organ.* 2002; 80: 839

VIVA VOCE QUESTIONS

Q1. What is the principle of Hb estimation?

Ans. In this method Hb is converted to acid haematin by N/10 HCl. The golden brown colour of the solution is matched with colour of a standard comparator to give rough estimate of Hb in gm%.

Q2. What is the function of N/10 HCl?

Ans. Hydrochloric acid acts with haemoglobin to form acid haematin.

Q3. What are the advantages and disadvantages of Sahli's method?

Ans. *The advantages of Sahli's method are:*

Sahli's haemoglobin meter is portable, easy to carry anywhere (bed side in case of critical patient, outpatient department in hospital, field visit during clinical studies, etc.) and it is easy to perform and handle.

Disadvantages of Sahli's method are:
a. The standard colouration on the haemoglobinometer fades away over the year and this will give wrong result.
b. It gives results in approximation only and not accurately and cannot be fully relied upon.

Q4. Which of the methods is most accurate method for haemoglobin estimation?

Ans. Cyanmethaemoglobin method is most accurate because estimation is done with photoelectric colorimeter.

Q5. Enlist three main causes for error reporting while estimating haemoglobin level.

Ans. *The error in reporting haemoglobin levels while estimating haemoglobin concentration in blood is*:
1. Technical errors—improper mixing of blood.
2. Errors in pipetting—tissue fluid contaminating capillary blood.
3. Visual errors—taking the reading is very subjective, as it is a comparison of colours. It can vary from person to person. Hence the results may not be accurate.
4. Quality of the colour comparators can affect the reading—if the glass blocks are old or faded it can cause wrong results.

Q6. What is the adequate time required for conversion of Hb to acid haematin?

Ans. Minimum time period of ten minutes is required for complete conversion of Hb to acid haematin; otherwise it will lead to false negative result. The 95% of Hb is converted acid haematin at the end of 10 minutes, 98% at the end of 20 minutes, and the maximum colour is reached in about 1 hour.

Q7. What are the types of haemoglobin which do not get converted to acid haematin?

Ans. The types of haemoglobin which do not get converted to acid haematin are carboxyhaemoglobin, methaemoglobin and sulphaemoglobin.

Q8. What will time delay in noting the haemoglobin levels by Sahli's method lead to?

Ans. The golden brown colour of acid haematin is unstable, hence undue delay in reading the test result will lead to false result.

Q9. What are the precautions to be taken while making the reading for haemoglobin value with that of comparator?

Ans.
1. The most important precaution to be taken is that the glass rod should not be left inside the haemoglobin tube.
2. Note the reading only when the colour of the solution in the haemoglobin tube is same as that of the comparator.
3. The matching should be done against natural light.

Q10. Hb concentration of a given subject was found to be 14 gm%. Calculate its oxygen carrying capacity %.

Ans. The normal oxygen carrying capacity of blood per gram of haemoglobin is 1.34 ml; hence the oxygen carrying capacity of the subject is 14 × 1.34 = 18.76 ml/dl.

Q11. What are the functions of haemoglobin?

Ans. *The functions of haemoglobin are*: Haemoglobin transports oxygen from the lungs to the tissues and carbon dioxide from the tissues to the lungs. It also acts as a buffer in and helps maintaining the blood pH. Haemoglobin in tissue regulates iron metabolism and mediates antioxidant effects.

Q12. What is the name of the molecule that transports oxygen in red blood cells?

Ans. The respiratory pigment of the red blood cells is haemoglobin.

Q13. What is the molecular composition of haemoglobin? Does the functionality of haemoglobin as a protein depend upon its tertiary or upon its quaternary structure?

Ans. Haemoglobin is a molecule made of four polypeptide chains, each bound to an iron-containing molecular group called a haem group. Thus, the molecule contains four polypeptide chains and four haem groups. As a protein it is composed of association of polypeptide chains, the functionality of haemoglobin depends upon the integrity of its quaternary structure.

Q14. What is the molecular weight of haemoglobin?

Ans. Haemoglobin is a globular molecule having a molecular weight of 68,000 daltons.

Q15. **What is the normal blood haemoglobin level in adult male and adult female?**

Ans. The normal haemoglobin concentration in adult male is 15.5 g/dl (range 14–18 g/dl) and females it is 14 g/dl (range 12–15.5 g/dl).

Q16. **What is the normal haemoglobin concentration at birth and 1 year of age?**

Ans. At birth the concentration of haemoglobin increases and may reach up to 23 g/dl. After two days of birth the Hb level starts decreasing and stabilizes at the end of three months to 10.5 g/dl. At 1 year of age the Hb concentration rises to 12 g/dl.

Q17. **Enlist the normal variant of haemoglobin.**

Ans. The normal variants of haemoglobin are adult haemoglobin (Hb A) and haemoglobin A2 (Hb A2) and foetal haemoglobin (Hb F2).

Q18. **Enlist the various methods of estimation of haemoglobin concentration.**

Ans. *Haemoglobin can be estimated by various methods and categorically can be classified as:*

1. Visual methods include Sahli's method, Wintrobes method, Haldane's method and tallquists method.
2. Gasometric method includes cyanmethaemoglobin method, Van Slyke method, spectrophotometric method and oxyhaemoglobin method.
3. Automated haemoglobinometry
4. Other methods include alkaline-haematin method, specific gravity method and comparator method.

Q19. **Describe the various methods of estimation of haemoglobin.**

Ans. *The various methods of estimation of haemoglobin are:*

Other Methods

A. Spectrophotometry (photoelectric colorimeter method): It measures the amount of light which gets absorbed by a solution. The wave band of light corresponds with portion of the spectrum which is absorbed to maximum in the test solution. These methods are rapid and give accurate results.

1. **Oxyhaemoglobin method:** Principle—ammonium hydroxide (0.04 ml/dl) haemolyse the red cells and converts the haemoglobin to oxyhaemoglobin and the absorbance of the solution, then it measures in the spectrophotometer (photoelectric colorimeter). This conversion is immediate, and the resulting colour is stable.

2. **Cyanmethaemoglobin method:** In this method blood is diluted in a solution containing Drabkin's reagent (1 gm of sodium bicarbonate, 50 mg potassium cyanide, 200 mg potassium ferricyanide in one liter of distilled water). Hb is oxidized to methaemoglobin by potassium ferricyanide and combined with potassium cyanide to form cyanmethaemoglobin. The absorbance of the solution measures in a spectrophotometer at wavelength 540 nm against Drabkin's solution as a blank. The result is expressed in gm/litre or mg/dl.

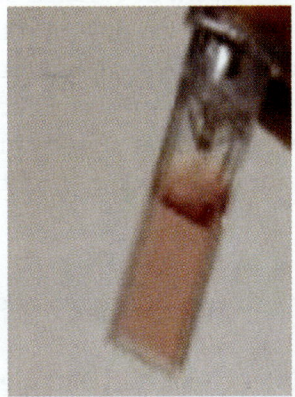

Fig. 4.3

Note: Measure the absorbance of this solution (Reaction of blood with Drabkin's solution) at 540 nm for estimating haemoglobin concentration.

B. **Gasometric method:** Gasometric method of estimation of haemoglobin is by using Van Slyke apparatus. This method is not used routinely in clinical laboratories as it is time-consuming, and the process of estimation is complex.

C. **Automated haemoglobinometry:** Various automated techniques have been employed to measure haemoglobin. Nowadays with developing health technology automated haemoglobinometer are also being used for haemoglobin estimation due to its simple and quick method of assessment.

D. **Tallquists method:** The method involves direct matching of the red colour of a drop of whole fresh blood on a filter paper with colour standards on the paper. Depending on the colour haemoglobin concentration value as depicted in the standard is noted as result.

E. **Comparator method:** This is a visual method and diluents used are an alkali solution (ammonia solution 0.04 percent). After mixing with dilute ammonia solution, the intensity of the colour of the haemolysed solution of red blood cells is compared against a standard colour disc in the comparator.

F. **Haldane method using** *Haldane's haemoglobinometer* (Haldane's modification of Gower's method): The instrument consists of two tubes, one of which contains 20 cu mm of blood haemolysed with distilled water and saturated with CO gas. The colour of this tube is used as standard. In the other tube a little distilled water is taken and 20 cu mm of patient's blood, collected from the fingertip by a special pipette, is added. When blood becomes fully haemolysed, it is saturated with CO by passing coal gas through it. The colour developed is compared against that of the standard. If the colour of the unknown is stronger, it is diluted with distilled water until the tinge is same in both. The graduation up to which the blood has been diluted gives the percentage haemoglobin.

G. **Alkaline haematin method:** In this method 50 ml of blood is added to an alkaline solution of 4.95 ml N/10 NAOH. The mixed solution is kept warmed at 37°C and kept in cold bath. The haemoglobin is converted to alkaline haematin and a stable colour compound is formed. The absorbance of alkaline haematin is measured using photoelectric colorimeter.

> **Note:** The student should refer Appendix 1 for colorimetry.

Q20. What are the types of haemoglobin and its variant?

Ans. *The types of haemoglobin and its variants are:*

In the embryo haemoglobin types are: Gower 1 ($\zeta_2\varepsilon_2$) and Gower 2 ($\alpha_2\varepsilon_2$) haemoglobin Portland I ($\zeta_2\gamma_2$) and Haemoglobin Portland II ($\zeta_2\beta_2$).

In the fetus haemoglobin type is: Haemoglobin F ($\alpha_2\gamma_2$)

In the adult haemoglobin types are: Haemoglobin A ($\alpha_2\beta_2$), Haemoglobin A2 ($\alpha_2\delta_2$) and Haemoglobin F ($\alpha_2\gamma_2$).

Haemoglobin variant forms that cause disease:
- Haemoglobin H (β_4)—which may be present in variants of α thalassemia.
- Haemoglobin Barts (γ_4)—may be present in variants of α thalassemia.
- Haemoglobin S ($\alpha_2\beta_2^S$)—a variant form of haemoglobin found in patients of sickle cell anaemia.
- Haemoglobin C ($\alpha_2\beta_2^C$)—this variant causes a mild chronic haemolytic anaemia.
- Haemoglobin E ($\alpha_2\beta_2^E$)—this variant also causes a mild chronic haemolytic anaemia.
- Haemoglobin AS—a heterozygous form in sickle cell traits and has one adult gene and one sickle cell disease gene.

Q21. Define anaemia.

Ans. The decrease oxygen carrying capacity due to decreased haemoglobin and red blood cell count is called anaemia.

Q22. How foetal haemoglobin (HbF) does differ chemically and spectroscopically than adult haemoglobin (HbA) and what is the advantage of foetal haemoglobin in terms of oxygen carrying capacity?

Ans. Foetal haemoglobin differs chemically and spectroscopically from the adult haemoglobin. It has a greater affinity for oxygen and releases CO_2 more readily. This is due to some difference in the globin fraction. This property helps to compensate the relative anoxia of foetal blood. At low O_2 pressure foetal haemoglobin can take up larger volumes of O_2 than adult haemoglobin.

Advantage of foetal haemoglobin: HbF (foetal haemoglobin) is 70% saturated at 20 mm Hg of PO_2 pressure, whereas adult haemoglobin is only 20% saturated at this pressure.

Q23. What is haemoglobinuria and what are causes for the condition?

Ans. *Haemoglobinuria* is the condition when free haemoglobins excreted through the urine. If Hb is free in the plasma, then it is excreted through the urine. In plasma, haemoglobinuria may be caused under the following conditions:

1. In strenuous exercise.
2. Due to mismatched blood transfusion.
3. Black water fever due to virulent type of malaria and red water fever due to another type of parasite which invades the erythrocyte causing release of Hb in the plasma.
4. Paroxysmal nocturnal haemoglobinuria
5. Hypotonicity of plasma
6. Thermal or chemical injuries
7. Paroxysmal cold haemoglobinuria.

Q24. Who shared the Nobel Prize for the studies of the structures of haemoglobin and myoglobin?

Ans. Max Ferdin and Perutz Wasan Austrian-born British molecular biologist who shared the Nobel Prize for Chemistry with John Kendrew for their studies of the structures of haemoglobin and myoglobin in 1962.

Q25. Discuss the causes for variation in haemoglobin concentration.

Ans. *The causes for variation in haemoglobin concentration are:*

1. *Age:* In the foetus, the concentration is highest. At birth, the average concentration is about 23 g per 100 ml. By the end of the third month it falls below normal, probably, because of deficiency of iron in milk. After this gradual recovery takes place and at the end of the first year, the average amount is 12.5 g. Then it rises gradually up to normal adult (physiological) range.
2. *Sex:* In females, the amount of haemoglobin is slightly lower than in males. In adult females, the average is 14 gm%, in adult males the average is 15.5 gm%.
3. *Diurnal variation:* Variation of at least 10% occurs throughout the day. In the morning it is the lowest; in the evening it is the highest.
4. *Altitude:* At higher altitude haemoglobin percentage rises.
5. *Exercise, excitement, adrenaline injection,* etc. increase the amount of haemoglobin.

> **Note:** It should be noted from the above that normal variation of haemoglobin is mostly due to alteration of number of red cells and not due to any change in the absolute quantity of haemoglobin in each cell. Anything that alters the red cell count will alter the percentage of Hb proportionally.

26. Describe the various derivatives of haemoglobin compound.

Ans. *The various derivatives of haemoglobin are:*

a. **Oxyhaemoglobin:** It is a compound of haemoglobin with oxygen. Iron remains in the ferrous (Fe^{++}) state in haemoglobin. It is not a stable compound.

b. **Methaemoglobin:** It is metalloprotein haemoglobin. It has iron in the heme group which is in the Fe^{3+} (ferric) state and not the Fe^{2+} (ferrous) state as in normal haemoglobin. It can be produced after treating the blood with potassium ferricyanide. It is chocolate brown in colour. It is a stable compound.

c. **Carbohaemoglobin:** It is a compound of haemoglobin with CO_2. The compound is formed by union of CO_2 with the globin portion.

d. **Carboxyhaemoglobin or carbon monoxyhaemoglobin:** Haemoglobin combined with CO instead of oxygen. The affinity of human haemoglobin at 38°C, for CO is 210 times greater than oxygen, and is extremely poisonous.

e. **Sulphaemoglobin:** It is formed by the reaction of haemoglobin with a sulfide in the presence of oxygen or hydrogen peroxide and found in putrefied organs and cadavers.

f. **Nitric oxide haemoglobin:** Haemoglobin combined with NO instead of oxygen.

Bibliography

1. Gamperling N, Mast B, Hagbloom R, Houwen B: Performance Evaluation of the Sysmex KX-21 [TM] Automated Hematology Analyzer. Sysmex J Int. 1998, 8: 96–101.

2. Morris SS, Ruel MT, Cohen RJ, Dewey KG, de la Briere B, Hassan MN: Precision, accuracy, and reliability of haemoglobin assessment with use of capillary blood. Am J Clin Nutr. 1999, 69 (6): 1243–1248.

3. Sari M, dePee S, Martini E, Herman S, Bloem MW, Yip R: Estimating the prevalence of anaemia: A comparison of three methods. Bull World Health Org. 2001, 79: 506–511.

4. Zhou X, Yan H, Xing Y, Dang S, Zhuoma B, Wang D: Evaluation of a portable haemoglobin photometer in pregnant women in a high altitude area: A pilot study. DMC Public Health. 2009, 9 (1): 228–10.1186/1471–2458–9–228.

EXERCISE FOR STUDENTS: OBSERVATIONS: NOTE YOUR RESULTS

Results

1. The Hb concentration in the volunteer subject is _____ by Sahli's method.

2. Oxygen carrying capacity —1 gm of haemoglobin carries 1.34 ml of oxygen, hence the oxygen carrying capacity in the subject is

....

....

....

....

....

....

....

....

....

....

....

....

....

....

....

....

....

....

....

5

Determination of Red Blood Cells Count

Learning Objectives

After learning the practical the students should be able to:
1. Discuss the significance of performing red blood cell count.
2. Describe the principle of estimation of red blood cell count.
3. Determine the red blood cell count under haemocytometer.
4. Describe the rule for counting of cells.
5. Enlist precautions while conducting red blood cell count.
6. Discuss the physiological and pathological conditions of variation in red blood cell count.

Aim of the experiment: Enumeration of the number of erythrocytes in one cubic millimeter of blood.

Principle: As red blood cell count is in million, the red blood cell diluting fluid is used to dilute the blood so that red blood cells can be counted under magnification in a known volume of fluid and thereafter the observe count is multiplied by the diluting factor to determine the total red blood cell count.

Materials and chemicals: Neubauer chamber with coverslip, red cell pipette, and microscope and diluting fluid. [The diluting fluid is the Hayem's fluid and it contains sodium sulphate 2.5 gm, mercuric chloride 0.25 gm, sodium chloride 0.5 gm, dissolved in 100 ml of distilled water].

The functions of contents of Hayem's fluid are:

Sodium sulphate: It prevents red blood cell aggregation and rouleaux formation.

Sodium chloride: It is responsible for maintaining isotonocity of Hayem's fluid, thereby aiding red blood cells suspension in solution.

Mercuric chloride: It acts as preservative and prevent contamination and preservation against bacteria and fungi.

Procedure
1. Take a clean and dry pipette.
2. Pour the RBC diluting fluid (Hayem's fluid) in a clean and dry watch glass.
3. Wipe the middle finger or the index finger with methylated spirit before pricking.
4. Give a finger prick using lancet, allow free flow of blood, discard the first drop and then suck blood up to the 0.5 mark. No air bubbles should accumulate during the process.
5. Wipe the tip of the pipette using sterile gauze, and then suck Hayem's fluid up to the 101 mark.
6. Keep the pipette initially at an acute angle while sucking in the Hayem's fluid and then gradually make it vertical as the fluid reaches the 101 mark.
7. Place the pipette in a horizontal position and firmly hold it between your palms.
8. Mix the contents of the bulb between the palms of the two hands gently.

9. Charge the Neubauer chamber
   A. Clean the haemocytometer and its coverslip with a sterile gauze piece and wait for 2 minutes to make it dry.
   B. Discard first few drops of fluid from the RBC pipette in order to expel the diluents from the stem.
   C. The drop of fluid appears at the tip of the pipette; thereafter the tip of the pipette is placed on the central platform near the edge of the coverslip. The fluid is drawn under coverslip by capillary action.
   D. Ensure that no air bubbles are present (it occurs if undercharged) and there is no overflow of fluid into the grooves (this occurs if overcharged).
   E. After charging allow the cells to settle and then focus the cells under low power to ensure uniform distribution.
10. Conduct RBC count in the central square of the Neubauer chamber under high power objective in the four medium-sized corner square and one medium-sized central square.
11. **Counting:** Count the total number of RBCs in the four corner squares and in the central square. (Total of 5 medium-sized squares or 16 × 5 = 80 small squares.) Ensure that you count all cells on upper and left border in that square; the cells on lower and right border are not to be counted in that square.

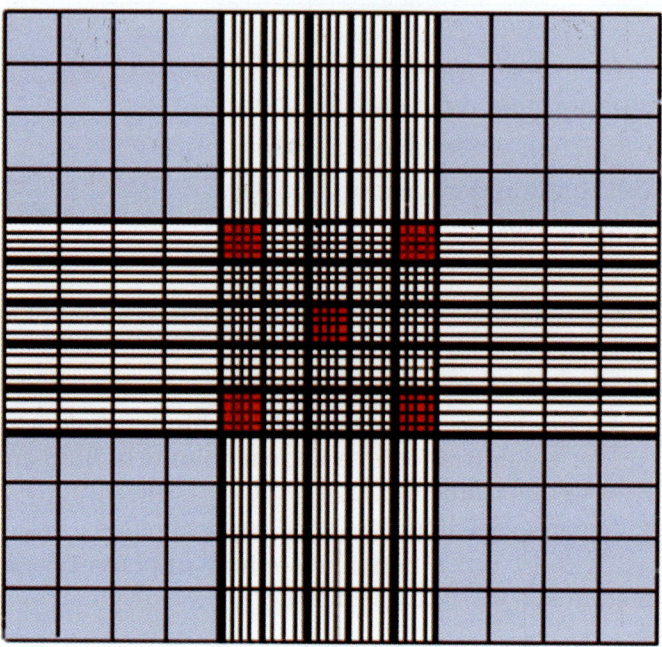

Fig. 5.1: Grid area of RBC count (shown in red)

Calculations

1. Dilution Factor

0.5 parts of blood is diluted in 100.5 parts of red blood cell diluting fluid. Note that during mixing of blood the diluting fluid which remains in stem do not participate in dilution while one which is in bulb does. Hence 0.5 part of blood gets mixed with 99.5 parts of diluting fluid forming 100 parts of solution, thereby dilution factor will be **Final Volume** (100 parts)/**Original Volume** (0.5 parts)…, that is, the blood being diluted 200 times.

2. Volume of Fluid

Area of 5 medium-sized RBC squares = 5 × 1/5 × 1/5 sq.mm.

Depth under the coverslip = 1/10 mm.

Thus volume of 5 medium-sized squares = 1/5 sq.mm. × 1/10 mm = 1/50 cu.mm.

3. Total RBC Count

Number of cells in 1/50 cu. mm volume of diluted blood = n RBCs

Therefore, 1 cu. mm of diluted blood contains = n (No. of RBCs) × 50.

The dilution factor is 1:200. (0.5 parts of blood in 100 parts of Hayem's fluid makes the blood diluted 200 times)

Therefore, 1 cu. mm of undiluted blood contains = $n \times 50 \times 200$.

= $n \times 10000$ RBCs

Results: Record your observations and results.

Precautions

1. Ensure that the Neubauer chamber, pipette, fingertip, lancet and coverslip are clean and dry.
2. The diluted blood sample after pipetting should be thoroughly mixed.
3. The air bubble should not be present in charging pipette or under coverslip of the counting chamber.
4. The chamber should be uniformly charged and ensure that there is no overflowing in the chamber.
5. Note that cells touching the left and lower borders are to be considered for counting while those at right and upper borders are omitted.
6. Cell count should be started after they get equally distributed.

Sources of Error

1. Improper collection of blood sample: Blood collected less than that required for counting may give error in results.
2. Wet or contaminated pipettes: This may result in improper results.
3. Poor pipetting technique, for example, under collection below desired line with blood or diluting fluid or over collection above desired line with blood or diluting fluid or presence of air bubble in the pipette, etc.
4. Failure to discard 2 or 3 drops from the pipette tips before charging the haemocytometer.
5. Overcharging or undercharging the haemocytometer.
6. If wet or contaminated coverslip and haemocytometer is being used for cell count.
7. The cells in the counting chamber are unevenly distributed.
8. Error while counting cell.

Results: Record your observations and results.

> **Note:** Nomal red blood cell count in adult is: Males: It is 5–6 million/μL (average 5.5 million/μL) and females: 4.5–5.5 million/μL (average value in female is 4.8 million/μL).

EXERCISE FOR STUDENTS

OSPE Skilled

Q1. Dilute the given sample of blood for RBC count.

Ans.

1. Draws blood up to the 0.5 mark; ensure no air bubbles accumulates during the process. (Yes/No)
2. Wipes the tip of the pipette using sterile gauze, and then sucks hayem's fluid up to the 101 mark. (Yes/No)
3. Keeps the pipette initially at an acute angle while sucking in the Hayem's fluid and then gradually makes it vertical as the fluid reaches the 101 mark. (Yes/No)
4. Places the pipette in a horizontal position and firmly holds it between palms. (Yes/No)
5. Mixes the contents of the bulb between the palms of the two hands gently. (Yes/No)
6. Places back the RBC pipette in the tray. (Yes/No)

Q2. Charge the Neubauer chamber.

Ans.

1. Ensures that the haemocytometer and its coverslip are clean and dry. (Yes/No)
2. Discards the first two drops from the RBC pipette in order to expel the diluents from the stem. (Yes/No)
3. Gently applying pressure along the rubber tubing of pipette allows the drop of blood to be formed at the tip of the pipette; thereafter places the tip of the pipette on the central platform near the edge of the coverslip. The fluid is drawn under coverslip by capillary action. (Yes/No)

4. Ensures that no air bubbles are present and there is no overflow of fluid into the grooves. (Yes/No)
5. After charging allow the cells to settle and then focus the cells under low power to ensure uniform distribution. (Yes/No)
6. Places back the RBC pipette in the tray. (Yes/No)

SPOTTERS—NON-SKILLED OSPE QUESTION I

Q1. Enlist the elements and source required for red blood cell production.

Ans. *The elements and dietary sources for increasing red blood cell production are*:
- Iron—Lentils and legumes.
- Folic acid—Lentils, cereals fortified with folic acid and dark green leafy vegetables.
- Copper—Shellfish, poultry, liver, beans, cherries, whole grains, nuts and chocolate.
- Vitamin B$_{12}$—Meat, eggs and fortified cereals.
- Vitamin B$_6$—Meats, fish, whole grains, vegetables and legumes.
- Vitamin A—Grapefruit, watermelon, plums, mangoes and apricots.

SPOTTERS—NON-SKILLED OSPE QUESTION II

Q1. Enlist any three measures for increasing red blood cells.

Ans. *The three measures for increasing red blood cells are*:
1. Exercise.
2. Blood transfusions.
3. Erythropoietin hormone therapy stimulates the bone marrow to increase red blood cells production. It is especially useful in patients who are in kidney failure or receiving chemotherapy treatment.

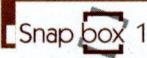 Snap box 1

JAN SWAMMERDAM (1637–1680)

He was a biologist and microscopist. As part of his anatomical research, he carried out experiments on contraction of muscle. In 1658, he was the first to observe and describe the red blood cell. He was one of the first people to use the microscope in dissections, and his techniques remained useful for hundreds of years.

VIVA VOCE QUESTIONS

Q1. What is the principle of determination of red blood cell count?

Ans. *The principle of determination of red blood cell count is*: As red blood cell count is in million, the red blood cell diluting fluid is used to dilute the blood so that red blood cells can be counted under magnification in a known volume of fluid and multiplied by the diluting factor to determine the red blood cell count.

Q2. When a blood sample is to be collected from inpatient ward for RBC count? Which anticoagulant is used?

Ans. The preferred anticoagulant for collecting blood for red blood cell count is EDTA. Heparinized whole blood or citrate is the other anticoagulant being used; but moreover citrate solution dilutes the blood by 10% so necessary correction should be made while reporting.

Q3. What are the features of RBC diluting pipette?

Ans. *The features of RBC diluting pipette are*:
a. The markings on the pipette include 0.5, 1 and 101.
b. The luminal diameter of the stem of RBC pipette is smaller when compared to that of WBC pipette.
c. The bulb contains a red bead.
d. The volume of the bulb of the RBC pipette is larger than that of the WBC pipette.

Q4. Why do we discard the first two drops from the RBC pipette before charging the Neubauer chamber?

Ans. The first two drops from the RBC pipette are discarded before charging the Neubauer chamber as they contain only the diluting fluid.

Q5. What is the role of bead of the RBC pipette?

Ans. It helps in recognizing the RBC pipette while especially helping in thorough mixing of blood with the diluting fluid.

Q6. What are the precautions to be taken while estimating red blood cell count?

Ans. *The precautions to be taken while estimating red blood cell count are*:
1. Ensure that the Neubauer chamber, pipette, fingertip, lancet and coverslip is clean and dry.
2. The diluted blood sample after pipetting should be thoroughly mixed.
3. The air bubble should not be present in charging pipette or under coverslip of the counting chamber.
4. The chamber should be uniformly charged and ensure that there is no overflowing in the chamber
5. Note that cells touching the left and lower borders are to be considered for counting while those at right and upper borders are omitted.
6. Cell count should be started after they get equally distributed.

Q7. What are the various sources of errors while estimating red blood cell count?

Ans. *The various sources of errors while estimating red blood cell count are*:
1. Improper collection of blood sample—blood collected less than that required for counting may give error in results.
2. Wet or contaminated pipettes—this may result in improper results.
3. Poor pipetting technique, for example, under collection below desired line with blood or diluting fluid or over collection above desired line with blood or diluting fluid or presence of air bubble in the pipette, etc.
4. Failure to discard 2 or 3 drops from the pipette tips before charging the haemocytometer.
5. Overcharging or undercharging the haemocytometer
6. If wet or contaminated coverslip and haemocytometer is being used for cell count.
7. The cells in the counting chamber are unevenly distributed.
8. Error while counting cell.

Q8. How will you calculate the volume of blood in RBC count?

Ans. *The volume of fluid is calculated as follows*:
- Area of 5 medium-sized RBC squares = $5 \times 1/5$ sq.mm $\times 1/5$ sq.mm.
- Depth under the coverslip = $1/10$ mm.
  Thus volume of 5 medium-sized squares = $1/5$ sq.mm $\times 1/10$ mm = $1/50$ μL.

Q9. Describe the structure of red blood cells and its normal range in circulation in males and females.

Ans. Red blood cells are biconcave oval disc shape and 7.2 μm in diameter. The red blood cell per micro litre of blood ranges between 5 and 6 million in males and in-between 4.5 and 5.5 million in females. A normal red blood cell count for children is between 3.8 and 5.5 million.

Q10. What are the main functions of red blood cells?

Ans. *The main functions of red blood corpuscles are*:
1. They carry oxygen and deliver it to the tissue and carbon dioxide from tissue is carried to lung and expired out.
2. They maintain acid–base balance by the buffering action of haemoglobin.
3. They help to maintain the viscosity of blood.

Q11. What is the site of synthesis of red blood cell after birth and in adult age?

Ans. The bone marrow is the main site of erythropoiesis after birth. Then up to twenty years of age all bones contribute towards formation of red blood cells but after twentieth year most of the long bones are replaced with yellow marrow and upper ends of femur and humerus which contain red marrow continue to form red cells throughout life. Similarly, the vertebrae, the ribs and the flat bones are the site for production of red cells in adult life.

Q12. What is the average life span of the red blood cells? Where are they destroyed?

Ans. The average life span of red blood cells live is around 120 days. The spleen is the main organ where old red blood cells are destroyed.

Q13. What factors are required for conversion of pro-erythroblast into early normoblast?

Ans. Intrinsic castle factor; Vitamin B_{12} (extrinsic factors) and folic acid are required for the conversion of pro-erythroblast into the early normoblast.

Q14. What is the role of metals in erythropoiesis?

Ans. *The role of metals in erythropoiesis is:*

    1. Iron: It is required for synthesis of haem.

    2. Copper and manganese: They help in the conversion of iron into haemoglobin by catalytic action.

    3. Cobalt: As a component of vitamin B_{12} they help in maturation of red blood cells.

    4. Calcium: It helps in directly by conserving more iron and its subsequent assimilation.

    5. Bile salts: The presence of bile salts in the intestine is important for the proper absorption of these metals.

Q15. Discuss the various conditions in which red blood cell count is decreased and increased.

Ans. Red blood cell count is decreased in iron deficiency anaemia, sickle cell anaemia, haemolytic anaemia, thalassemia, pernicious anaemia, hereditary spherocytosis, pure red cell aplasia and aplastic anaemia. The increased in blood cell count leads to polycythemia. Polycythemia vera (PCV) is a condition in which the red blood count increases due to abnormality of the bone marrow. Secondary polycythemia also known as physiologic polycythemia is a condition in which the production of erythropoietin increases appropriately with increased production of red blood cells.

Q16. What is anaemia? What are the four main types of anaemia?

Ans. Anaemia is low concentration of haemoglobin in the blood.

    The four main types of anaemia are the nutrient-deficiency anaemia, blood loss anaemia, haemolytic anaemia and aplastic anaemia.

    Nutritional anaemia: It is caused due to deficiency of fundamental nutrients required for the development and maturation of the red blood cell. The nutrients required for maturation of red blood cells are iron, vitamin B_{12}, folic acid, vitamin C, cobalt, copper, zinc, manganese, nickel, etc.

    Blood loss anaemia: Mainly occurs in hemorrhagic conditions, peptic ulcerations

Q17. What are the symptoms observed in patients of anaemia?

Ans. The symptoms observed in patients of anaemia are fatigue, shortness of breath, palpitation, angina, intermittent claudicating legs, malaise, headache, etc.

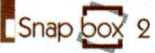

Snap box 2

In order to have an appropriate diagnosis and management of anaemia, a detailed clinical examination, i.e. examination of *peripheral blood smear of the patient, determination of red* cell indices, red cell diameter width (RDW), and red blood cell histograms are the preferred mode of investigations today.

EXERCISE FOR STUDENTS—OBSERVATIONS

Note your Results

Results: Total RBC count

Number of cells in 1/50 cu. mm volume of diluted blood (n) = ...

Therefore, 1 cu. mm of diluted blood contains = ... (n, No. of RBCs) × 50.

The dilution factor is 1:200. (0.5 parts of blood in 100 parts of Hayem's fluid makes the blood diluted 200 times)

Therefore, 1 cu. mm of undiluted blood contains = ... (n) × 50 × 200.

= ... (n) × 10000

Results: Thus total RBC count is ....…...………..............

...........................……...…..........…..............…………........................

6

Determination of Red Blood Cell Indices

Learning Objectives

After learning the practical the students should be able to:

1. Explain the significance of determining red blood cell indices.
2. Define and discuss regarding parameters concerned with determining red blood cell indices.
3. Calculate and report the red blood cell indices.
4. Discuss the clinical significance of each red blood cell indices.

Aim of experiment: Determination of red blood cell indices.

Principle: The parameters such as haemoglobin, RBC count, haematocrit value, packed cell volume helps to evaluate certain blood indices which indicate haemoglobin concentration in red blood cell and red blood cell size that aids in accurate diagnosis of the type of anaemia which the patient is suffering from.

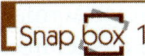 Snap box 1

This vital information can be obtained from blood indices:

1. Mean corpuscular volume (MCV)
2. Mean corpuscular haemoglobin (MCH)
3. Mean corpuscular haemoglobin concentration (MCHC)
4. Colour index (CI)
5. Red blood cell distribution width (RDW)

Mean corpuscular volume (MCV) determines the average size of the RBCs; Mean corpuscular haemoglobin (MCH) states the average amount of oxygen-carrying haemoglobin inside a red blood cell; and mean corpuscular haemoglobin concentration (MCHC) denotes the average concentration of haemoglobin inside a red blood cell. The variation in size of RBC can be ascertained by calculating the red cell distribution width (RDW). In pernicious anaemia the variation in RBC size (anisocytosis) along with variation in shape (poikilocytosis) increases the RDW.

Apparatus: Same as that described in chapters of estimation of haemoglobin, RBC count, haematocrit and packed cell volume.

Method

The parameters such as haemoglobin, RBC count, haematocrit value, packed cell volume are calculated by manual method or automated method and red blood cell indices are then determined.

Calculation

1. Mean corpuscular volume (MCV): It is the average volume of single red blood cells. The normal MCV averages in between 78 and 94 µm³. MCV is increased in pernicious anaemia and megaloblastic anaemia. MCV is decreased in iron deficiency anaemia.

Calculation of the MCV: For example, RBC count is 5 millions/μL of blood; and haematocrit reading is 40%.

$$MCV = \frac{PCV \text{ per } 100 \text{ ml of blood}}{RBC \text{ count in millions/μL}} \times 10$$

$$MCV = 40/5 \times 10$$
$$MCV = 80 \ \mu m^3$$

Physiological Significance—MCV

A. **Macrocytes:** When the MCV is higher than normal, the red blood cells are called macrocytes and the clinical condition which patient develops is macrocytic anaemia. The macrocytic anaemia can be caused by: Vitamin B_{12} deficiency, folate deficiency, chemotherapy and preleukemias.

B. **Microcytes:** When the MCV is lower than normal, the red blood cells are called microcytes and the clinical condition which patient develops is microcytic anaemia. Microcytic anaemia may be caused by iron deficiency (secondary to poor dietary intake of iron, menstrual bleeding, or gastrointestinal bleeding), chronic diseases, thalassemia and lead poisoning.

C. **Normocytes:** Normocytic normochromic red blood cells are seen in after acute haemorrhage, aplastic anaemia and in all haemolytic anaemia with thalassemia as exception.

2. Mean corpuscular haemoglobin (MCH): This is the quantity or amount of haemoglobin present in one red blood cell. The normal value of MCH averages around 28 to 32 pg ($1pg = 10^{-12}$).

Calculation of the MCH: For example, RBC count is 5 millions/μL; and haemoglobin level is 15 gm/dl

$$MCH = \frac{Haemoglobin \text{ in gm/dl}}{RBC \text{ in millions/μL}} \times 10$$

$$MCH = \frac{15}{5} \times 10$$

Thus, MCH = 30 pg or micro microgram.

Physiological Significance—MCH

Decreased MCH occurs in microcytosis associated with chronic infections (microcytic normochromic anaemia) but the decreased in MCH is more significant in iron deficiency anaemia and thalassemia as they are associated with hypochromia.

3. Mean corpuscular haemoglobin concentration (MCHC): MCHC is the concentration of haemoglobin in one red blood cell. It is the amount of haemoglobin expressed in relation to the volume of one red blood cell. The normal value of MCHC is 30% (30 to 38%).

Calculation of the MCHC: For example, haemoglobin level is 15 gm/dl

And haematocrit reading is 40%

$$MCHC = \frac{Haemoglobin \text{ in gm/dl}}{PCV \text{ per } 100 \text{ ml of blood}} \times 100$$

$$MCHC = 15/40 \times 100$$

Thus, MCHC = 37.5%

Physiological Significance—MCHC

It is decreased in iron deficiency anaemia in which, red blood cells are hypochromic and microcytic. The increased MCHC may occur during dehydration in patient of hereditary spherocytosis.

4. Colour index (CI): This is the ratio between the percentage of haemoglobin and the percentage of red blood cells in the blood. The normal colour index is 1.0 (0.8 to 1.2).

Calculation of colour index: Haemoglobin is 14.8 μ/dl and RBC count is 5 million/μL of blood.

$$Colour \ index = \frac{Haemoglobin\%}{RBC \ \%}$$

Note: For standard reference: Haemoglobin of 14.8 µ/dl is 100%; and RBC count of 5 million /µL of blood is 100%.

Colour index = 100/100 = 1

Physiological Significance—Colour Index

It determines the type of anaemia. Colour index is normal in normocytic normochromic anaemia, lower in iron deficiency anaemia and higher in pernicious anaemia and megaloblastic anaemia,

5. Red blood cell distribution width (RDW): It is an index of the variation in cell volume within the red blood cell population. The normal range of RDW is 11.5 to 14.5%.

The red blood cell distribution width percentage is calculated as follows:

$$RDW\ (\%) = (Standard\ deviation \div mean)\ cell\ volume \times 100$$

Physiological significance: Red blood cell distribution width (RDW): It may be used to quantitate the amount of anisocytosis on peripheral blood smear.

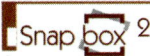 Snap box 2

The first textbook of haematology was written by the French physician Gabriel Andral in 1843 but then the fact that decreased RBC count leads to anaemia was not known. In the early part of nineteenth century, the term anaemia was a clinical term used by physician referring to pallor of the skin and mucous membranes. The technical method for white blood cells count was discovered in 1852 by Karl Vierordt. H. Welcher who was Vierordt's student in 1854, counted the blood cells in a patient with chlorosis and found that an anaemic patient had significantly lesser red blood cells than a normal individual. The clinical and biological science of haematology gain significant importance between 1878 and 1888, when the microscopic details of blood cells could be evaluated. As gradually haematology studies achieved advancement, the blood indices started being used as an important investigation in morphological classification of anaemia.

VIVA VOCE QUESTIONS

Q1. What is mainly indicated by the results of red blood cell indices?

Ans. The red blood cell mainly indicates
   a. MCV reveals the average size of the RBCs
   b. RDW reveals a variation in size among the RBCs
   c. MCHC reveals how much of the cell is being taken up by haemoglobin. Together can reveal anaemia or physiologic disorders that affect quality of life.

Q2. What does increased, decreased and normal MCV indicate?

Ans. *The increased, decreased and normal MCV indicate type of anaemia and is explained below:*
   1. Macrocytic anaemia: When the MCV is higher than normal the red blood cells are called macrocytes and the clinical condition which patient develops is macrocytic anaemia. The macrocytic anaemia can be caused by: Vitamin B_{12} deficiency, folate deficiency, chemotherapy and preleukemias.
   2. Microcytic anaemia: When the MCV is lower than normal, the red blood cells are called microcytes and the clinical condition which patient develops is microcytic anaemia. Microcytic anaemia may be caused by iron deficiency (secondary to poor dietary intake of iron, menstrual bleeding, or gastrointestinal bleeding), chronic diseases, thalassemia and lead poisoning.
   3. Normocytic anaemia: Normocytic normochromic red blood cells are seen in after acute haemorrhage, aplastic anaemia and in all haemolytic anaemia with thalassemia as exception.

Q3. What are the causes for decreased MCH?

Ans. The decreased MCH occurs in microcytosis associated with chronic infections (microcytic normochromic anaemia) but the decreased in MCH is more significant in iron deficiency anaemia and thalassemia as they are associated with hypochromia.

Q4. What are the causes for decreased and increased in MCHC?

Ans. It is decreased in iron deficiency anaemia in which, red blood cells are hypochromic and microcytic. The increased MCHC may occur during dehydration in patient of hereditary spherocytosis.

Q5. What does colour index indicate?

Ans. It determines the type of anaemia. Colour Index is normal in normocytic normochromic anaemia, lower in iron deficiency anaemia and higher in pernicious anaemia and megaloblastic anaemia.

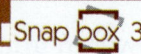 Snap box 3

Nowadays all clinical laboratories prefer using automated machines to perform blood counts, complete blood count which includes red cell indices as part of the profile. Two types of advance automated machines used are Coulter S model which employs the principle of electric impedance; and hemalog system analyzer, which use optical methods in performing cell counts. More advance machines are able to calculate RDW or red cell morphology index, mean platelet volume, differential white cell count and absolute lymphocyte count.

EXERCISE FOR STUDENTS

Spotters—OSPE: Non-Skilled—Calculations

1. **Calculate the MCV from given data:** RBC count is 6 millions/µL of blood; and haematocrit reading is 42%

$$MCV = \frac{PCV \text{ per } 100 \text{ ml of blood}}{RBC \text{ count in millions/µL}} \times 10$$

MCV = ... × 10

Thus MCV = ... µm³

2. **Calculate the MCH value from given data:** RBC count is 5 millions/µL of blood; and haemoglobin level is 10 gm/dl

$$MCH = \frac{Haemoglobin \text{ in gm/dl}}{RBC \text{ in millions/µL}} \times 10$$

Thus, MCH = ... × 10

Thus, MCH = ... pg or micro microgram.

3. **Calculate the MCHC value from given data:** For example, haemoglobin level is 15 gm/dl and haematocrit reading is 40%.

$$MCHC = \frac{Haemoglobin \text{ in gm/dl}}{PCV \text{ per } 100 \text{ ml of blood}} \times 100$$

MCHC = ... × 100

Thus MCHC = ... %

4. **Calculate colour index:** Haemoglobin is 14.8 µ/dl and RBC count is 5 million/µL of blood.
Colour index = Haemoglobin%/RBC %

Note: For standard reference: Haemoglobin of 14.8 µ/dl is 100%; and RBC count of 5 million /µL of blood is 100%.

Colour index = ...

....

....

....

....

....

....

....

GENESIS OF WHITE BLOOD CELLS AND RED BLOOD CELLS

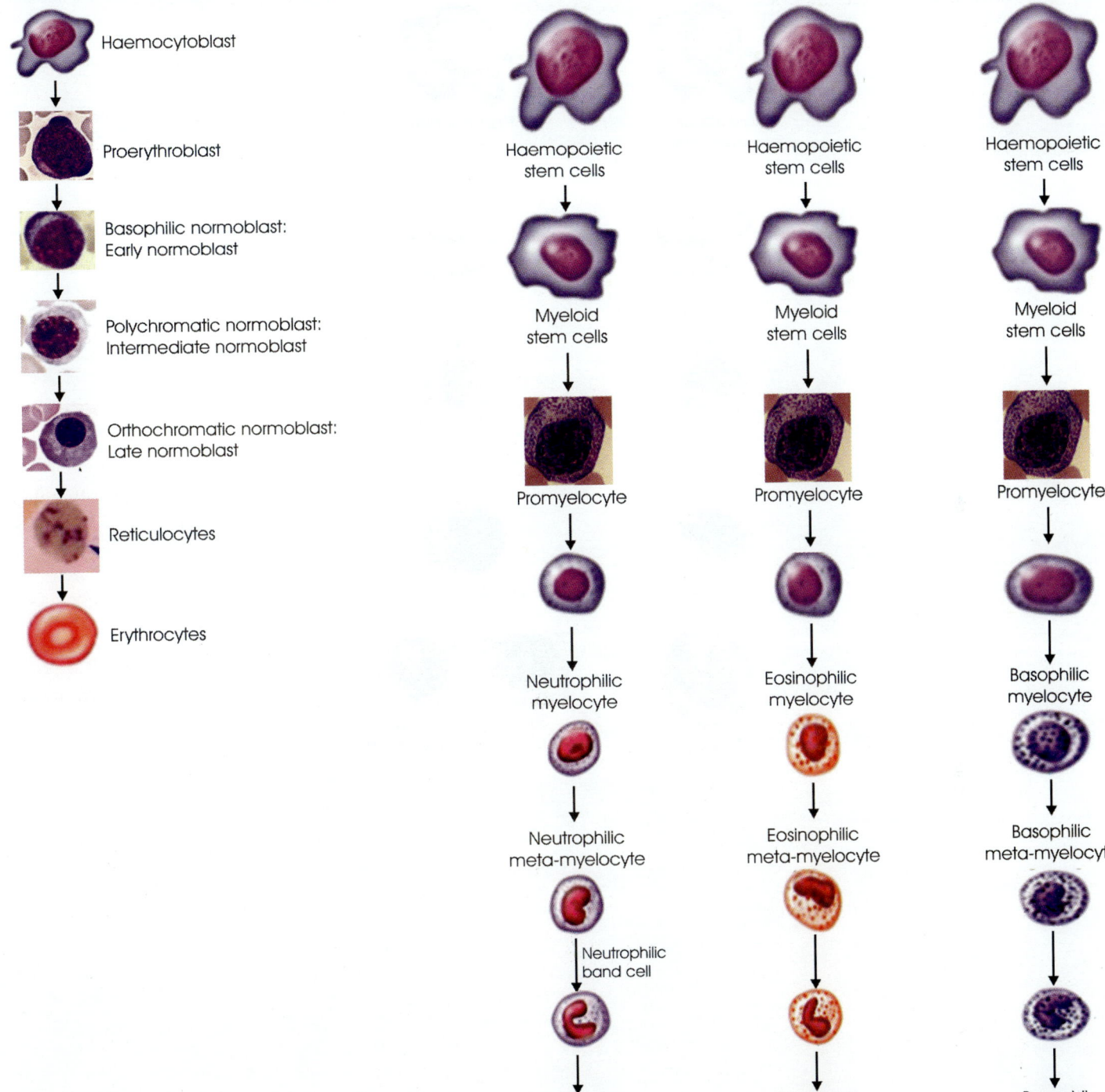

Haemocytoblast

Proerythroblast

Basophilic normoblast:
Early normoblast

Polychromatic normoblast:
Intermediate normoblast

Orthochromatic normoblast:
Late normoblast

Reticulocytes

Erythrocytes

Haemopoietic stem cells

Myeloid stem cells

Promyelocyte

Neutrophilic myelocyte

Neutrophilic meta-myelocyte

Neutrophilic band cell

Neutrophil

Haemopoietic stem cells

Myeloid stem cells

Promyelocyte

Eosinophilic myelocyte

Eosinophilic meta-myelocyte

Eosinophil

Haemopoietic stem cells

Myeloid stem cells

Promyelocyte

Basophilic myelocyte

Basophilic meta-myelocyte

Basophil

GENESIS OF MONOCYTES AND LYMPHOCYTES

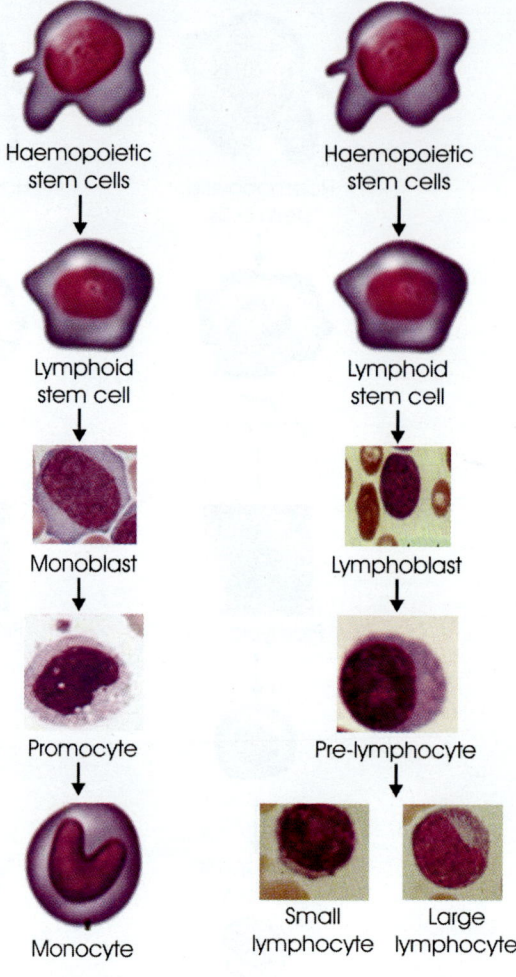

STRUCTURE OF PLATELET AND ITS GENESIS

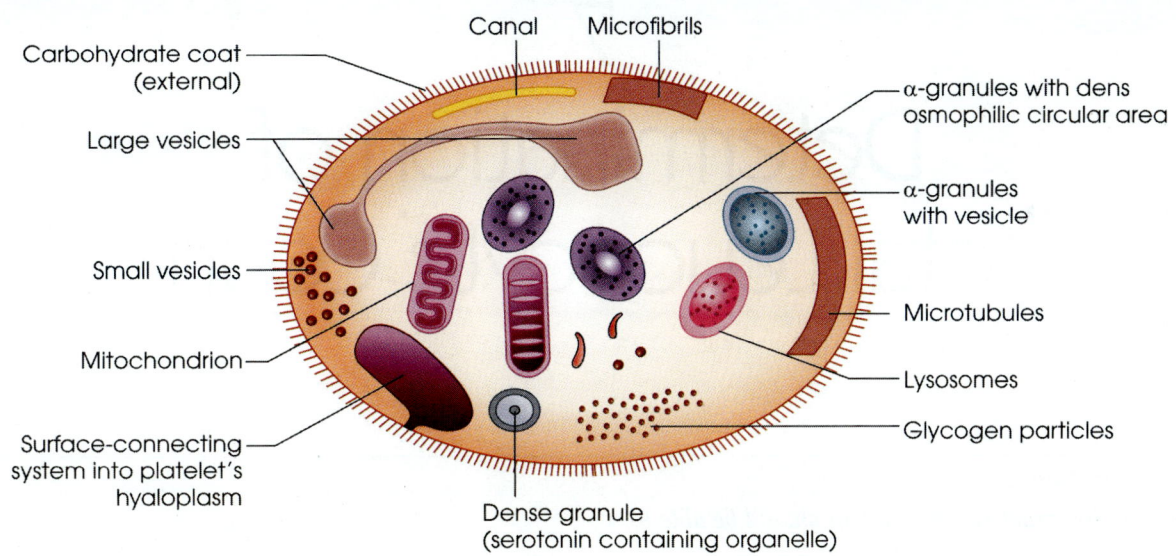

Carbohydrate coat (external)

Canal   Microfibrils

Large vesicles

α-granules with dens osmophilic circular area

α-granules with vesicle

Small vesicles

Mitochondrion

Microtubules

Lysosomes

Surface-connecting system into platelet's hyaloplasm

Glycogen particles

Dense granule (serotonin containing organelle)

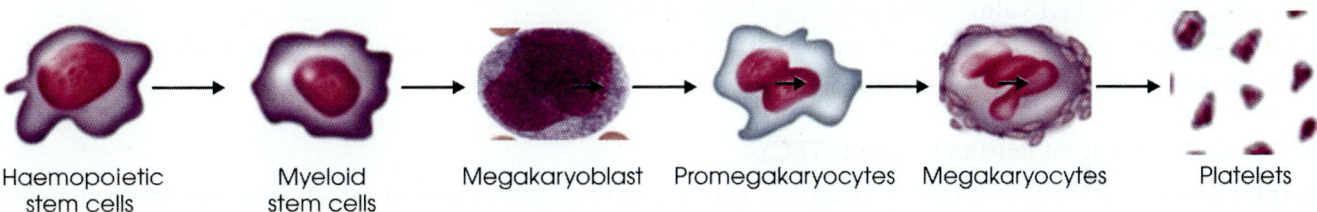

Haemopoietic stem cells → Myeloid stem cells → Megakaryoblast → Promegakaryocytes → Megakaryocytes → Platelets

7

Determination of Total Leucocyte Count

Aim: Determine the total leucocyte count (TLC).

Principle: The blood sample which is drawn is diluted with a diluting fluid which destroys the red cells and stains the nuclei of the leucocytes. The cells are then counted in a counting chamber and leucocyte count in undiluted blood is reported as number of WBCs/mm^3.

Materials and chemicals: Blood lanced/pricking needle, sterile cotton swabs, spirit, microscope, coverslip, haemocytometer, WBC pipette and WBC diluting fluid (Turk's fluid).

Composition of WBC Diluting Fluid (Turk's Fluid)

Glacial acetic acid (3%): 3 ml (glacial acetic acid lyses the red blood cell and the platelets).

Gentian violet (1%): 1 ml (stain the nuclei of the WBCs).

Distilled water: 100 ml (acts as solvent for preparing WBC diluting fluid amounting to 100 ml).

Method

1. Take 1 ml of Turk's fluid in a watch glass.
2. Clean the finger with spirit using gauze. Give a finger prick (any one of the middle, ring or index finger). Wait till free flow of blood is there (do not squeeze finger)
3. Wipe out the first drop of blood as it contains tissue fluids; while as subsequent drop appears then draw blood into the pipette up to 0.5 mark.
4. The tip of the pipette is to be placed in the diluting fluid and then draw the diluting fluid up to 11 mark.
5. Hold the WBC pipette horizontally and gently rotate the pipette between the palms for three minutes so that the blood and diluting fluid are mixed evenly in the bulb. During this three minutes duration the lysis of the red blood cell also occurs.
6. After discarding the first two drops charge the Neubauer chamber and wait for 3–4 minutes for the cells to settle. Do not overcharge or undercharge.
7. Check for even distribution of cells in the four corner squares under the low power objective.

8. Count the total number of WBCs in the four corner large squares (these are divided into 16 squares) using the low power objective.
9. Note your count for all four corner large squares (total 64 squares) and note the total cell count as *n*.
10. Calculate the total leucocyte count as below: First calculate the volume of fluid in four white blood cells square, then proceed for total leucocyte count.

Calculation

A. Volume of fluid which is used for estimating total leucocyte count:

Area of the four WBC squares = 4×1 mm $\times 1$ mm = 4 sq.mm.

Depth under the coverslip (distance between coverslip and glass of Neubauer chamber) = 1/10 mm (0.1 mm).

Thus the volume of fluid in four white blood cells square is = 4 sq mm $\times 0.1$ mm = 0.4 mm^3

Total Leucocyte Count

The number of WBCs in 0.4 mm^3 of diluted blood = *n* cells.

The dilution factor = 1: 20 (0.5 parts of blood in 10 parts of Turk's fluid)

Therefore, the number of WBCs in 1 mm^3 of undiluted blood

$$= \frac{n \times 20 \text{ (dilution factor)}}{0.4}$$

$$= n \times 50 \text{ cells.}$$

Results: Record your observation and result:

The WBC count is ....

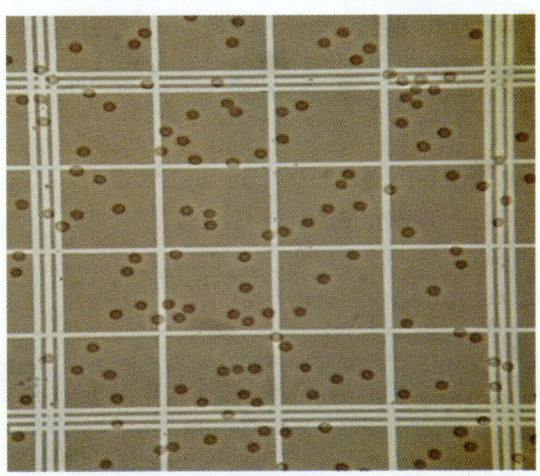

Fig. 7.1: WBC cells as seen under microscope

Note: You may have to lower the light on the microscope to visualize the WBCs. They will be refractile and round with a definite outline

Precautions

1. Ensure that the Neubauer chamber, pipette, fingertip, lancet and coverslip is clean and dry.
2. The diluted blood sample after pipetting should be thoroughly mixed.
3. The air bubble should not be present in charging pipette or under coverslip of the counting chamber.
4. The chamber should be uniformly charged and ensure that there is no overflowing in the chamber
5. Note that cells touching the left and lower borders are to be considered for counting while those at right and upper borders are omitted.
6. Cell count should be started after they get equally distributed.

Sources of Error

1. Improper collection of blood sample: Blood collected less than that required for counting may give error in results.
2. Wet or contaminated pipettes: This may result in improper results.
3. Poor pipetting technique, for example, under collection below desired line with blood or diluting fluid or overcollection above desired line with blood or diluting fluid or presence of air bubble in the pipette, etc.
4. Failure to discard 2 drops from the pipette tips before charging the haemocytometer.
5. Overcharging or undercharging the haemocytometer
6. If wet or contaminated coverslip and haemocytometer is being used for cell count.
7. The cells in the counting chamber are unevenly distributed.
8. Error while counting cell.

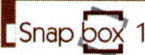 Snap box 1

Gabriel Andral (1797–1876) was a distinguished French pathologist and a Professor at the University of Paris. Gabriel Andral and William Addison simultaneously discovered white blood cell in 1843. They believed that both red and white cells were altered in disease.

Bibliography

Doyle L. Gabriel Andral (1797–1876) and the first reports of lymphangitis carcinomatosa. J R Soc Med. 1989 Aug; 82(8): 491–3.

OSPE 1

Q1. Draw the blood from the given sample in WBC pipette.

STUDENT 1

1. Draws the blood up to 0.5 marks in the WBC pipette. (Yes/No)
2. Holding the pipette almost vertical place into the fluid, draws the diluting fluid into the pipette slowly until the mixture reaches the 11 mark. (Yes/No)
3. Places the pipette in a horizontal position and firmly hold it between the palms. (Yes/No)
4. Mixes the contents of the bulb between the palms of the two hands gently for at least 3 minutes to facilitate haemolysis of RBCs. (Yes/No)
5. Places the pipette in the examination tray. (Yes/No)

OSPE 2

Q1. Charge the Neubauer chamber.

STUDENT 2

Steps

1. Ensures that the haemocytometer and its coverslip are clean and dry. (Yes/No)
2. Discards the first two drops from the WBC pipette in order to expel the diluents from the stem. (Yes/No)
3. Gently applying pressure along the rubber tubing of pipette allows the drop of blood to be formed at the tip of the pipette; thereafter places the tip of the pipette on the central platform near the edge of the coverslip. The fluid is drawn under coverslip by capillary action. (Yes/No)
4. Ensures that no air bubbles are present and there is no overflow of fluid into the grooves. (Yes/No)
5. After charging allows the cells to settle and then focus the cells under low power to ensure uniform distribution. (Yes/No)

VIVA VOCE QUESTIONS

Q1. What is the principle of the determination of total leucocyte count?

Ans. *The principle of the determination of total leucocyte count is as follows*: The blood sample is diluted with a diluting fluid which destroys the red cells and stains the nuclei of the leucocytes. The cells are then counted in a counting chamber and leucocyte count of undiluted blood is reported as number of leucocyte/mm^3.

Q2. What is the composition of Turk's fluid?

Ans. *The composition of WBC diluting fluid (Turk's fluid) is*:
- **Glacial acetic acid 3%:** 3 ml (glacial acetic acid lyses the red blood cell and the platelets).
- **Gentian violet (1% solution):** 1 ml (stain the nuclei of the WBCs).
- **Distilled water:** 100 ml (acts as solvent for preparing WBC diluting fluid amounting to 100 ml).

Q3. What is the function of the bead in white cell pipette bulb?

Ans. The bead in white cell pipette bulb aids mixing the blood with the diluents, informs whether the pipette is dry or not and helps in identifying the pipette.

Q4. What are the uses of WBC pipette?

Ans. WBC pipette can be used for counting WBC, platelets and sperms.

Q5. What precaution should be taken while making white blood cell count?

Ans. The cells that touch any of the upper and left borders should be counted while cells that touch the lower or right border should be excluded.

Q6. How is the dilution factor calculated?

Ans. The dilution factor = 1: 20 (As 0.5 parts of blood is diluted in 10 parts of Turk's fluid, the dilution of blood in Turk's fluid is 20).

Q7. Enlist the precautions to be taken while conducting WBC count.

Ans. Precautions are stated above under heading precaution.

Q8. What is the normal total leucocyte count?

Ans. The normal total leucocyte count in blood ranges between 4000 and 11000 WBC per mm^3 of blood.

Q9. What is leucopoiesis? Which cells produce WBC?

Ans. The process of development and maturation of the white blood cells is termed leucopoiesis. They develop from the pluripotent haemopoietic stem cell which differentiates into colony forming units which are the progenitor cells.

Q10. What are the types of leucocytes and how are they classified into granulocytes and agranulocytes?

Ans. The types of leucocytes are lymphocytes, monocytes, neutrophils, eosinophils and basophils. The neutrophils, eosinophils and basophils are granulocytes in whose cytoplasms have granules (when viewed under electronic microscopy). Lymphocytes and monocytes are the agranulocytes.

Q11. Discuss the physiological and pathological causes of leucocytosis and leucopenia.

Ans. **Leucocytosis:** It is due to increase in the number of WBCs beyond 11000/mm^3 of blood.
- a. **Physiological leucocytosis** is observed in normal infants, after intake of food and after digestion, physical exercise, pregnancy, mental stress, parturition, etc.
- b. **Pathological leucocytosis** occurs in bacterial and viral infections, whooping cough, tuberculosis, myelofibrosis, rheumatoid arthritis, acute and chronic myelogenous leukemia (AML), chronic lymphocytic leukemia, smoking, secondary to emotional and physical stress, post-administration of drugs such as corticosteroid and epinephrine, allergic reactions, etc.

Leucopenia: It is a decrease in the number of white cells below the normal lower limit of 4000/mm^3 of blood.
- a. **Physiological leucopenia** is rare and marginal decrease may occur in extreme cold conditions as in arctic environment exposure.

b. Pathological leucopenia occurs in aplastic anaemia, hypersplenism, lupus, leukemia, HIV AIDS, post-chemotherapy and radiotherapy, Kostmann's syndrome (congenital disorder in which there is low production of neutrophils), tuberculosis, myelodysplastic syndromes, rheumatoid arthritis, etc.

Q12. Enlist the functions of white blood cells.

Ans. *The main functions of white blood cells are*:

1. **Phagocytosis:** The neutrophil and the monocytes engulf foreign particles and bacteria.

2. **Antibody formation:** Lymphocytes manufacture β- and γ-fractions of serum globulin.

3. **Manufacture of trephones:** They exert great influence on the nutrition growth and repair of tissues.

4. **Secretion of heparin:** The basophils secrete 'heparin'; which prevents intravascular clotting.

5. **Antihistamine function:** The eosinophil cells are very rich in histamine. They defend against allergic conditions in which histamine like body are present in excess.

Q13. Enlist the functional characteristic activities of white blood cell.

Ans. The functional characteristic activities of white blood cell are diapedesis and margination, chemotaxis, opsonisation and phagocytosis.

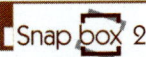 **Snap box 2**

A new class of white blood cells was discovered by the scientist in the year 2013 in human lung and gut tissues. The dendritic cells are a specialized group of white blood cells which present tiny fragments from micro-organisms, vaccines or tumors to the T cells. T helper 17 (Th17) cells play a key role in activating a protective response crucial for our body to eliminate harmful bacteria or fungi.

Bibliography

I Mellman. Dendritic cells: Master regulators of the immune response. Cancer Immunol Res. 2013 Sep; 1(3): 145–9.

OBSERVATIONS: EXERCISE FOR STUDENTS

Note your calculations ....

The number of WBCs in 0.4 mm^3 = ... (n)

The dilution factor is 1.20

Therefore, the number of WBCs in 1 mm^3

Undiluted blood $= \dfrac{n \times 20 \text{ (diluting factor)}}{0.4}$

    $= n \times 50$

    = ... × 50 (note your value n)

Thus total WBC count is ....

....

....

....

....

....

....

....

....

8
Preparation of Peripheral Blood Smear and Determination of Differential Leucocyte Count

Learning Objectives

After learning this practical the students should be able to:

1. Enlist the content of the Leishman stain and discuss their functions.
2. Make an ideal smear and describe the criterion for grading a smear as ideal smear.
3. Stain the smear for differential leucocyte count.
4. Evaluate the quality of smear.
5. Identify the neutrophil, eosinophil, basophil, monocytes and lymphocyte in smear slide.
6. Determine the number of each type of white blood cell present in the blood and expressed them as a percentage of each type among the total hundred cell counted.
7. Enlist the precautions while preparing the smear for differential leucocyte count.

Aim: To stain and study the different types of white blood cells in the smear. Determine the number of each type of white blood cell present in the blood.

Principle: The drop of blood is used to make a peripheral smear which is fixed and stained with Leishman's stain and examined under oil immersion lens of microscope to conduct the differential leucocyte count.

Material and chemicals: Lancet, clean dry glass slides, cedar wood oil, Leishman's stain and microscope.

The constituent of Leishman stain is:

1. Eosin—it is a negatively charged acidic dye staining positively charged basic particles which include eosinophil granules and red blood cells.
2. Methylene blue—it is a positively charged basic dye staining negatively charged acidic particles such as basophil granules, cytoplasm and nuclei of the white blood cells.
3. Acetone free methyl alcohol which acts as a fixative and helps in fixing the blood smear over the slide and so also preserves the morphological characteristic of the white blood cells.

Note: Leishman stain is readily available in crystal form, 0.15 gm of Leishman stain powder is dissolved in 100 ml of acetone free methyl alcohol.

Procedure

I. Preparation of an Ideal Blood Smear

1. Make a sterile finger prick under aseptic precaution. Discard the first drop of blood and allow the blood to free flow.
2. Place a drop of blood at one of the ends of each of the glass slides.
3. Place the spreader slide at an angle of 45° just in front of the blood drop. (Fig. 8.1A)
4. Move the spreader slide backwards to touch the blood drop.
5. The drop must spread out along the line of contact of the spreader slide. (Fig. 8.1B)

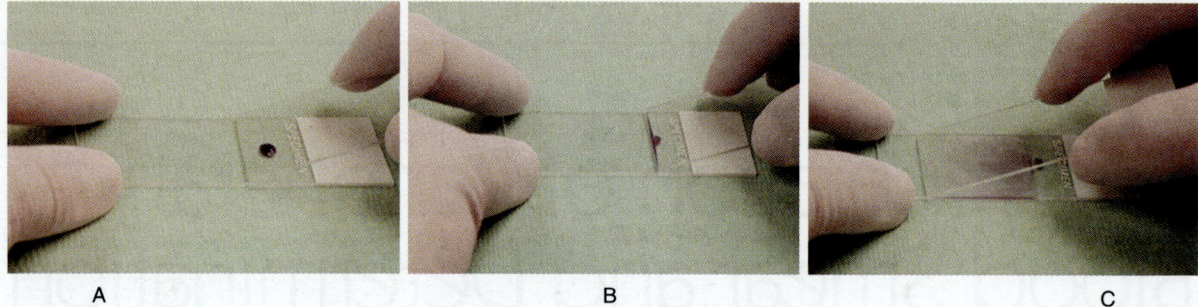

     A   B   C

Fig. 8.1: Technique of making the peripheral blood smear. A. The spreader slide placed at an angle of 45 degrees just in front of the blood drop. B. The drop spreads out along the line of contact of the spreader slide. C. Move the spreader slide smoothly and evenly in forward direction maintaining an angle of 45 degrees; to make the blood smear.

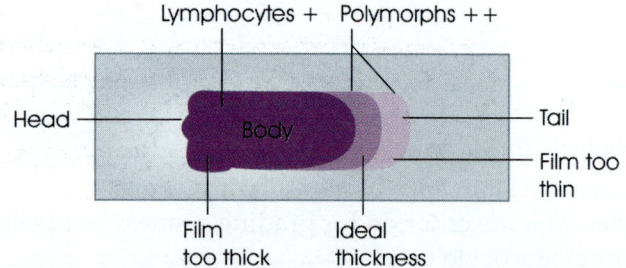

Fig. 8.2: Ideal peripheral blood smear should be ideally thick

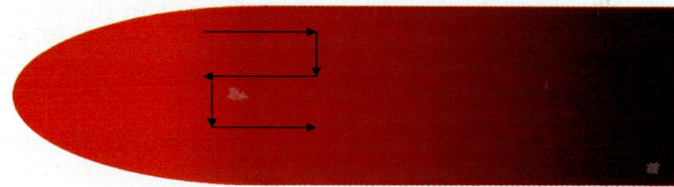

Fig. 8.3: Counting of cells in blood smear

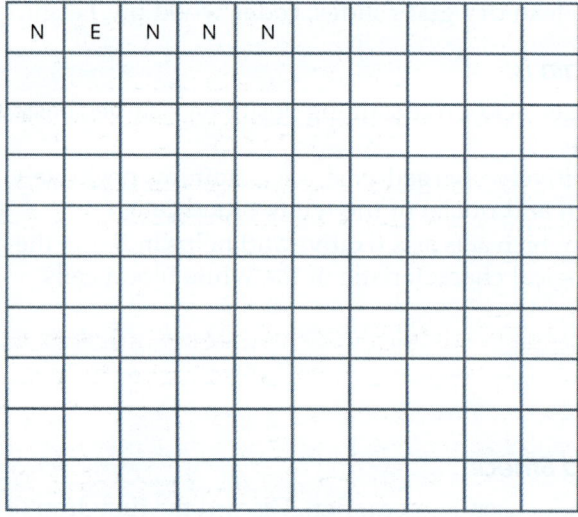

Fig. 8.4

6. Move the spreader slide smoothly and evenly in forward direction maintaining an angle of 45 degrees; to make the blood smear. (Fig. 8.1C)
7. Let the smear dry in air. Repeat the procedure and make three more blood smears.

A smear is described as having a head, body and tail.

Note: An ideal smear is uniform without any striations or vacuoles and neither too thin nor too thick.

Precautions for preparation of a blood smear:
1. Ensure that the complete drop of blood is uniformly spread along the edge of the spreader slide.
2. The gentle pressure should be constantly maintained when drawing the slide forward.
3. The spreader slide should be moved smoothly and evenly in forward direction maintaining an angle of 45 degrees; to make the ideal blood smear.
4. If spreader slide is moved slowly, the leucocytes will be unevenly distributed.
5. Place the slide on glass rods and let it dry.

Note: There should be no delay in making the smear after placing the drop of blood on the slide because delay will result in non-uniform distribution of the white blood cells, and most of the white cells will be visible at the thin edge of the smear.

Causes of Poor Blood Smear
1. If small drop of blood is taken it will produce thin slide; while large drop of blood will make the slide too thick.
2. If the spreader slide is not pushed smoothly and gently across the slide.
3. Failure to maintain an angle of 45 degrees with the slide while moving the spreader slide at a 30° angle.
4. The spreader slide is incompletely moved across the slide.
5. Use of contaminated greasy slide.

II. Fixing and Staining of Blood Smear
1. Place the slide on the staining stand rack in the washing sink.
2. Pour 10–12 drops of Leishman stain on the slide so as to cover it under the stain and wait for two minutes and this is the fixation time.
3. Add adequate amount of distilled water so that it spreads over the smear uniformly. Mix the water and stain by holding slide in hand and making a rocking movement or blowing over it gently. Ensure that the stain is completely covered with distilled water so as to clear any overstained portion.
4. Wait for another 8–10 minutes allowing time for proper staining.
5. After interval of 10 minutes wash the slide, holding it horizontally with tap water. Ensure water does not hit the smear directly, otherwise the stained portion may get removed.
6. Allow slide to dry placing it over the staining stand rack.

Note: The characteristic features of ideal blood smear.

1. An ideal smear covers around ¾ the entire slide area.
2. Ideal smear is tongue shaped, slightly rounded or curved at the feathery edge tail region. It is thick at head end, and thin at tail end.
3. The upper and lower edges of the smear are clear and visible.
4. The smear is smooth without any streaks or vacuoles.
5. It is single cell layer thick.

Examination of a blood film
1. The dry and stained film is examined without a coverslip under oil immersion objective.
2. Place a drop of cedar wood oil over the chosen area and move the oil immersion objective into position; making the lower end of the objective touch the drop of oil.
3. Focus the cell using fine adjustment knob.
4. The differential cell count is done by moving the slide along the central and periphery of the smear. A total of 100 cells are to be counted in which every white cell seen must be recorded as neutrophil, basophil, eosinophil, monocytes and lymphocyte appropriately.
5. White blood cells are found more in numbers along the upper edge, lower edge and tail but are poorly stained. The lymphocytes are more along body area while monocytes and neutrophils along the edges and tail of the smear.

Precaution while counting WBC under smear: Make your observation in one field and record the number of WBC according to its type; then move to another field in the snake-liked direction as shown in Fig. 8.3.

PRECAUTIONS

1. Clean and dry the slides before use.
2. The glass-spreader must have a smooth and clean edge for uniform spreading of the blood drop.
3. Prepare 2–3 slides at a time for practice and obtain an ideal smear.
4. Well-stained slide should be examined under the oil-immersion lens for appropriate results.

Then Find the Percentage of Each Type

Results

N = ... %, E = ... %, B = ... %, L = ... %, M = ... %

Observe the cells and note them successively in the squares below.

> **✎ Key Notes**
>
> *Avoid delay while making blood smear after drop of blood is placed on slide. The delay may lead to abnormal distribution of the white blood cells, and a few large white cells may accumulate at the thin edge of the smear. Pressure to the spreader slide—the fingers should be positioned on the spreader slide as far towards edge as possible and then apply moderate and even pressure along the spreader slide.*

CHARACTERISTICS OF DIFFERENTIAL LEUCOCYTES

Granulocytes

Neutrophil (Fig. 8.5)

1. They are also known as polymorphonuclear leukocytes.
2. They are ten to fourteen micron in diameter.
3. The nucleus is multilobed (1–6 lobes), cytoplasm is bluish pink in colour with plenty of red brown or purple colour granules.
4. Their main function is phagocytosis of bacteria. They are the first cells to reach an injured tissue and their count increases in the acute phase of any infections.
5. The increase in neutrophil is called neutrophilia. It is commonly seen in acute bacterial infections, lung abscesses, burns, acute haemorrhage and in physiological conditions such as after muscular exercise, after meals, pregnancy, lactation, etc.
6. The decrease in neutrophil is called neutropenia. It is seen in typhoid, paratyphoid fever, viral infections, malaria, aplastic anaemia and in bone marrow destruction due to irradiation.

Eosinophil (Fig. 8.5)

1. Eosinophil is 10–14 micron in diameter.
2. The nucleus is purple in colour and has bilobed and spectacle-shaped or horseshoe shaped nucleus.
3. The cytoplasm is pink in colour having large coarse brick red coloured granules.
4. The eosinophil helps in phagocytosis and they release toxins from the granules and kill the pathogens especially parasites and worms.
5. The eosinophil count is increased in allergic condition and then by degrading mediators of inflammation such as bradykinin and histamine limit allergic reactions. The increase in eosinophil count is known as eosinophilia. It occurs in allergic conditions like urticaria and bronchial asthma, parasitic infestations (round worm, dermatitis and tropical eosinophilia).
6. The decrease in eosinophil count is known as eosinopenia. It is seen in Cushing syndrome, ACTH or steroid treatment, acute infections, etc.

Basophil (Fig. 8.5)

1. The basophil is 10–14 micron in diameter.
2. The nucleus is bilobed and purplish blue in colour.
3. The cytoplasm is bluish, granular and basophilic in nature and has large coarse purple or blue coloured granules overlying the nucleus.
4. They have mild phagocytic action. They are functional against hypersensitivity reactions. They liberate eosinophil chemotactic factor and histamine in response to allergy. The anticoagulant histamine is secreted by basophils. They also contain the vasodilator histamine which dilates blood vessel. Basophils have receptors

Revise the characteristic features of WBC			
Differential leucocytes	Percentage of white blood cells	Morphology	Function
Neutrophils 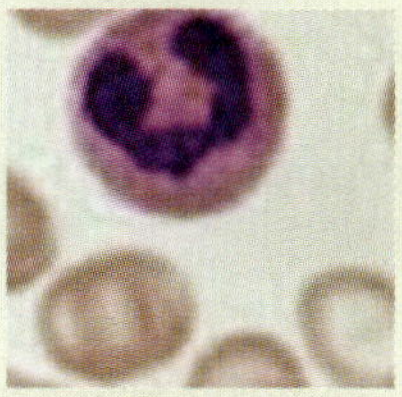	50–70%	10–14 μm in diameter, multilobed nucleus (2–6 lobes) purple in colour, cytoplasm is blue in colour and fine sand like red brown coloured granules are present	Phagocytosis—engulf and destroy bacterial pathogens and also act as mediators of pyrexia response
Eosinophils 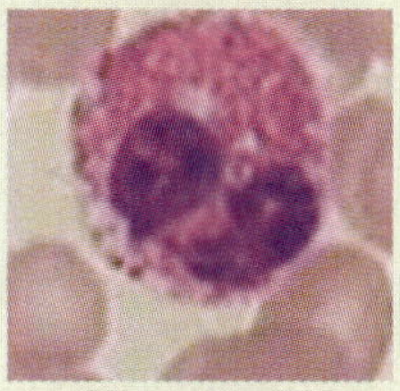	1–4%	10–14 μm in diameter, nucleus purple in colour and has bilobed nuclei; eosinophilic pink coloured cytoplasm with large, coarse brick red coloured granules	Play a role in limiting allergic reactions. Mild phagocytic action and provides local mucosal immunity
Basophils 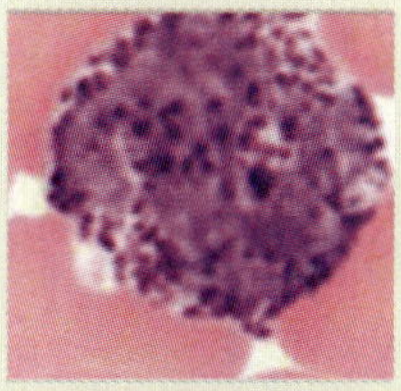	< 1%	10–14 μm in diameter, purple coloured bilobed nuclei, basophilic blue coloured cytoplasm, coarse, large purplish blue granules overlying the nucleus	Function as mediators of inflammation, mild phagocytic action and contains heparin which is an anticoagulant
Lymphocytes 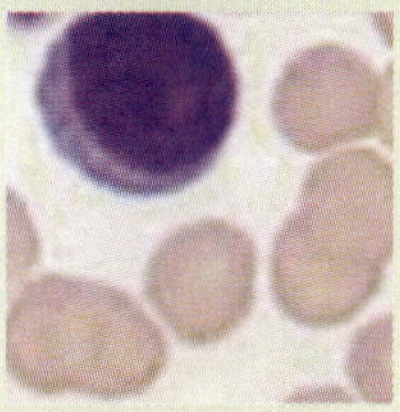	20–40%	Small lymphocyte: 7–10 μm in diameter, large lymphocyte: 10–14 μm in diameter, dense, purple staining, oval or round nucleus; little cytoplasm	The most important cells of the immune system; effective in fighting infectious organisms; act against a specific foreign molecule (antigen)
Monocytes 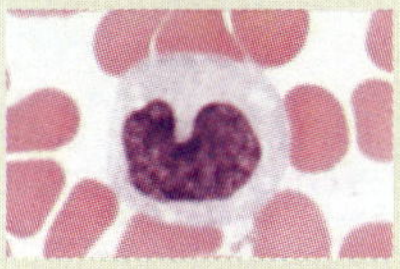	2–8%	10–18 μm in diameter indented kidney-shaped nucleus, pale in colour, cytoplasm abundant pale blue in colour and cell is agranular	Transform into macrophages; phagocytic cells and detoxify killing tumor cells

Fig. 8.5: Characteristic features WBC (neutrophil, eosinophils, basophils, lymphocytes, monocytes)

on their cell surface which bind IgE (immunoglobulin). The receptor bound IgE antibody that confers a selective response of the basophils to pollutants such as pollen proteins or helminth antigens.

5. The increase in basophil count is known as basophilia. It is seen in chronic myeloid leukemia, smallpox and polycythemia.

Agranulocytes: Lymphocytes and Monocytes

Lymphocyte (Fig. 8.5)

1. They are of two types—small and large lymphocytes.

2. The small lymphocyte is 7–10 micron in diameter; having single large oval or round-shaped nucleus which is purple in colour and scanty bluish coloured cytoplasm.

3. The large lymphocytes are 10–14 micron in diameter. The nucleus is mostly indented, and occupies almost entire cell. Nucleus is oval or round-shaped and is purple in colour. The cytoplasm is sky blue and cytoplasm to nucleus ratio is more than small lymphocyte.

4. B lymphocytes produce antibodies. T lymphocytes are differentiated in the thymus and play important role in cell-mediated immunity.

5. The increase in lymphocyte count is known as lymphocytosis. It is seen in tuberculosis, whooping cough, Lymphatic leukemia and in physiological conditions in infancy and childhood. The decrease in lymphocyte count is known as lymphopenia: It is seen in acquired immune deficiency syndrome and hypoplasia of the bone marrow which may be secondary to chemotherapy or irradiation.

Monocyte (Fig. 8.5)

1. They are 14–18 micron in diameter.
2. They are the largest in size amongst the WBC.
3. Nucleus is large round, oval or kidney shape and deeply indented, it is pale purplish blue in colour and its location is usually eccentric.
4. The cytoplasm is abundant and greyish blue in colour.
5. The increase in monocytes count is known as monocytosis. It is seen in tuberculosis, brucellosis, malaria and infectious mononucleosis.

Normal Differential Leucocyte Count

1. **Neutrophils:** 50–70%
2. **Lymphocytes:** 20–40%
3. **Eosinophils:** 1–4%
4. **Basophils:** 0–1%
5. **Monocytes:** 2–8%

OSPE SKILLED

Q1. Prepare a blood smear.

I. Preparation of an ideal blood smear

1. Makes a sterile finger prick under aseptic precaution. Discards the first drop of blood and allows the blood to free flow. (Yes/No)
2. Places a drop of blood at one of the end of each of the glass slides. (Yes/No)
3. Places the spreader slide at an angle of 45 degrees just in front of the blood drop. (Yes/No)
4. Moves the spreader slide backwards to touch the blood drop. (Yes/No)
5. The drop spreads out along the line of contact of the spreader slide. (Yes/No)
6. Moves the spreader slide smoothly and evenly in forward direction maintains an angle of 45 degrees. (Yes/No)
7. Let the smear dry in air. (Yes / No)

II. Fixed and stain the blood smear

Fixing and staining of blood smear:

1. Places the slide on the two glass rods which are placed parallel in the arrangement made in the washing sink. (Yes/No)
2. Pours 10–12 drops of Leishman stain on the slide so as to cover it under the stain and waits for two minutes. (Yes/No)
3. Adds adequate amount of buffered water so that it spreads over the smear uniformly. Mixes the water and stain by rocking movement. Ensures that the stain is completely covered with distilled water so as to clear any overstained portion. (Yes/No)
4. Waits for another 10 minutes allowing time for proper staining. (Yes/No)
5. After interval of 10 minutes washes the slide holding it horizontally with tap water. Ensures water does not hit the smear directly, otherwise the stained portion may get removed. (Yes/No)

Focus the peripheral blood smear under microscope and identify a single neutrophil, eosinophil, lymphocytes and monocyte.

Examination of a blood film:

1. Keeps the peripheral blood smear slide under oil immersion objective. (Yes/No)
2. Places a drop of cedar wood oil over the chosen area and move the oil immersion objective into position; making the lower end of the objective touch the drop of oil. (Yes/No)
3. Focuses the cell using fine adjustment knob. (Yes/No)
4. Identifies a single neutrophil, eosinophil, lymphocytes and monocyte (the differential cell count is done by moving the slide along the central and periphery of the smear). (Yes/No)

VIVA VOCE QUESTIONS

Q1. What are the components of Romanowsky stain? What are their prime functions?

Ans. *The components of a Romanowsky stain are*:
1. A basic or cationic dye (methylene blue or azure B), which binds to anionic sites and imparts a blue-grey colour to nucleic acids, nucleoproteins, granules of neutrophils and granules of basophils.
2. An anionic or acidic dye such as eosin Y or eosin B, which binds to cationic sites on proteins and imparts an orange-red colour to eosinophil granules and haemoglobin.

Q2. What are the types of Romanowsky stains?

Ans. *The types of Romanowsky stains are*: May-Grunwald-Giemsa, Giemsa stain, Wright's stain, Leishman's stain and Field's stain (malarial parasites).

Q3. What are the constituents of Leishman stain?

Ans. *The composition of Leishman's stain is*: Powdered Leishman's stain 0.15 gm is dissolve in 100 ml methyl alcohol. Leishman's stain belongs to the Romanowsky group of stains. It is a mixture of methylene blue and eosin in acetone free methyl alcohol.

Q4. What is the function of methylene blue and eosin in Leishman stain?

Ans. Methylene blue which is a basic dye stains cytoplasm, nucleus and granules of basophils. Eosin is an acidic dye which stains the granules of the eosinophils and RBCs.

Q5. What is the function of acetone free methyl alcohol?

Ans. The acetone free methyl alcohol is a fixative; it causes precipitation of the proteins thus aiding the blood smear to get fixed to the slide and is prevented from being washed off.

Q6. Why there should not be any delay in making smear after placing drop of blood on slide?

Ans. There should be no delay in making the smear after placing the drop of blood is placed on the slide because delay will result in non-uniform distribution of the white blood cells, and most of the white cells will be visible at the thin edge of the smear.

Q7. Describe the characteristic features of ideal blood smear.

Ans. *The characteristic features of ideal blood smear are*:
1. An ideal smear covers around ¾ the entire slide area.
2. Ideal smear is tongue shaped, slightly rounded or curved at the feathery edge tail region. It is thick at head end, and thin at tail end.
3. The upper and lower edges of the smear are clear and visible.
4. The smear is smooth without any streaks or vacuoles.
5. It is single cell layer thick.

Q8. Enlist the precautions for preparation of a blood smear.

Ans. *The precautions for preparation of a blood smear are*:
1. Ensure that the complete drop of blood is uniformly spread along the edge of the spreader slide.
2. The gentle pressure should be constantly maintained when drawing the slide forward.

3. The spreader slide should be moved smoothly and evenly in forward direction maintaining an angle of 45 degrees; to make the ideal blood smear.

4. If spreader slide is moved slowly, the leucocytes will be unevenly distribute.

5. Place the slide on glass rods and let it dry.

Q9. What are the biological causes of poor smear?

Ans. *The biological causes of poor smear are*:

A. **Cold agglutinin:** In which RBCs clumps together. This can be resolved by warming the blood at 37° C for 5 minutes, and then remaking the smear.

B. **Lipemia:** It produces vacuoles like holes in the smear. This cannot be corrected.

C. **Rouleaux:** RBCs form stacks resembling coins. This also cannot be corrected.

Q10. Enlist the causes for increased and decreased in neutrophil count.

Ans. The increase in neutrophil is called neutrophilia. It is commonly seen in acute bacterial infections, lung abscesses, burns, acute haemorrhage and in physiological conditions such as after muscular exercise, after meals, pregnancy, lactation, etc. The decrease in neutrophil is called neutropenia. It is seen in typhoid, paratyphoid fever, viral infections, malaria, aplastic anaemia and in bone marrow destruction due to irradiation.

Q11. Enlist the causes for increased and decreased eosinophil count.

Ans. The eosinophil count is increased in allergic condition and they by degrading mediators of inflammation such as bradykinin and histamine limit allergic reactions. The increase in eosinophil count is known as eosinophilia. It occurs in allergic conditions like urticaria and bronchial asthma, parasitic infestations (round worm, dermatitis and tropical eosinophilia). The decrease in eosinophil count is known as eosinopenia. It is seen in Cushing syndrome, ACTH or steroid treatment, acute infections, etc.

Q12. What are the causes of increase basophil count?

Ans. The increase in basophil count is known as basophilia. It is seen in chronic myeloid leukemia, smallpox and polycythemia.

Q13. Enlist the causes lymphocytosis and lymphopenia.

Ans. Lymphocytosis (increase in lymphocytes) is seen in children (normal count 40–60%), lymphocytic leukemia, viral infection and tuberculosis. Lymphopenia (decrease in lymphocytes) is seen in hypoplastic bone marrow and acquired immune deficiency syndrome.

Q14. Enlist the causes of monocytosis and monocytopenia.

Ans. Monocytosis (increase in monocytes) seen in tuberculosis, syphilis and some leukaemias. Monocytopenia (decrease in monocytes) is seen in hypoplastic bone marrow.

Q15. What is the normal percentage range of differential leucocyte in peripheral blood smear?

Ans. The leucocytes are divided into five types on the basis of its morphological appearance under a light microscope and pictorial characteristics when stained: Neutrophils (50–70%), eosinophils (1–4%), basophils (less than 1%), monocytes (2–10%) and lymphocytes (20–40%).

Q16. What are fixed leucocytes?

Ans. Some white blood cells move and migrate into the tissues and permanently occupy stay at that location rather than remaining in the circulation. Examples are Kupffer cells of liver, mast cell in basophils, microglia and dendritic cells in central nervous system, and histiocytes (tissue microphages).

Q17. How do you classify proliferative disorders linked with leucocytes?

Ans. WBC proliferative disorders can be classed as myeloproliferative and lymphoproliferative.

Q18. Enlist the medication causing leucocytosis.

Ans. The medications, causing leucocytosis are corticosteroids, lithium and beta agonists, etc.

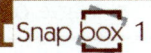 **Snap box 1**

Paul Ehrlich (1854–1915): He was a German Jewish physician and scientist who worked in the field of haematology, immunology, and chemotherapy. He invented the precursor technique to gram staining bacteria, and his methods of staining tissue made it possible to distinguish between different types of blood cells, and this helped to diagnose numerous blood diseases. Ehrlich used both alkaline and acid dyes, and also created new, "neutral" dyes. For the first time this made it possible to differentiate the lymphocytes among the leucocytes (white blood cells). He stained their granulation and could distinguish between non-granular lymphocytes, mononuclear and polynuclear leucocytes, eosinophil granulocytes, and mast cells.

Bibliography

Temkin. The era of *Paul Ehrlich*. Bull NY Acad Med. 1954 Dec; 30(12): 958–67.

OBSERVATIONS: EXERCISE FOR STUDENTS

Results:

N = ... %, E = ... %, B = ... %, L = ... %, M = ... %

Observe the cells and note them successively in the squares below.

N	E	N	N	N					

Fig. 8.6

....

....

....

....

....

....

....

....

....

9

Arneth Count

Learning Objectives

The students after learning the practicals should be able to:

1. Discuss the significance of segmentation of neutrophils
2. Prepare and stain the slide for Arneth count.
3. Describe the distribution of neutrophils depending on number of lobes.
4. Find out the percentage distribution in various stages and explain the significance of right and left shift.
5. Discuss the clinical significance of degenerative and regenerative shift.
6. Enlist the precaution while performing Arneth count.

Aim: To conduct Arneth count and study the distribution of neutrophils depending on number of lobes and clinically correlate the significance of segmentation of neutrophils.

Principle: The distribution of neutrophils depending on number of lobes is identified under smear prepared with Leishman stain and this aids in finding out the percentage distribution in various stages. The number of lobes of nucleus of the neutrophils helps to determine its age. The cells having more number of lobes are older whilst with less lobes are relatively younger. They typically have two or three lobes. The maximum number of lobes is five in general. The Arneth count thus indicates the state of bone marrow activity.

Materials and chemicals: Clean glass slides, lancet, microscope, cotton swab, dropper, glass rod, cedar wood oil, blow pipe and Leishman's stain.

Leishman stain: This stain is a Romanowsky group of stain and consists of eosinate of methylen blue which is dissolved in acetone and water-free methyl alcohol. This stain contains both basophilic and eosinophilic (acidophilic) staining components and thus helps to discriminate among the granules of the differential leucocytes.

The constituents of Leishman stain are:

1. Eosin—it is a negatively charged acidic dye staining positively charged basic particles which include eosinophil granules and red blood.
2. Methylene blue—it is a positively charged basic dye staining negatively charged acidic particles such as basophil granules, cytoplasm and nuclei of white blood cells.
3. Acetone-free methyl alcohol which acts as a fixative and helps in fixing the blood smear over the slide and so also preserves the morphological characteristic of the white blood cells.

Note: Leishman stain is readily available in crystal form 0.15 gm of Leishman stain powder is dissolved in 100 ml of acetone-free methyl alcohol.

Procedure

I. Preparation of Smear

1. Make a sterile finger prick under aseptic precaution. Clean the middle or ring fingertip with spirit swab and prick the finger. Discard the first drop of blood.
2. Place a drop of blood at one of the ends of each of the glass slides.

3. Place the spreader slide at an angle of 45 degrees just in front of the blood drop.
4. Move the spreader slide backwards to touch the blood drop.
5. The drop must spread out along the line of contact of the spreader slide.
6. Move the spreader slide smoothly and evenly in forward direction maintaining an angle of 45 degrees; to make the blood smear.
7. Let the smear dry in air.

II. Fixing and Staining of Blood Smear

1. Place the slide on the two glass rods which are placed parallel in the arrangement made in the washing sink.
2. Pour 10–12 drops of Leishman stain on the slide so as to cover it under the stain and wait for two minutes.
3. Add adequate amount of buffered water so that it spreads over the smear uniformly. Mix the water and stain by rocking movement. Ensure that the stain is completely covered with distilled water so as to clear any overstained portion.
4. Wait for another 10 minutes allowing time for proper staining.
5. After interval of 10 minutes wash the slide holding it horizontally with tap water. Ensure water does not hit the smear directly otherwise the stained portion may get removed.
6. Place the slide on stand and let it dry.
7. Examine minimum of 100 neutrophils and observe the number of lobes in each cell.

Discussion: Inferring your observations.

Arneth count or **Arneth index** describes the nucleus of a neutrophil in terms of number of lobes. The number of lobes of nucleus of the neutrophils helps to determine its age. The cells having more number of lobes are older whilst with less lobes are relatively younger. They typically have two or three lobes. The maximum number of lobes is five in general. The Arneth count thus indicates the state of bone marrow activity.

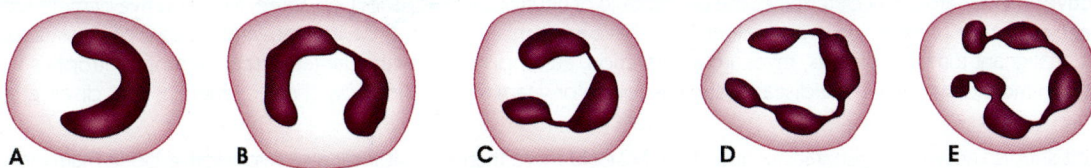

Fig. 9.1: Diagrammatic representation of lobes of neutrophil: A. Stab or Schaf cell; B. Two Lobes; C. Three Lobes; D. Four Lobes; E. Five lobes

Description

The various stages of Arneth count include:

Stage I—1 (Nucleus is C or U-shaped the two limbs connected by thick band of chromatin)—5–10%

Stage II—N2 (Nucleus is bilobed and connected by thin band of chromatin)—20–30%

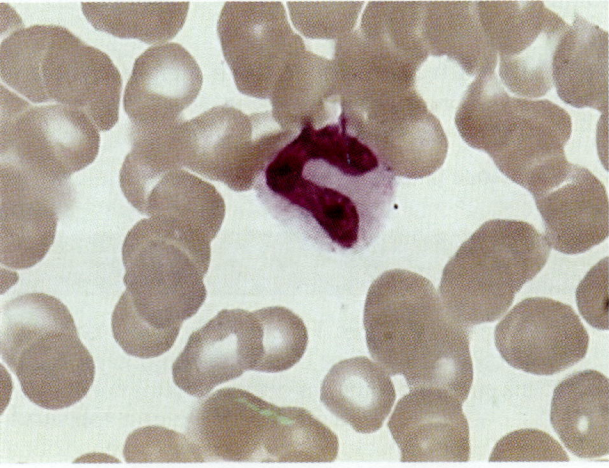

Fig. 9.2: Band neutrophil (left shift)

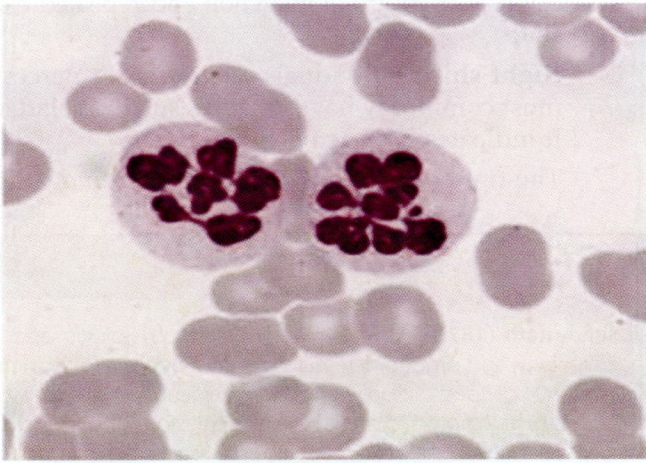

Fig. 9.3: Hypersegmented neutrophils (right shift)

Stage III—N3 (Three lobes and connected by chromatin filament)—40–50%

Stage IV—N4 (Four Lobes and connected by thin band of chromatin)—10–15%

Stage V—N5 (Five lobes with unclear outline)—3–5%.

Results

> **NOTE THE RESULTS**
>
> Stage I—N1 (Nucleus is C or U-shaped the two limbs connected by thick band of chromatin)—Percentage ....
>
> Stage II—N2 (Nucleus is bilobed and connected by thin band of chromatin)—Percentage ....
>
> Stage III—N3 (Three lobes and connected by chromatin filament)—Percentage ....
>
> Stage IV—N4 (Four Lobes and connected by thin band of chromatin)—Percentage ....
>
> Stage V—N5 (Five lobes with unclear outline) Percentage ....

Precautions

1. Draw blood under aseptic precaution and stain appropriately as described in method above.
2. The blood film should be thin and smooth.
3. The slides used must be clean.
4. The staining and blowing should be as gentle as possible.
5. Count the lobes and note carefully.

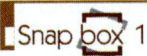 **Snap box 1**

Clinical Perspective: The Arneth count determines the percentage of neutrophils with one, two, three, four, and five or more lobes. Individuals who have a larger percentage of neutrophils with fewer lobes have a left shift which may be indicative of disease processes such as infection, haemolytic crisis, malignant tumors, acidosis, myocardial infarction, etc. Individuals with a larger percentage of neutrophils with more lobes have a right shift and most commonly have diseases such as foliate or vitamin B_{12} deficiency, chronic uraemia, liver disease, aplasia of bone marrow, etc.

Left shift: The left shift is known as regenerative shift—N1+ N2+ N3 more than 80%. It indicates hyperactive bone marrow.

Right Shift: The right shift is known as degenerative shift—N4+ N5+ N6 is more than 20%. The increased number of hypersegmented neutrophils is seen in right shift.

OSPE SKILLED

Q1. Explain regarding right and left shift.

Ans. Left shift: Individuals who have a larger percentage of neutrophils with fewer lobes have a left shift which may be indicative of disease processes such as pyogenic infection, haemolytic crisis, malignant tumors, acidosis, myocardial infarction and repeated exposure to radiation, etc. The left shift is known as regenerative shift.

Right shift: Individuals with a larger percentage of neutrophils with more lobes have a right shift and most commonly have diseases such as folate or vitamin B_{12} deficiency, chronic uraemia, liver disease, etc. It indicates hypoactive bone marrow.

The right shift is known as degenerative shift—N4+ N5+ N6 is more than 20%.

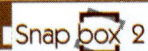 **Snap box 2**

Josef Arneth (1873–1955): He was German physiologist and his credited to naming the Arneth Count. He published several books on haematology, and produced research on neutrophils and their changes in reaction to infection for which he is remembered. Joseph Arneth in year 1904 divided the polymorphonuclear leucocytes into five classes according to the number of divisions or lobules in the nucleus. On this basis he attempted to draw certain conclusions of diagnostic importance. In the first class he included myelocytes and neutrophils with horseshoe-shaped or indented nuclei; in the second, neutrophils were classified as having bilobed nuclei; in third were those with trilobed nuclei; in the fourth those with four-lobed nuclei; in the fifth those with five or more lobes in the nuclei.

VIVA VOCE QUESTIONS

Q1. **What does Arneth count indicates?**

Ans. The state of development of neutrophil is indicated by Arneth count.

Q2. **Are number of neutrophil lobes development a programmed process?**

Ans. The number of lobes in a neutrophil nucleus is supposed to be predetermined and programmed at the band stage. As neutrophil are released, the nuclear segmentation continues till the cell achieves the number of lobes it is programmed to reach.

Q3. **What are the average numbers of lobes of neutrophil in a normal peripheral smear?**

Ans. The average number of lobes of neutrophil in a normal peripheral smear is 2.5–3.3.

Q4. **What does drumstick appendages indicate?**

Ans. In women one of the X chromosomes gets inactivated and appears as the drumstick appendage. It is seen in 0.5–2.6% of the neutrophils.

Q5. **Describe the various stages of Arneth count.**

Ans. *The various stages of Arneth count includes*:

Stage I—N1 (Nucleus is C or U-shaped the two limbs connected by thick band of chromatin)—5–10%

Stage II—N2 (Nucleus is bilobed and connected by thin band of chromatin)—20–30%

Stage III—N3 (Three lobes and connected by chromatin filament)—40–50%

Stage IV—N4 (Four lobes and connected by thin band of chromatin)—10–15%

Stage V—N5 (Five lobes with unclear outline)—3–5%

Q6. **What do you understand by shift to right or shift to left in Arneth count?**

Ans. *The shift to right or shift to left in Arneth Count indicates state of bone marrow activity. The details are as follows*:

1. Individuals who have a larger percentage of neutrophils with fewer lobes have a left shift which may be indicative of disease processes such as pyogenic infection, haemolytic crisis, malignant tumours, acidosis, myocardial infarction, repeated exposure to radiation, etc. The left shift is known as regenerative shift.

2. Individuals with a larger percentage of neutrophils with more lobes have a right shift and most commonly have diseases such as foliate or vitamin B_{12} deficiency, chronic uraemia, liver disease, aplasia of bone marrow, etc. The right shift is known as degenerative shift.

3. Left shift or regenerative shift when N1+ N2+ N3 more than 80%. It indicates hyperactive bone marrow. Right shift or degenerative shift when N4+ N5+ N6 is more than 20%. The increased number of hyper-segmented neutrophils is seen in right shift.

Q7. **What are the conditions in which you see increased nuclear lobulation or hypersegmentation?**

Ans. The increased nuclear lobulation or hypersegmentation are seen in megaloblastic anaemia, iron deficiency anaemia, uraemia, infection, myelodysplastic syndromes and hereditary neutrophil hypersegmentations.

Q8. **Define neutrophilia. What are its causes?**

Ans. Increase in neutrophil count above normal is called neutrophilia. Physiological neutrophilia is seen after exercise, acute mental stress, after meals, during pregnancy, etc. The pathological causes of neutrophilia included acute infections, tissue necrosis (occurs in pulmonary, renal or myocardial infarction), after surgery, burns, acute haemorrhages, etc. and may be drug induced (adrenaline, glucocorticoids, etc.).

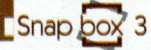 Snap box 3

RECENT UPDATES

Arneth count (ANC) is a more accurate measure for risk of infection than WBC alone. ANC can indicate whether a patient is suitable candidate for specific treatments like inducement of growth factors (also called granulocyte-colony stimulating factors or G-CSFs). ANC measures the status of immune system in patients undergoing radiation, chemotherapy, or a bone marrow or stem cell transplant.

Results

Note the Results

Stage I—N1 (Nucleus is C or U-shaped the two limbs connected by thick band of chromatin)—Percentage.............................

Stage II—N2 (nucleus is bilobed and connected by thin band of chromatin)—Percentage ....

Stage III—N3 (three lobes and connected by chromatin filament)—Percentage ....

Stage IV—N4 (four lobes and connected by thin band of chromatin)—Percentage ....

Stage V—N5 (five lobes with unclear outline) Percentage ....

10

Determination of Absolute Eosinophil Count

Learning Objectives

After learning the practical the students should be able to:

1. Explain the significance of conducting absolute eosinophil count.
2. Describe the composition and functions of pilot solution.
3. Prepare a peripheral blood smear and stain the smear.
4. Identify and conduct the eosinophil count under haemocytometer.
5. Enlist the precautions while conducting absolute eosinophil count.
6. Discuss the reason for altered eosinophil count.

Aim: Determination of absolute eosinophil count.

Principle: Absolute eosinophil count is the number of circulating eosinophils in the peripheral blood and is altered in various disease conditions. Blood is diluted with Pilot's solution. The Pilot's solution lyses red and white blood cells except eosinophil thus aiding in eosinophil count.

Materials and Chemicals

Lancet, WBC pipette, counting chamber, coverslip and Pilot's diluting fluid.

Contents of Pilot's Diluting Fluid

The 100 ml of Pilot's solution consists of phyloxine 10 ml (it stains eosinophil granules); propylene glycol 50 ml (it lyses RBC cells and acts as a solvent for stain); and sodium carbonate 1 ml (it further enhances staining of granules); heparin 100 units (it acts as anticoagulant); distilled water to make the solution to 100 ml. The student should note that eosin may be used instead of phyloxine.

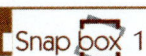 Snap box 1

It is estimated by multiplying the total white blood cell (WBC) count by the percentage of eosinophils. The absolute eosinophil count aids in evaluation and confirmation of role of eosinophils in aetiology of clinical manifestations in the infectious or inflammatory diseases such as allergies, parasitic infections, collagen-vascular diseases, skin diseases, bacterial infections and myeloproliferative disorders, etc. The normal observed absolute eosinophilic count is 150–400/µL.

Methods

The test for absolute eosinophilic count can be done by two methods.

1. **Indirect method:** The percentage of eosinophil can be derived from slide prepared for differential leucocyte count. The total leucocyte count is measured. The absolute eosinophilic count is estimated by multiplying the total white blood cell (WBC) count by the percentage of eosinophils.

2. **Direct method:** Haemocytometry is carried out for the absolute eosinophilic count.

Procedure

1. Make a gentle finger prick under aseptic precaution. Discard the first drop as it may contain tissue fluid. Wait till a fresh drop of blood appears. Draw it up to mark 1 of WBC pipette.
2. Further draw the diluting fluid up to mark 11 of the WBC pipette. Gently mix for two to three minutes.
3. Place the pipette on moist filter paper and cover the Petridish; wait for 10 minutes for lysis of the red and white blood cells and for appropriate staining.
4. Mix the content of pipette gently for a minute and then charge the chamber. The fluid in the stem must be discarded.
5. Count the eosinophil under high power in four corner WBC squares, each having 16 squares (i.e. in total of 64 squares).

Calculation

1. The volume of fluid in four WBC square is calculated as follows:
   Area of four corner WBC squares = 4 × 1 mm × 1 mm
   (as each cover square is 1 mm × 1 mm)
   - Area of four square = 4 sq mm.
   - The chamber depth is of 0.1 mm
     Thus the volume of fluid in four, WBC square = 4 sq. mm × 0.1 mm
     $$= 0.4 \; \mu L$$
2. Let eosinophil count in 0.4 μL of diluted blood be N.
   - Thus the number of eosinophil in

     $$1 \; \mu L \text{ of undiluted blood} = \frac{N \times \text{dilution factor}}{0.4}$$
   - The dilution factor = 20 (Refer to practical determination total).

   Thus total number of eosinophil in μL of undiluted blood $= \dfrac{N \times 20}{0.4}$

   $$= N \times 50$$

The normal observed absolute eosinophilic count is 150–400/μL

Indirect Method

Calculate the percentage of eosinophil from slide prepared for differential leucocyte count. Count for the total leucocyte count. The absolute eosinophilic count is estimated by multiplying the total white blood cell (WBC) count by the percentage of eosinophils.

Results: Absolute eosinophilic count is.

Direct method..

Indirect method.................................

Precautions

1. Ensure that the Neubauer chamber, pipette, fingertip, lancet and coverslip is clean and dry.
2. The diluted blood sample after pipetting should be thoroughly mixed.
3. Wait for suitable time as mentioned in the method after adding diluting fluid so as to hemolyze other cells except eosinophil.
4. The air bubble should not be present in charging pipette or under coverslip of the counting chamber.
5. The chamber should be uniformly charged and ensure that there is no overflowing in the chamber.
6. Note that cells touching the left and lower borders are to be considered for counting while those at right and upper borders are omitted.
7. Cell count should be started after they get equally distributed.
8. Complete your cell count before thirty minutes as cell starts to disintegrate then.

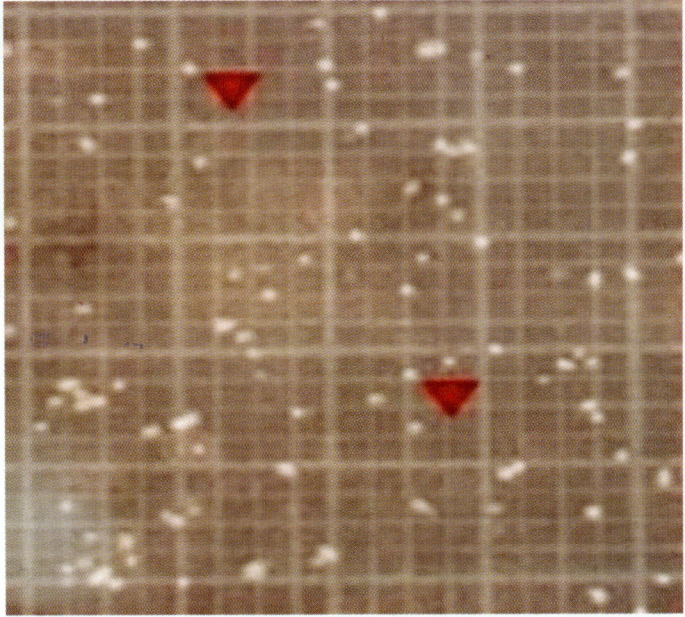

Fig. 10.1: Eosinophils in WBC square after staining with Pilot solution

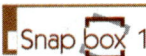 **Snap box 1**

Clinical perspective: Eosinophils play a role in immune defense in cases of parasitic, viral, and bacterial infections. The increased count of eosinophils (eosinophilia) is usually associated with allergic diseases, hay fever, asthma, autoimmune diseases, eczema and leukemia. A lower-eosinophil count may be due to aplastic anemia, Cushing syndrome, alcohol intoxication, or overproduction of certain steroids such as cortisol, acute pyogenic infections, etc.

OSPE NON-SKILLED

Q1. **Name the diluting fluid used for absolute eosinophil count.**

What are its contents? What is the principle basis of the test for absolute eosinophil count?

Ans. Pilot diluting fluid.

The 100 ml of Pilot's solution consists of phyloxine 10 ml (it stains eosinophil granules); propylene glycol 50 ml (it lyses RBC cells and acts as a solvent for stain); and sodium carbonate 1 ml (it further enhances staining of granules); heparin 100 units (it acts as anticoagulant); distilled water to make the solution to 100 ml.

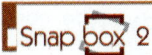 **Snap box 2**

Max Schultze was first to identify the eosinophil in the year 1865. The staining property of eosinophil was described by P. Ehrlich in the year 1879. Mayer described his eosin-glycerine method in late 80s. Dunger established the eosinophil counting method using the counting chamber in the year 1910.

VIVA VOCE QUESTIONS

Q1. **Describe the contents of Pilot's solution.**

Ans. Kindly refer OSPE non-skilled above.

Q2. **What is principle behind conducting absolute eosinophil count?**

Ans. The Pilot's solution lyses red and white blood cells except eosinophil, thus aiding in eosinophil count.

Q3. What is the normal absolute eosinophil count?

Ans. The normal absolute eosinophil count is 150–400/µL.

Q4. Describe the methods of estimating absolute eosinophil count.

Ans. *The two methods of estimating absolute eosinophil count are*:

1. **Indirect method:** The percentage of eosinophil can be derived from slide prepared for differential leucocyte count. The total leucocyte count is measured. The absolute eosinophil count is estimated by multiplying the total white blood cell (WBC) count by the percentage of eosinophils.

2. **Direct method:** Haemocytometry is carried out for the absolute eosinophil count.

Q5. What are the causes for increased and decreased absolute eosinophil count?

Ans. The increased count of eosinophils (eosinophilia) is usually associated with allergic diseases, hay fever, asthma, autoimmune diseases, eczema and leukaemia. A lower eosinophil count may be due to aplastic anaemia, Cushing syndrome, alcohol intoxication, or overproduction of certain steroids such as cortisol, acute pyogenic infections, etc.

Q6. Enlist the conditions in which absolute eosinophilic count is recommended.

Ans. *Absolute eosinophilic count is useful in diagnosis of*:

a. Parasitic infections

b. Bacterial infections

c. Myeloproliferative disorders and other malignancies

d. Collagen vascular diseases

e. Side effects of medications ex-ACTH Therapy

Q7. Define hypereosinophilia.

Ans. **Hypereosinophilia:** Hypereosinophilia is defined as moderate to severe eosinophilia (i.e. ≥1500 eosinophils/µL). The end-organ manifestations help to diagnose the cause. If the cause of the eosinophilia is unknown and no clinical manifestations are seen, then such patients are considered to having hypereosinophilia of unknown significance.

Q8. How do you confirm the diagnosis of eosinophilic esophagitis?

Ans. The esophageal biopsy demonstrates more than 20 epithelial eosinophils per high-power field in patients of eosinophilic esophagitis.

Q9. How do you confirm the diagnosis of allergic etiology in skin disease?

Ans. Skin biopsy demonstrates a few to large numbers of eosinophils indicating eosinophil-associated skin disease. The biopsy staining reveals extracellular major basic protein, which is out of proportion to the numbers of intact eosinophils.

Bibliography

1. Brewer, BD "Max Schultze (1865), G. Bizzozero (1882) and the discovery of the platelet". *British Journal of Haematology.* 2006.

2. Lehrer, Steven. *Explorers of the Body: Dramatic Breakthroughs in Medicine from Ancient Times to Modern Science.* Doubleday. 1979: 295.

3. Rothenberg ME, Hogan SP. "The eosinophil". *Annual review of Immunology.* 2006; 24 (1): 147–74.

OBSERVATIONS: EXERCISE FOR STUDENTS

Results

Results: Absolute eosinophilic count is:

Direct method ....

Indirect method ....

....

....

Determination of Blood Groups (A, B, O and Rh System)

Learning Objectives

After learning the practical the students should be able to:

1. Discuss the principle of blood group determination.
2. Determine the blood group using anti-A, anti-B and anti-D.
3. Enlist the precautions while carrying blood grouping.
4. Classify blood groups.
5. Explain the Landsteiner law.
6. Explain the significance of blood typing and crossmatching.
7. Describe the indications for blood transfusion.
8. Explain the hazards of mismatched blood transfusion.

Aim: Determination of blood group.

Principle: Antigens (agglutinogens) are present on red blood cell surface membrane and antibodies (agglutinins) are present in plasma. Blood group determination is done by using specific agglutinins (antibodies) to confirm the presence or absence of the corresponding agglutinogen (antigen) on the RBC membrane.

Materials and chemicals: Lancet, spirit, cotton, normal saline, glass marking pencil, anti-A serum, anti-B serum, anti-D, test tubes, slides, 0.9% saline, applicator sticks, compound microscope, capillary dropper and glass marking pencil.

Procedure

1. Take four clean slides, and label them as A, B, D and C using glass marking pencil.
2. Place anti-sera A on slide labelled A, anti-sera B on slide labelled B, anti-sera D on slide labelled D and A drop of 0.9% saline on slide labelled C (that is considered as control).
3. Take 3 ml of isotonic 0.9% saline in a clean porcelain dish.
4. The finger then should be pricked under aseptic conditions till free flow of blood is obtained and wipe away the first drop of blood.
5. Add the drop of capillary blood to the saline to make a red blood cell suspension (to obtain 1 to 2 volumes of cells in 100 ml of saline).
6. Add a drop of red blood cell suspension to each of anti-A, anti-B, anti-D sera and saline.
7. Mix the anti-sera and red cell suspension by using separate sticks.
8. Wait for 7–10 minutes and observe the agglutination (clumping).
9. Compare it with the saline standard.
10. Record your findings.

Note: If there is doubt regarding agglutination, confirm it under the microscope.

Result

The blood group of the subject is ....

Interpret the results as follows

Observe for presence of agglutination in slide A, B, D, and C.

Slide A	Slide B	Agglutinogens present	Blood group
Present	Absent	A	A
Absent	Present	B	B
Present	Present	A, B	AB
Absent	Absent	Neither	O

Observe: Slide D and observe for agglutination of cells, the clumping of cell confirms presence of antigen D and blood group is recognized as Rh+ and absence of clumping indicates that the blood group is recognized as Rh−.

Note: Slide C is control and shows no clumping or agglutination of cells and this slide is for comparison.

PRECAUTIONS

1. The slides should be cleaned and dried.
2. Aseptic precaution should be followed while pricking and the finger should not be squeezed for obtaining blood drop. The prick should be bold and blood allowed to freely flow.
3. The slide should be labelled before placing the antisera A, B and Rh and isotonic saline.
4. Examine the slide for agglutination before the solution dries up. The findings should be confirmed under the low power of the microscope.

Note: False positive reaction can occur due to use of antisera contaminated with bacterial growth or due to loss of potency of the antisera because of improper storage.

OSPE

Q1. Perform the blood group typing steps and prepare slides for observing agglutination.

Ans.

1. Takes four clean slides, and label them as A, B, D and C using glass marking pencil. (Yes/No)
2. Places anti-sera A on slide labeled A, anti-sera B on slide labeled B, anti-sera D on slide labeled D and a drop of 0.9% saline on slide labeled C. (Yes/No)
3. Takes 3 ml of isotonic 0.9% saline in a clean porcelain dish. (Yes/No)
4. The finger is pricked under aseptic conditions till free flow of blood is obtained and wipe away the first drop of blood. (Yes/No)
5. Adds the drop of capillary blood to the saline to make a red blood cell suspension (to obtain 1 to 2 volumes of cells in 100 ml of saline). (Yes/No)
6. Adds a drop of red blood cell suspension to each of anti-A, anti-B, anti-D sera and saline
7. Mix the anti-sera and red cell suspension by using separate sticks.

   The slide is ready for observation after 7–10 minutes for agglutination confirmation and identification of blood group.

Q2. Identify the blood groups from the figure in which results of four slides were snipped and placed side by side for identification testing.

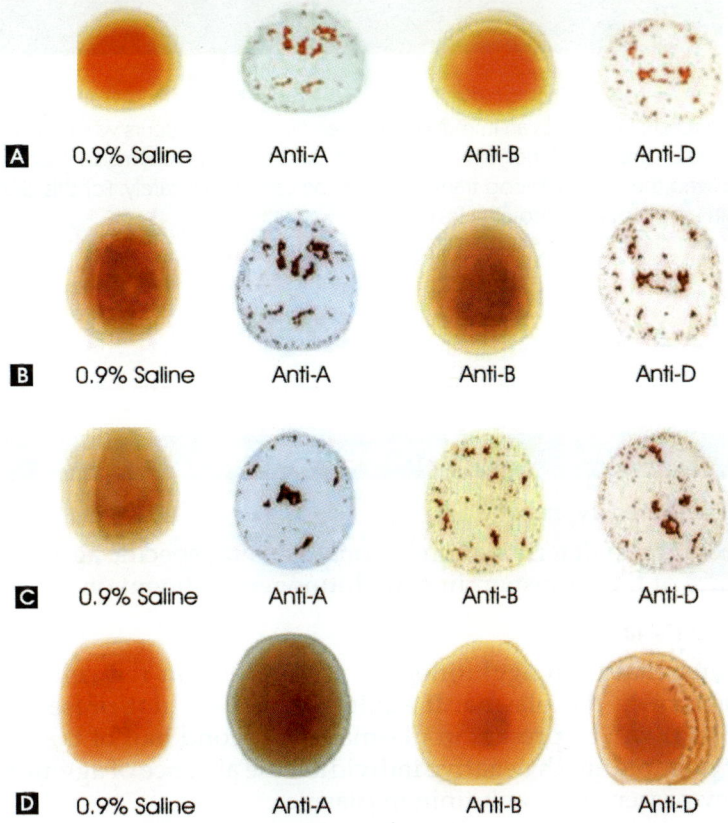

Ans. A-blood group as clumping of cells is seen after addition of anti-sera, anti-A, B-blood group as clumping of cells is seen after addition of anti-sera, anti-B and AB blood group as clumping of cells is seen after addition of anti-sera, anti-A and anti-B and D as there is no clumping of cells the blood group is O.

Q3. Draw a table showing blood types with their genotypes.

Ans. *Blood types with their genotypes*:

Genotypes	Blood types	Agglutinogen	Agglutinin
OO	O	–	Anti-A and Anti-B
OA or AA	A	A	Anti-B
OB or BB	B	B	Anti-A
AB	AB	A and B	–

Q4. Identify the bottles.

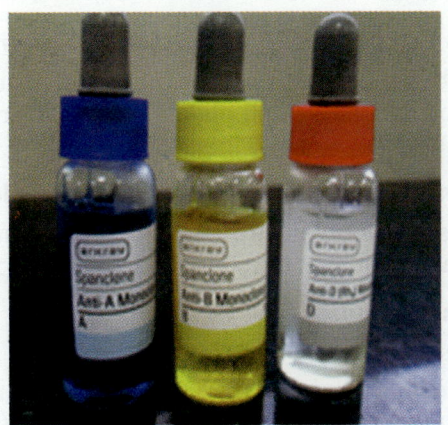

Ans. These are anti-sera A, B and D bottles containing anti-sera and is used for ABO blood typing.

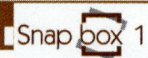

Snap box 1

Karl Landsteiner (1868–1943)

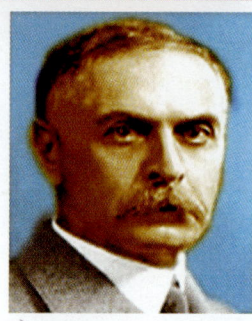

Karl Landsteiner discovered that blood clumping was an immunological reaction which occurs when the receiver of a blood transfusion has antibodies against the donor blood cells. Karl Landsteiner's work made it possible to determine blood types and thus paved the way for blood transfusions to be carried out safely. For this discovery he was awarded the Nobel Prize in Physiology or Medicine in 1930.

VIVA VOCE QUESTIONS

Q1. What is the principle of blood typing?

Ans. **The principle is:** Blood group determination is done by using specific agglutinins (antibodies) to confirm the presence or absence of the corresponding agglutinogen (antigen) on the RBC membrane.

Q2. Describe the Landsteiner's law.

Ans. Landsteiner's law states that if an agglutinogens are present on red cell membrane the corresponding agglutinin may be absent in the plasma. If agglutinogens are not present on red cell membrane, the corresponding agglutinin will be present in plasma. The second half of the definition is not applicable to all blood groups. For example, in Rh negative individual the absence of agglutinogen on red cell membrane is not accompanied by presence of agglutinin in plasma.

Q3. Name a few blood group systems.

Ans. The commonly known blood group systems are ABO system, MNS system, Kell system, Lewis system. These blood group systems were named after the patients in whom the corresponding antibodies were initially encountered.

Q4. Why ABO incompatibilities rarely produce haemolytic disease of the newborn?

Ans. ABO incompatibilities are rare because A and B antibodies are of IgM type and cannot cross the placenta.

Q5. Discuss the clinical application of blood grouping.

Ans. *The blood grouping is useful for*:
1. Safe blood transfusion.
2. Preventing haemolytic disease
3. Resolving paternity disputes.
4. Arriving at conclusion in medicolegal cases.
5. Knowing susceptibility to diseases.

Q6. Which methods and procedures can be used in performing blood grouping?

Ans. Three manual methods that can be used when performing blood grouping are glass slide or white porcelain tile method, glass test tube method and microwell plate method. The newer techniques are column technique (sephadex gel) and solid phase tests.

Q7. Name the methods for detection of antigen–antibody reaction serologically.

Ans. The antigen–antibody reactions in blood group serology are usually detected by haem-agglutination, complement fixation, neutralization, absorption, elution and precipitation.

Q8. Discuss the hazards of blood transfusion.

Ans. *Hazards of mismatched blood transfusion are*:
1. *Mismatched transfusion reactions include*: Tissue ischemia, haemolytic jaundice, circulatory shock, haemoglobinuria, renal tubular damage, acute renal shut down (anuria) and uraemia.
2. Circulatory overload due to hypervolemia.

3. Transmission of blood-borne infections such as AIDS, viral hepatitis, malaria, syphilis, etc.
4. Pyogenic reactions
5. Allergic reactions
6. Hyperkalemia and
7. Hypocalcaemia.

Q9. If an Rh negative mother carries Rh positive foetus, discuss the likely complications?

Ans. When an Rh negative mother carries Rh positive fetus, RBCs containing D-antigen may enter the maternal circulation at the time of delivery. The mother shall form anti-D and during second pregnancy the antibodies will enter the foetal circulation and tend to destroy foetal red blood cell causing hemolytic disease of the newborn.

Q10. Enlist the various forms of clinical manifestation of haemolytic disease of the newborn.

Ans. *The various forms of clinical manifestation of haemolytic disease of the newborn are*:
   i. Hydrops foetalis.
   ii. Icterus gravis neonatorum (haemolytic jaundice).
   iii. Kernicterus.
   iv. Erythroblastosis foetalis.

Q11. Which safety procedures should be followed to prevent blood transfusion complication?

Ans. Direct crossmatching of the blood is the only safeguard against blood transfusion complication. It involves matching the serum of the recipient directly against the RBCs of the donor and again to match the RBCs of the recipient against the serum of the donor.

Q12. What will happen if individual is transfused with an incompatible blood group?

Ans. If an individual is transfused with an incompatible blood group, destruction of the red blood cells will occur and this may result in the death of the recipient mainly due to disseminated intravascular coagulation.

Q13. What is major crossmatching?

Ans. Matching the serum of the recipient directly against the RBCs of the donor.

Q14. Who was awarded the Nobel Prize in Physiology or Medicine in 1930 for his discovery of blood types?

Ans. Karl Landsteiner was awarded the Nobel Prize in Physiology or Medicine in 1930 for his discovery of blood types.

Q15. Which element shows a little change in stored blood?

Ans. Sodium shows a little change in stored blood.

Q16. Which are the important ABO blood group systems?

Ans. There are around 30 known blood group systems out of which ABO and Rh systems are important. ABO system has A and B antibodies in individual from birth with corresponding antigen being absent in the individual. Based on the experiment they are classified as blood group A, B, AB and O.

Q17. What is Rh system?

Ans. Rh antigens also known as D antigens are trans-membrane proteins with loops exposed at the surface of red blood cells. Rh antigen when present on red cell membrane of an individual, the blood group is said to be Rh D positive, if not the individuals blood group is Rh D negative. They are name 'Rhesus' comes from the rhesus monkey in which they were first discovered. 85% of the population is Rh D positive, the other 15% of the population Rh D negative.

Q18. What are merits and demerits of ABO blood group testing?

Ans. ABO blood group testing system is accurate and identifies the common blood grouping system A, B, O, AB and Rhesus (D) but the unusual blood groups and rare sub-types are not detected by this method. Crossmatching followed by a Coombs' test helps detect these minor antigens and is done before transfusions. Further exploration by a blood transfusion laboratory and pharmaceutical company for better designed test identification kit is necessary to recognize such groups.

Q19. Who discovered MN blood group system and when?

Ans. Landsteiner, with Philip Levine, discovered the MN blood group system in 1927.

Q20. What is Bombay blood group?

Ans. The h/h blood group is the Bombay blood group. It is rare found blood type and it has resulted due to mutation that leads to deficiency of H antigen. The H antigen is the precursor of O antigen. This blood type is characterized by the absence of O, A and B antigens.

Q21. What is para-Bombay blood group?

Ans. A weaker expression of h antigen is known as para-Bombay blood group.

Q22. Which anticoagulants are used to store blood in blood bank?

Ans. The commonly used anticoagulants to store blood in blood bank are acid-citrate-dextrose and citrate phosphate dextrose.

Q23. At what temperature is blood stored in blood bank?

Ans. The temperature at which blood is stored in blood bank is $4 \pm 2°$ Celsius.

Q24. What is ISBT?

Ans. ISBT is the International Society of Blood Transfusion (ISBT) and it promotes the study and research regarding blood transfusion, and health educate about the manner in which blood transfusion medicine and science best can serve the patient's interests.

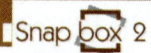 Snap box 2

Leonard Landois (1875)

He was born 1837 in Münster. A Medical student at the University of Greifswald and later Professor and Director of the Institute of Physiology at Greifswald studied blood transfusions and the phenomena of agglutination. In 1875 he published work titled 'Die Transfusion des Blutes'. He died 1902 in Greifswald.

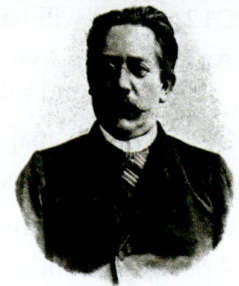

Bibliography

1. Colin Wilson, Damon wilson. *Written in Blood*. Carroll and Graf Publishers. 2003.
2. Karl Landsteiner. *Nobel Lectures, Physiology or Medicine 1922–1941*. Amsterdam: Elsevier Publishing Company. 1965.

OBSERVATIONS: EXERCISE FOR STUDENTS

Results

The blood group of the subject is

....

....

....

....

....

....

....

....

12

Determination of Bleeding Time (BT) and Clotting Time (CT)

Learning Objectives

After learning the practical the student should be able to:

1. Determine his/her own bleeding and clotting time and to compare it with normal range of values expected for the bleeding and clotting time.
2. Interpret observed bleeding time and clotting time, and enlist the conditions in which bleeding time and clotting time is increased or decreased.
3. Recognize the importance of bleeding time and clotting time in haemostasis and in management of patient with haematological disorders.
4. List the precautions to be taken while determining the bleeding time and clotting time.

Bleeding Time

Principle: The time for bleed is noted after giving a deep prick over skin (fingers, ear lobe, forearm). There is stoppage of bleeding after a platelet plug is formed at site of injury in the vessel wall.

Methods for Determination of Bleeding Time

The two methods commonly used for determining the BT are:

1. Duke's Method
2. Ivy's Method

A. Duke's method: The Duke's method is the most commonly used method for estimating the bleeding time.

Principle: The time required for bleeding to stop from the time of giving deep skin puncture is the bleeding time.

Apparatus: Apparatus for sterile puncture (lancet) filter paper and stopwatch.

Procedure

1. Ask the subject to sit comfortably. After explaining the procedure to the subject, the tip of a finger is cleaned with spirit and the area is allowed to dry.
2. A deep puncture is made with the help of lancet so that blood flows freely and ensure not to squeeze the fingertip to obtain blood.
3. Start the stopwatch immediately and note the time of puncture of the finger.
4. The escaping blood is dried on the edge of a filter paper after thirty seconds.
5. The procedure of applying flowing blood on the fresh area of filter paper is continued every 30 seconds till blood ceases to flow.
6. The total number of blood spots on the filter paper is counted and multiplied by 30. This will give the BT in seconds which is converted in minutes. Normal bleeding time by this method is 2–6 minutes.

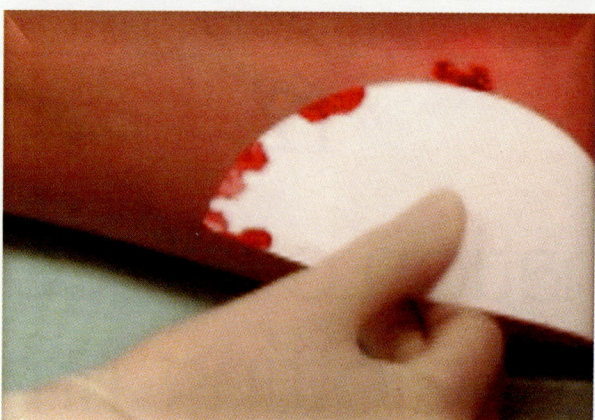

Fig. 12.1: Duke's method

B. Ivy's Method

1. The anterior surface of the forearm is cleaned with spirit.
2. A blood pressure cuff is tied over the subject upper arm and pressure of 40 mm Hg is maintained till the end of the experiment.
3. The anterior surface of forearm is cleaned with alcohol and a superficial incision (3 mm deep) is made with a sterile lancet avoiding visible blood vessels.
4. The blood drops are soaked up every 30 seconds with a piece of filter paper, until the blood no longer stains the paper.
5. The total number of blood spots on the filter paper is counted and multiplied by 30. This will give the bleeding time in seconds which is converted in minutes.

Normal value of bleeding time by IVY method is 3–6 minutes at 37°C.

Clotting Time (CT)

Principle: The time taken from the puncture of the blood vessel to the formation of a fibrin thread is the clotting time.

There are two methods commonly being used for determining the CT: Capillary glass tube method and Lee and White method.

A. Capillary Glass Tube Method

This is most commonly used method in practice.

1. Clean the tip of finger with spirit and allow the area to dry.
2. A deep puncture is made with help of lancet so that blood flows freely and ensure not to squeeze the fingertip to obtain blood.
3. As the blood freely flows, a large drop will appear at the fingertip. The capillary tube is to be placed in the drop and hold obliquely so that its other end is at lower level. The blood moves into capillary by capillary action.
4. The capillary tube filled with blood is hold in the palm of the hand so that it remains warm as the body temperature (37°C).
5. Break the capillary tube at 1 cm distance every 30 seconds starting from one end and break over till you notice for thread of fibrin at the broken ends of the tube. The fibrin thread of about 5 mm length when observed indicates that the blood has clotted.
6. The total time taken from the time of puncture (zero time) till the formation of a fibrin thread is the clotting time. Normal value of clotting time by this method is 1–5 minutes at 37°C.

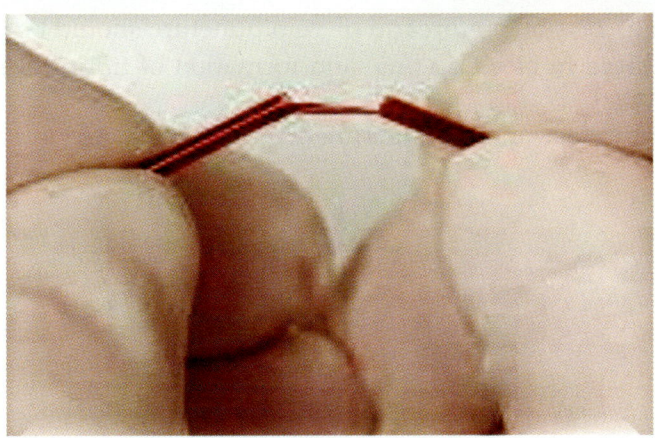

Fig. 12.2: Capillary tube method

B. Lee-White Method

1. 3 ml of venous blood is collected under aseptic precaution. The time of vein puncture is noted.
2. The blood is immediately transferred into three glass tubes and amount is 1 ml in each tube.
   They are kept in a 37°C water bath.
3. Wait for three minutes and then tilt the tubes one by one at interval of 30 sec.
   Blood clotting is tested by tilting the tube back and forth every 30 seconds.
4. The clotting time is measured when the blood does not flow out of the test tubes when tilted horizontally.
   The clotting time is noted. The normal value by this method is 5–10 minutes. The normal clotting time by using silicon tubes varies between 20 and 60 minutes.

Precautions

1. The finger pricking, incision on forearm or vein puncture should be done under aseptic precaution. The first drop of blood is not wiped out.

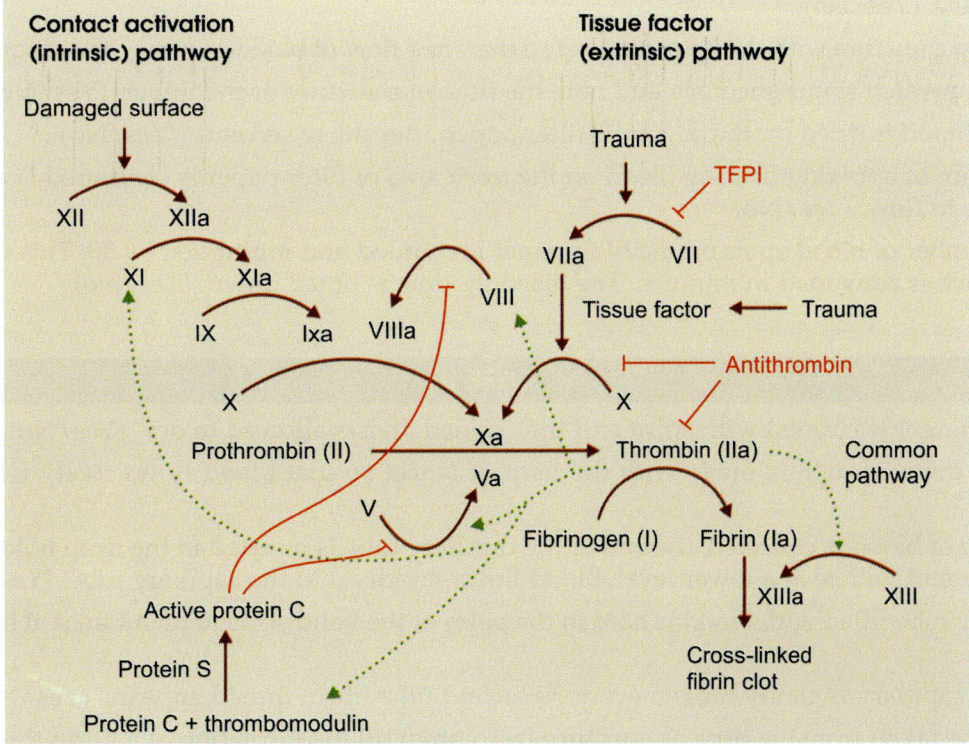

Fig. 12.3: Extrinsic and intrinsic mechanism of coagulation

2. The time of finger pricking, incision on forearm or vein puncture should be noted as starting time.

3. The time of stoppage of bleed in bleeding time and formation of fibrin thread in clotting time estimation should be meticulously noted.

4. Strictly follow the procedure steps and the experiment should be carried out at normal body temperature of 37°C.

Results

Note:

Bleeding time as per Duke's method: ....

Bleeding time as per IVY method: ....

Clotting time as per capillary tube method: ....

Clotting time as per Lee-White method: ....

Snap box 1
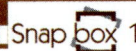

Blood coagulation refers to the process of forming of a clot which arrest bleeding. Three mechanisms involved in clotting are vasoconstriction, platelet plug formation and platelet clot formation. The clotting cascade occurs through two separate pathways that interact, the intrinsic and the extrinsic pathway.

Extrinsic pathway: The extrinsic pathway is activated by external trauma that causes blood to escape from the vascular system. This pathway is quicker than the intrinsic pathway. It involves factor VII.

Intrinsic pathway: The intrinsic pathway is activated by trauma inside the vascular system, and is activated by platelets, exposed endothelium, chemicals, or collagen. This pathway is slower than the extrinsic pathway, but more important. It involves factors XII, XI, IX, and VIII.

Common pathway: Both pathways meet and finish the pathway of clot production in what is known as the common pathway. The common pathway involves factors I, II, V and X.

OSPE I

1. The subject is explained the procedure and then the tip of a finger is cleaned with spirit and the area is allowed to dry. (Yes/No)

2. Makes a deep puncture with the help of lancet so that free flow of blood occurs without squeezing. (Yes/No)

3. Starts the stopwatch simultaneously and note the time of puncture of the finger. (Yes/No)

4. The oozing blood is dried on the edge of a filter paper after thirty seconds. (Yes/No)

5. The procedure of applying flowing blood on the fresh area of filter paper is continued every 30 seconds till blood ceases to flow. (Yes/No)

6. The total number of blood spots on the filter paper is counted and multiplied by 30. This will give the BT in seconds which is converted in minutes. The bleeding time is noted down. (Yes/No)

OSPE II

1. The tip of a finger is cleaned with spirit and the cleaned area is allowed to dry. (Yes/No)

2. A puncture deep enough is made with the help of lancet so that blood flows freely without squeezing. (Yes/No)

3. A large drop of blood is collected, the end of the capillary tube is inserted in the drop holding the tube such that its other end will be at a lower level. Blood flows rapidly into the capillary tube. (Yes/No)

4. The capillary tube filled with blood is hold in the palm of the hand so as to maintain it at body temperature. (Yes/No)

5. The 1 cm of capillary is gently broken every 30 second till a fibrin thread appears. (Yes/No)

6. The total time taken from the time of puncture (zero time) till the formation of a fibrin thread is the clotting time. The clotting time is noted down. (Yes/No)

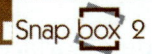
Snap box 2

Historical Aspect—William Howell and Jay McLean: William Howell studied the pro-coagulant effects on experimental animals at Johns Hopkins in 1915. Jay McLean joined the lab to assist his research work of isolating a thromboplastic material then. Jay McLean found that a phosphatide from the liver, initially pro-coagulant lost this property and became anticoagulant. McLean informed his mentor Dr. Howell that he has discovered anti-thrombin. McLean named this substance heparphosphatide. Meanwhile, Howell pursued studies on the substance. In 1918 he renamed it heparin.

VIVA VOCE QUESTIONS

Q1. Define bleeding time and clotting time.

Ans. Bleeding time is the time taken from puncture of blood vessel to the stoppage of bleeding. The clotting time is the time taken from puncture of blood vessel to formation of a fibrin thread.

Q2. How much is the bleeding time as per Duke's method?

Ans. The normal bleeding time as per Duke's method is 2–6 minutes.

Q3. How much is the clotting time as per capillary glass tube method?

Ans. The normal clotting time as per capillary glass tube method is 3–8 minutes at 37°C.

Q4. Explain the series of events involved in haemostasis.

Ans. *Three major events which get involved during arrest of bleeding are*:

　i. Constriction of injured blood vessel due to release of 5-HT from the damaged platelets.

　ii. Formation of a haemostatic plug of platelets.

　iii. Seal of damaged blood vessel by the blood clot.

Q5. Enlist two conditions each in which bleeding and clotting time is prolonged.

Ans. The two conditions in which bleeding time is prolonged are thrombocytopenic purpura and purpura haemorrhagica.

The two conditions in which clotting time is prolonged are haemophilia and vitamin K deficiency.

Q6. What are the clinical implications of bleeding time and clotting time?

Ans. The bleeding time and clotting time are estimated to evaluate the integrity of the haemostatic mechanism.

Q7. Enlist the clotting factors.

Ans. *The coagulation factors are*:

- Factor I—fibrinogen.
- Factor II—prothrombin.
- Factor III—tissue thromboplastin (tissue factor).
- Factor IV—ionized calcium (Ca^{++}).
- Factor V—labile factor or proaccelerin.
- Factor VII—stable factor or proconvertin.
- Factor VIII—antihemophilic factor.
- Factor IX—plasma thromboplastin component, Christmas factor.
- Factor X—Stuart-Prower factor.
- Factor XI—plasma thromboplastin antecedent.
- Factor XII—Hageman factor.
- Factor XIII—fibrin-stabilizing factor.

Q8. What are the essential components for coagulation to occur?

Ans. The coagulation process requires coagulation factors, calcium and phospholipids.

Q9. What is the role of phospholipid in coagulation?

Ans. Phospholipids are prominent components of cellular and platelet membranes. They provide a surface upon which the chemical reactions of coagulation can take place.

Q10. What is the role of vitamin K in coagulation?

Ans. Vitamin K is required for formation of factors II, VII, IX and X, as well as protein S, protein C and protein Z.

Q11. What is the role of plasmin in coagulation?

Ans. Plasmin proteolytically cleaves fibrin into fibrin degradation products, thereby inhibiting excessive fibrin formation.

Q12. Where is Protein S synthesized and what is its function?

Ans. It is synthesized by liver, platelets, osteoblast and Leydig cells. Protein S forms a complex with protein C and this complex inactivates factor Va and factor VIIIa.

Q13. What are factors that hastens coagulation?

Ans. *The factors that hastens coagulation are*:

1. Warmth.
2. Contact with water-wettable surface and contact with rough surface.
3. Addition of thrombin.
4. Addition of thromboplastin.
5. Vitamin K injection or oral administration in high doses increases the prothrombin content of blood and increases the coagulability.
6. Addition of calcium chloride, both *in vivo* and *in vitro*.
7. Adrenaline injection produces constriction of blood vessels and helps in haemostatis mechanism.

Q14. What is von Willebrand disease and discuss its types?

Ans. *von Willebrand disease*:

The deficiency in the formation of quality or quantity of von Willebrand factor (vWF) leads to this disease. The von Willebrand factor (vWF) is required for platelet adhesion. The three forms of von Willebrand factor (vWF)/disease are hereditary, acquired, and pseudo or platelet type. The types of hereditary von Willebrand factor (vWF)/disease are: vWD type 1, vWD type 2, and vWD type 3. The platelet type of von Willebrand factor (vWF)/disease is also an inherited condition.

Q15. What are the causes of haemophilia A, B and C?

Ans. Haemophilia A is due to factor 8 deficiency, haemophilia B is due to factor 9 deficiency and haemophilia C is due to factor 11 deficiency.

Q16. What is disseminated intravascular coagulation (DIC)?

Ans. Disseminated intravascular coagulation (DIC) is a pathological condition in which there is widespread activation of the clotting cascade and this leads to formation of blood clots in the small blood vessels.

Q17. What are the common causes of disseminated intravascular coagulation (DIC)?

Ans. *The common causes of DIC are*:

1. Septicaemia
2. Massive tissue injury in cases of severe trauma, burns, rhabdomyolysis, extensive surgery
3. Snakebite
4. As a complication of mismatched blood transfusion
5. Giant haemangiomas (Kasabach-Merritt syndrome)
6. Large aortic aneurysms
7. Secondary to obstetric complications such as abruptio placentae, pre-eclampsia or eclampsia, septic abortion.

OBSERVATIONS: EXERCISE FOR STUDENTS

Results

Note:
Bleeding time as per Duke's method: ....
Bleeding time as per IVY method: ....
Clotting time as per capillary tube method: ....
Clotting time as per Lee-white method: ....

....
....
....
....
....
....
....
....
....
....
....
....
....
....
....
....
....
....
....
....
....
....
....
....
....
....
....
....

13

Platelet Count

Learning Objectives

After learning the practical the students should be able to:

1. Understand the significance of doing a platelet count
2. Know the methods of performing a platelet count.
3. Perform and estimate the platelet count.
4. Identify the sources of error and precautions while conducting a platelet count.
5. Know the normal values.
   - Explain and enlist the causes for altered platelet counts.

Aim: Determination of platelet count.

Material and chemicals: Lancet, cotton, spirit, RBC pipette, Neubauer's chamber, compound microscope, cover-slips and platelet diluting fluid (using 1% ammonium oxalate).

Principle: The diluents contain ammonium oxalate which completely lyses the red cells. It also acts as anti-coagulant. The platelets are then counted with a phase—haemocytometer and phase contrast microscope to enhance the refractileness of the platelets.

Method

1. Under aseptic precaution give a gentle finger prick. The blood sample is drawn to the 1 mark of a red blood cell diluting pipette.
2. The diluting fluid (1% ammonium oxalate) is drawn to the 101 mark, and gently mixed for 3–4 minutes.
3. Wait for 15–20 minutes so as red blood cell hemolysis occurs and the platelets settle down.
4. Charge the counting chamber. Focus under high power as done for RBC count. Observe for the platelets carefully. Platelets appear as highly refractile blue rounded bodies with silvery appearance.
5. Count the platelet in all 25 RBC square each (in central square area, i.e. 1 mm × 1 mm).

Calculations

Volume of fluid under which platelet cells are counted is 1 mm × 1 mm × 0.1 mm (= 1 μL).

Dilution factor as determined for dilution using RBC pipette is 200.

Let the count be N for total number of cells in 25 RBC square, i.e. it represents total number of cells in 1 mm³ of undiluted blood.

Thus number of platelets in 1 mm³ of undiluted blood = $N \times 200/0.1 = N \times 2000$.

Advantages

Identification is easier and the error involved is low. The use of ammonium oxalate as diluents ensures clearing of the background by haemolysis.

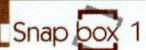

Snap box 1

Other Common Method of Platelet Count: Rees-Ecker Method

Materials: Thoma pipette, haemocytometer and reagent (Rees-Ecker diluting fluid).

Composition of Rees-Ecker solution

1. Sodium citrate (3.8 g) which prevents coagulation.
2. Formalin 2 ml—it acts as fixative and fixes platelets and prevents premature haemolysis.
3. Brilliant cresyl blue (0.1 g)—allows the platelets to be observed more clearly under a microscope
4. Distilled water 100 ml

Procedure

1. Draw the diluents up to the 0.5 mark, then the blood sample up to the 1 mark of the red blood cell diluting pipette
2. Further draw the diluents up to the 101 mark of the red blood cell diluting pipette and gently mix for 3–5 minutes by keeping the pipette in the palm.
3. Wait for 10–15 minutes so as red blood cell hemolysis occurs and the platelets settle down.
4. Charge the counting chamber (preferably spencer-briteline chamber). Focus under high power as done for RBC count. Observe for the platelets carefully. Platelets appear as highly refractile blue rounded bodies with silvery appearance.
5. Count the platelet in all 25 RBC square each (in central square area, i.e. 1 mm × 1 mm).

Calculations

Volume of fluid under which platelet cells are counted is 1 mm × 1 mm × 0.1 mm (= 1 µL)

Dilution factor as determined for dilution using RBC pipette is 200

Let the count be N for total number of cells in 25 RBC square, i.e. it represents total number of cells in 1 mm³ of undiluted blood.

Thus number of platelets in 1 mm³ of undiluted blood = $N \times 200/0.1 = N \times 2000$.

The structure of platelet and genesis of platelet are given below for orientation of students to viva voce questions and easy understanding.

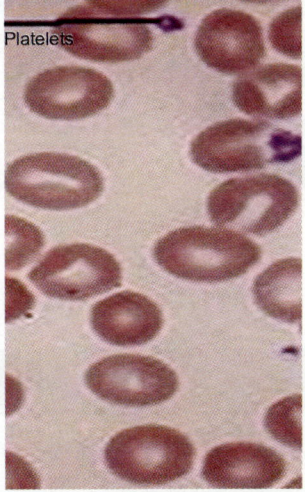

Fig. 13.1: Platelets as observed under peripheral smear

Note: A drop of 14% magnesium sulphate (prevent clumping of cells) is applied on sterilised fingertip. Blood is obtained then and smear is prepared using the Leishman stain. Total number of platelet/1000 cells are counted.

Precautions

1. Carry all aseptic measures and precaution during the procedure of filling the pipette. Do not over or under charge the chamber.
2. Wait for suitable time as mentioned in the method after adding diluting fluid so as to haemolyze other cells except platelets.
3. Identify platelets and maintain accuracy as you conduct the cell count.

OSPE SKILLED

Q1. Using 14% MgSO₄ as anticoagulant prepare a smear.

Ans.

   1. Finger is wiped with spirit and dried. A drop of the $MgSO_4$ mixture is to be applied on the fingertip. (Yes/No)

   2. Given a gentle prick where 14% $MgSO_4$ was applied. (Yes/No)

   3. Adds a drop of blood, spreads and make an ideal smear. (Yes/No)

Q2. Draw a well-labelled diagram of platelet formation.

Ans. The stages of formation of blood platelets are:

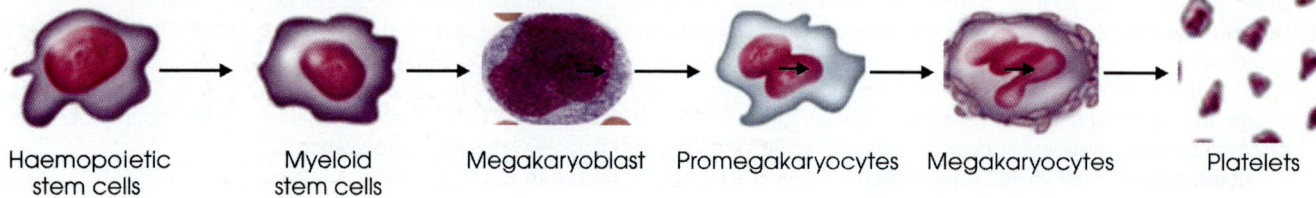

Haemopoietic stem cells → Myeloid stem cells → Megakaryoblast → Promegakaryocytes → Megakaryocytes → Platelets

Q3. Draw a well-labelled diagram of platelet.

Ans.

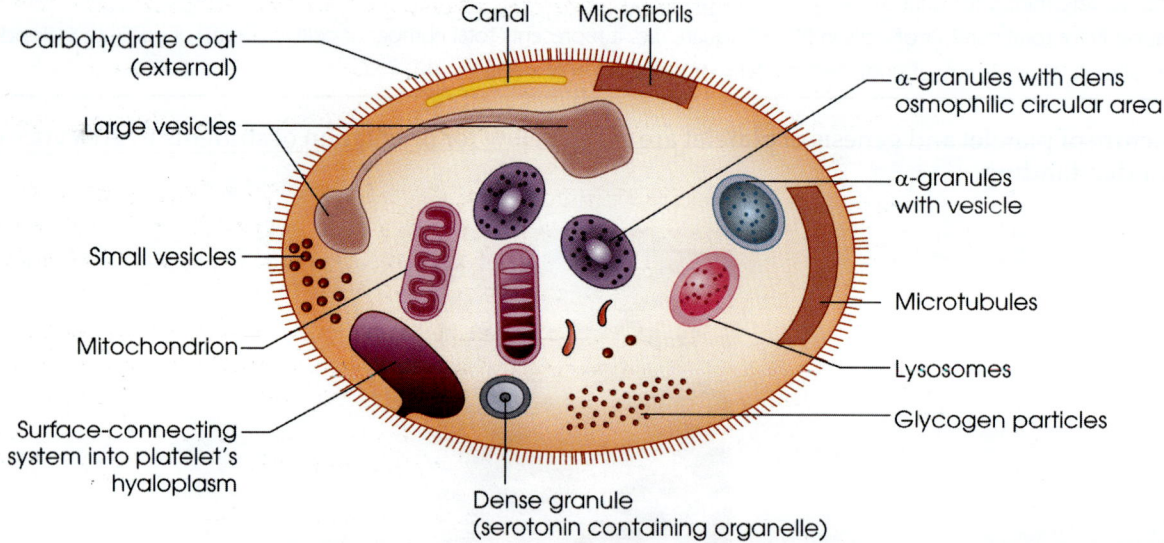

Labels: Carbohydrate coat (external); Canal; Microfibrils; Large vesicles; Small vesicles; Mitochondrion; Surface-connecting system into platelet's hyaloplasm; Dense granule (serotonin containing organelle); α-granules with dens osmophilic circular area; α-granules with vesicle; Microtubules; Lysosomes; Glycogen particles

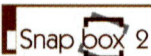

Snap box 2

Historical Time Line and Discovery of Platelets

In 1841 George Gulliver first drew pictures of platelets using compound microscope after its invention in 1830 by Joseph Jackson Lister.

In 1842 William Addison drew pictures of a platelet-fibrin clot.

In 1864 Lionel Beale first time in history published a drawing showing platelets.

In 1880 Dr Richard Hill Norris was the first to describe the action of platelets.

In 1886 William Osler published lectures in 1886, called them a *third corpuscle* and described them as a colourless protoplasmic disc.

In 1906 James Wright examined blood smears using the stain named and described them as **plates** in his 1906 publication but later changed its name to **platelets** in his 1910 publication which is now the universally accepted term.

VIVA VOCE QUESTIONS

Q1. What is the size of platelet cell?

Ans. Platelets are nearly about 20% of the diameter of the red blood cells. Platelets are on an average 2–3 microns in diameter.

Q2. What is the survival rate of platelets?

Ans. Platelets survive for 8–10 days.

Q3. What is the relation of platelets to circadian rhythm?

Ans. The relation of platelets to circadian rhythm is its circadian periodicity; and platelet count increases during miday.

Q4. How are platelets formed?

Ans. Platelets also known as megakaryocytes are produced in the bone marrow. Megakaryocyte develops into giant cells and undergoes a process of fragmentation that results in the release of over thousand platelets per megakaryocyte. The megakaryocyte development is controlled by thrombopoietin.

Q5. Enlist a few reasons for recommending platelet count in a patient.

Ans. *Platelet count is indicated and may be recommended in patients presenting with*:
  1. Bruising marks over the body without any injury
  2. Bleeding from the nose, mouth, or rectum without obvious injury
  3. Excessive or prolonged menstrual periods
  4. Delayed bleeding time from an injury site or wound.

Q6. What are giant platelets?

Ans. Giant platelets are abnormally large and are similar to size of a normal red blood cell. They are seen in disorders such as immune thrombocytopenic purpura (ITP) or also in rare inherited disorders such as Bernard-Soulier disease.

Q7. Enlist a few causes of thrombocytopenia.

Ans. Thrombocytopenia is lowered platelet count because of impaired production, increase destruction of platelets and splenic sequestrations.
  1. **Impaired production:** It occurs in viral infections—HIV, rubella, mumps, hepatitis C, Epstein-Barr virus, parovirus, etc. Aplastic anaemia, as adverse effect of medications such as chloramphenicol, gold, phenytoin, valproic acid, etc. after radiation therapy, congenital disorders (Fanconi's anaemia) and in patients on chemotherapeutic drugs, etc.
  2. **Increased platelet destruction:** Immunological causes of increased platelet destruction are: (a) Adverse effect of drugs such as sulfonamide, carbamazepine, digoxin, quinine, acetaminophen, rifampin, etc; (b) Due to transfusion reactions and (c) In patients of systemic lupus erythematosus.
  3. **Splenic sequestration:** In condition such as cirrhosis or leukaemia, spleen captures and sequesters more platelets from the circulation than normal; leading to thrombocytopenia.

Q8. What is pseudothrombocytopenia?

Ans. In pseudothrombocytopenia there is a falsely low platelet count and may happen because of occasional clumping of the platelets together on drawing of blood.

Q9. Discuss the prime function of platelets.

Ans. Platelets because of their properties of aggregation and adhesiveness, they are directly involved in blood clotting as well as release substances that activate other haemostatic processes.

Q10. What is normal platelet count?

Ans. The normal platelet count is 150,000 to 450,000 per micro liter of blood.

Q11. What are the functions of platelet?

Ans. The functions of platelets are that they are important functionally for blood coagulation, haemostasis, clot retraction, they store 5HT and histamine (these are mediators of inflammation) and they engulf carbon particles, viruses and immune complexes.

Q12. What is thrombocytopenic purpura?

Ans. It is low platelet count with normal bone marrow and there are no other underlying causes for thrombocytopenia. Its characteristic feature includes appearance of purpuric rash and increased tendency to bleed.

Q13. Enlist the signs associated with thrombocytopenic purpura.

Ans. The signs associated with thrombocytopenic purpura include the spontaneous formation of bruises (purpura) and petechiae (tiny bruises), especially on the extremities, bleeding from the nostrils, bleeding gums, and menorrhagia and any of these signs occur when platelet count decreases below 20,000 per μl.

Q14. What will low count (<10,000 per μl) of platelet lead to?

Ans. A very low count (<10,000 per μl) may lead to spontaneous formation of hematomasin the mouth or on other mucous membranes. Bleeding time from minor lacerated bruised sites is usually prolonged.

Q15. What is gray platelet syndrome?

Ans. Gray platelet syndrome (GPS), is a rare congenital autosomal recessive bleeding disorder caused by a decreased or absence of alpha-granules in blood platelets. This affects the release of proteins from these granules into the marrow, causing myelofibrosis.

Q16. What is dengue fever and what happens to platelet count in it?

Ans. Dengue fever is a mosquito-borne tropical disease caused by the dengue virus and platelet count decreases in it.

Q17. What is purpura? How is it graded?

Ans. Purpura is the capillary abnormality leading to bleeding. Its characteristic features include spontaneous haemorrhages beneath the skin and mucous membrane. The purpura is graded depending on platelet count—fulminating purpura (platelet count less than 1000/μl), moderate purpura (platelet count less than 10000/μl) and mild platelet count (platelet count less than 50000/μl).

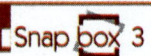 **Snap box 3**

Applied Clinical

Haemolytic uremic syndrome (HUS) —is a thrombocytopenic syndrome caused by infection with bacteria particularly certain types of *E. coli* which secretes a very potent toxin, named Shiga toxin. *E. coli* O157: H7 is commonly found in the normal intestinal bacteria in cattle. Therefore, consumption of undercooked beef or contact with cattle creates a risk for haemolytic uremic syndrome.

OBSERVATIONS: EXERCISE FOR STUDENTS

Results

Calculations

Volume of fluid under which platelet cells are counted is 1 mm × 1 mm × 0.1 mm (= 1 μL)

Dilution factor as determined for dilution using RBC pipette is 200

Let the count be N for total number of cells in 25 RBC square, i.e. it represents total number of cells in 1 mm³ of undiluted blood.

Thus number of platelets in 1 mm³ of undiluted blood = $N \times 200/0.1 = N \times 2000$

Thus number of platelets in 1 mm³ of undiluted blood = ...

....

....

....

....

....

....

....

Reticulocyte Count

Learning Objectives

After learning the practical the students should be able to:

1. Describe the morphology of a reticulocyte.
2. Discuss and explain stains being used and principle of the experiment.
3. Accurately calculate reticulocyte.
4. Explain the causes for altered reticulocyte count.
5. List the precautions to be followed while conducting reticulocyte count.

Aim: Determination of reticulocyte count.

Materials and chemicals: Lancet, pipettes, glass slides, Petridish, microscope, 12 × 75 mm tube, EDTA mediated whole blood, and new methylene blue staining solution (1 g of dye dissolved in 100 ml of citrate saline) or brilliant cresyl blue (1 g of dye dissolved in 100 ml of citrate saline).

Principle: The reticulocyte is a non-nucleated immature red cell containing residual RNA. A supravital stain, new methylene blue, is used to precipitate the RNA into dark-blue filaments or granules to identify reticulocytes. The new methylene blue stains residual RNA and ribosomes in cytoplasm of reticulocytes more deeply and uniformly than brilliant cresyl blue.

PROCEDURE

1. Add two drops of new methylene blue in the bottom of a 12 × 75 mm tube. Add 2 drops of well-mixed EDTA blood to the tube using a pipette.
2. Mix uniformly till smoky-gray mixture colour is observed.
3. Incubate mixture at least 10 minutes so that living conditions are simulated and stain is well taken by the reticulocyte.
4. After carefully mixing make 2 to 3 good quality smears and stain with Leishman stain as done in routine Leishman staining.
5. **Counting:** Conduct count for 500 RBC and record the number of reticulocytes seen.

Calculations

Percentage of reticulocyte = No. of reticulocytes/total no. of cells counted × 100.
Normal reticulocyte count = 0.2–2% in children and adult.

Results: The reticulocyte count of given sample is ....

Precautions

1. Carry all aseptic measures and precaution during the procedure of filling the pipette.
2. Ensure adequate mixing of new methylene blue with EDTA mediated whole blood prior to making smears
3. Do not count artifact or other inclusions as reticulocytes.
4. Ensure counting for 500 RBC and observe and note the number of reticulocytes seen.
5. Calculate precisely.

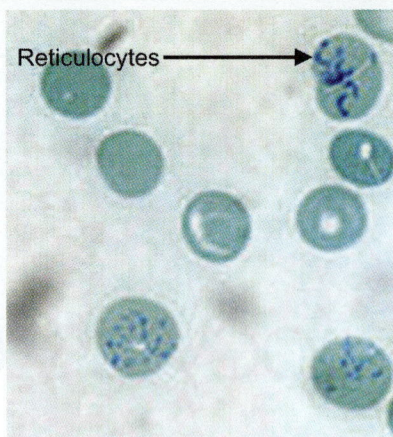

Reticulocytes ⟶

Fig 14.1: Reticulocytes as seen in peripheral smear

VIVA VOCE QUESTIONS

Q1. Discuss the characteristics of stains used for reticulocyte count.

Ans. A supravital stain, new methylene blue, is used to precipitate the RNA into dark-blue filaments or granules to identify reticulocytes. The new methylene blue stains residual RNA and ribosomes in cytoplasm of reticulocytes more deeply and uniformly than brilliant cresyl blue.

Q2. Enlist the causes for high reticulocyte count.

Ans. A high reticulocyte count is seen in newborn, i.e. 30–40% reaches to 1–2% in first week of life, high altitude, after haemorrhage, in patients of chronic haemolytic anaemia, in disorders of spleen and splenectomy, and as reticulocyte response to treatment of iron deficiency anaemia.

Q3. Enlist the causes for low reticulocyte count.

Ans. A low reticulocyte count is seen in hypopituitarism, aplastic anaemia, after splenectomy and myxedema.

Q4. Enlist the indications for reticulocyte count.

Ans. *The indications for reticulocyte count are*:
- Investigation of anaemia
- Monitoring the effect of haematinic or recombinant erythropoietin therapy
- Monitoring bone marrow regenerative capacity after chemotherapy or bone marrow transplantation

Q5. What are reticulocytes? How are they formed?

Ans. Reticulocytes are immature red blood cells. Reticulocytes develop and mature in the bone marrow and circulate for about a day in the blood stream as it develops into mature red blood cells. They are called reticulocytes because of a reticular (mesh-like) network of remnants of ribosomal RNA which becomes visible under a microscope with supravital stains.

Q6. How can accurate measurement of reticulocyte be done?

Ans. Accurate measurement of reticulocyte can be done with automated counters which employ a combination of laser excitation, detectors and a fluorescent dye that marks DNA and RNA.

Q7. How are reticulocytes distinguished from other cells?

Ans. Reticulocytes are easily distinguished from other circulating cells because they emit a signal that is neither weak (like red blood cells) nor strong (like lymphocytes).

Q8. What is the normal reticulocyte count?

Ans. The normal fraction of reticulocytes in the blood is usually 0.5% to 2.5% in adults and 2% to 6% in infants.

Q9. What does number of reticulocyte indicate?

Ans. The number of reticulocytes is a good indicator of bone marrow activity because it represents recent production and allows for the determination of the reticulocyte production index and reticulocyte count.

This value determines whether if a production problem is responsible for anaemia and is also useful in monitoring the progress of treatment for anaemia by the observed reticulocyte response.

Q10. What are the recent methods for estimation of reticulocytes?

Ans. Earlier reticulocyte count was carried out by microscopic examination of peripheral blood smears stained with a supravital dye. Today, reticulocyte counts are done with aid of automated hematology analyzers.

Q11. What are the advantages of automated methods in cell count?

Ans. Automated methods have several advantages such as it enumerates large numbers of cells, thereby greatly improves precision, accuracy and efficiency. Additional reticulocyte parameters such as reticulocyte maturation index and immature reticulocyte fraction can also be determined by automated analyzers.

Q12. What is the principle of functioning of automated analyzers?

Ans. Its functioning is based on flow cytometry technology and employs light scatter and immunofluorescence of a RNA specific dye, such as auramine-O for accuracy reporting.

Bibliography

1. Steren I hajdu. The discovery of blood cells. Ann Clin Lab SCi. 2003; 33(2): 237–238.

OBSERVATIONS: EXERCISE FOR STUDENTS

Results

Calculations

Percentage of reticulocyte = No. of reticulocytes/total no. of cells counted × 100

Normal reticulocyte count = 0–2% in children and adult.

Results—the reticulocyte count of given sample is ....

15
Determination of Erythrocyte Sedimentation Rate (ESR) and Packed Cell Volume (PCV)

Learning Objectives

The students should be able to:

1. Understand the procedure of determining erythrocyte sedimentation rate (ESR) and packed cell volume (PCV).
2. Explain the clinical importance of ESR and PCV in health and disease condition.

Aim: To determine the erythrocyte sedimentation rate (ESR) of the given sample of blood.

Principle and Theory

ESR is the rate at which RBCs settle down when blood to which an anticoagulant is added is allowed to stand in a specially designed narrow tube for one hour. The ESR is expressed in mm of clear plasma at the end of one hour.

The sedimentation occurs in three different stages:

a. **Stage I:** Rouleaux formation (piling of RBCs) and aggregation occurs in ten minutes. Rouleaux formation is determined largely by increased levels of plasma fibrinogen and globulins.

b. **Stage II:** Sinking of the aggregates takes place at approximately forty minutes.

c. **Stage III:** The aggregated cells pack at the bottom of the tube. This takes a period of ten minutes.

Materials and Chemicals

Wintrobe's haematocrit tube, Westergren's pipette, 3.8% sodium citrate solution as anticoagulant, anticoagulant mixture of potassium and ammonium oxalate, Pasteur pipette, spirit, cotton and syringe with 22 gauze needle.

Methods: ESR can be determined by Wintrobe's and Westergren's method.

Wintrobe's Method (Fig. 15.1)

Wintrobe's haematocrit tube: The Wintrobe's haematocrit tube is cylindrical in shape and approximately 11 cm in length having an internal bore diameter of 2.5 mm. The tube is graduated in mm in both directions from 0–10 cm. The markings 0 to 10 from above downwards are used for recording the ESR and markings 0–10 from below upwards are used for recording haematocrit (PCV).

Procedure

- Withdraw 5 ml of venous blood in penicillin bottle containing the anticoagulated powered mixture of double oxalate (6 mg of ammonium oxalate and 4 mg of potassium oxalate) and gently shake the bottle.
- Draw the blood with the Pasteur pipette and introduce the tip of the pipette down up to the bottom of the Wintrobe's tube in order to empty the blood into haematocrit tube.
- Empty the blood slowly out of the pipette into haematocrit tube, taking care to avoid air bubbles.
- The Wintrobe's tube is filled with blood up to the '0' mark and place the Wintrobe's tube vertically in its rack. At the end of one hour note the reading of clear plasma in the Wintrobe's tube.

0
1
2
3
4
5
6
7
8
9
10
9
8
7
6
5
4
3
2
1

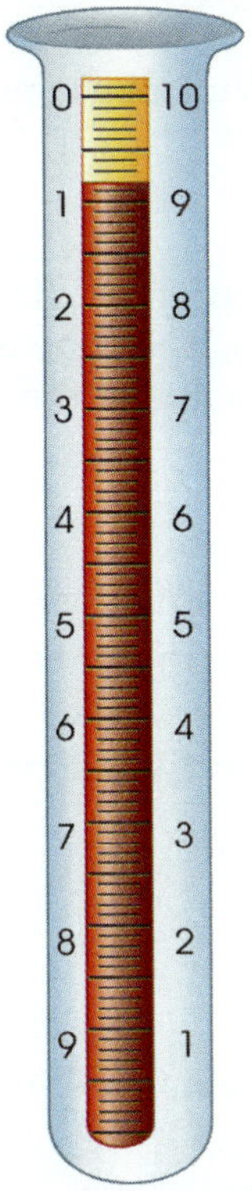

Fig. 15.1: Wintrobe's tube

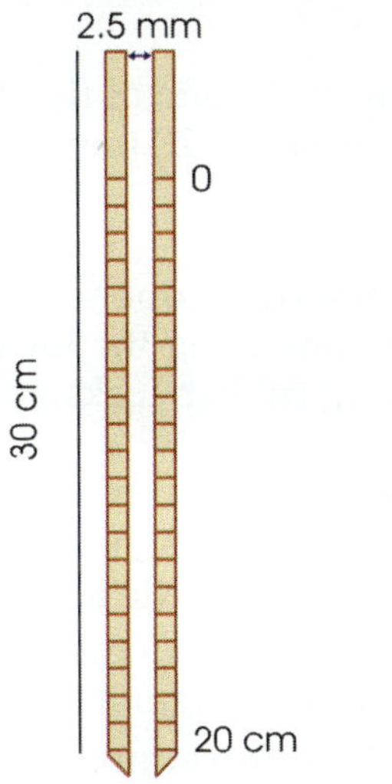

2.5 mm
0
30 cm
20 cm

Fig. 15.2: Westergren's tube

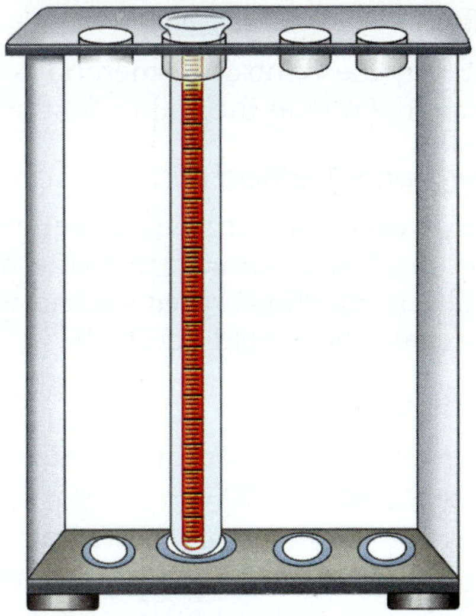

Fig. 15.3: Westergren's tube placed in rack

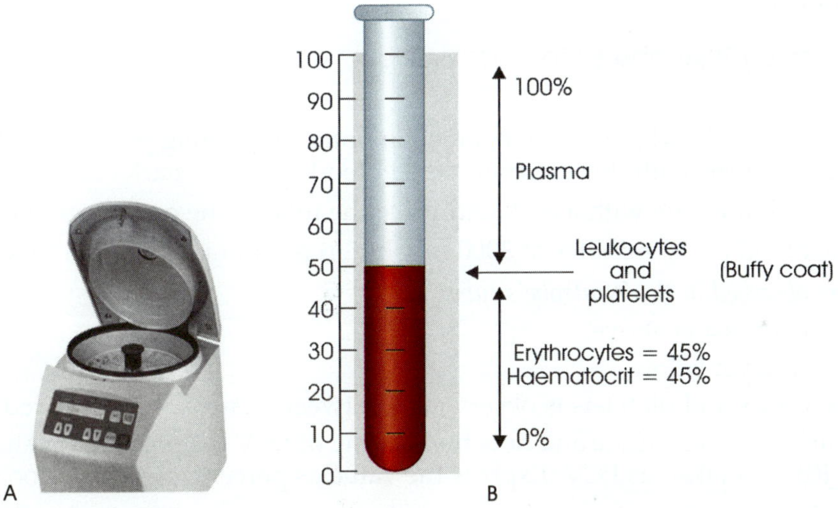

100
90
80
70
60
50
40
30
20
10
0
100%
Plasma
Leukocytes
and
platelets
(Buffy coat)
Erythrocytes = 45%
Haematocrit = 45%
0%
A
B

Fig. 15.4: A. Haematocrit centrifuge, B. Packed cell volume is 45%

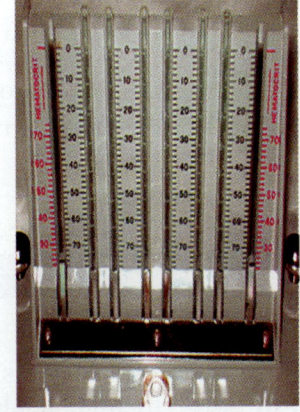

Fig. 15.5: Identify instruments (Q3)

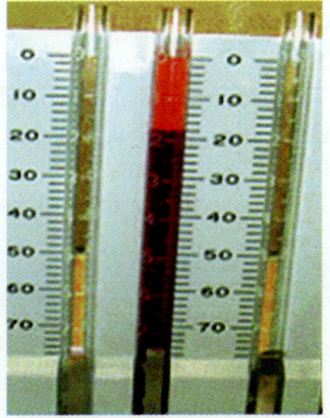

Fig. 15.6: Identify instruments (Q4)

Results

The ESR by the Wintrobe's method is .... mm at the end of first hour. (Normal values—Wintrobe's method: Males: 0 to 9 mm at the end of first hour and Females: 0 to 20 mm at the end of first hour).

Westergren's Method (Figs 15.2 and 15.3)

Descriptions: Westergren's pipette is 300 mm in length, opened at both ends and has an internal diameter of 2.5 mm. It is graduated marking from 0 to 200 mm along the lower two-thirds of its length. The tube is held vertically in the Westergren's stand which is having rubber corks at the lower end and metal clips at the upper end so that tube is held vertically.

Procedure

- Take 1 ml of 3.8% sodium citrate solution in penicillin bottle and add 4 ml of blood and then mix it gently.
- Draw the citrated blood into the Westergren's pipette up to the level of '0' mark and close the upper end with the finger immediately to prevent the blood from moving out of the pipette.
- Press the lower end tightly on the rubber cork of the Westergren's stand and fix the tube vertically with the clip at the upper end.
- Take the ESR reading at the end of one hour.

Result

The ESR by the Westergren's method is mm at the end of one hour.

Normal values as per Westergren's method—(Males: 3 to 5 mm at the end of first hour and Females: 4 to 7 mm at the end of first hour).

Packed Cell Volume by Wintrobe's Method (Fig. 15.4)

Method

1. Draw the venous blood and pour it in a penicillin bottle containing powder of double oxalate mixture. The Wintrobe's tube is filled with this anticoagulated blood up to 10 marks of the haematocrit readings.
2. Close the mouth of the tube with a cork and place the tube in the centrifuge machine.
3. Centrifuge the blood for 30 minutes at 3000 revolution per minutes. Watch till cells settle down at bottom.

   Three layers are observed in the Wintrobe's tube:
   a. A layer of clear plasma above.
   b. Red blood cell layer below.
   c. Buffy layer WBCs and platelets is observed in between plasma layer and red blood cell layer.
4. Remove the tube from centrifuge and note the reading of PCV (haematocrit) value from the tube. The height of column of RBCs is taken as PCV. Express the value as percentage of the blood.

Normal Values

Wintrobes's method: Adult men: Average 45% (range 40–50%) and Adult women: Average 42% (range 37–47%).

Precautions

1. Take dry clean glass apparatus like tubes, pipette, dropper, etc. for conducting the test.
2. The drawn venous blood should be immediately transferred into the penicillin bottle to prevent haemolysis.
3. Care should be taken that while filling blood the Wintrobe's tube or Westergren's pipette there is no air bubble appearing.
4. Take note of the time of fixing the tube/pipette and of observed readings exactly after one hour.

OSPE NON-SKILLED

Q1. Enlist the causes of increase or decrease in ESR.

Ans. The ESR is increased in anaemia, acute or chronic infections, renal disorders, auto immune diseases such as rheumatoid arthritis, malignancies, nephrosis, etc. The ESR is decreased in polycythemia, sickle cell anaemia, leukaemia, congestive heart failure, burns, dehydration, severe allergic reactions, etc.

Q2. Enlist the conditions where PCV is increased and decreased.

Ans. The causes of increased packed cell volume are polycythemia, congestive heart failure, burns and dehydration. Packed cell volume is decreased in anaemia, aplastic anaemia and severe leucopenia.

Q3. Identify the instrument shown in Fig. 15.5.

Ans. The instrument is Westergren's pipette in erythrocyte sedimentation rack.

Q4. Read the results shown in Fig. 15.6.

Ans. Figure 15.6 shows ESR value of 18 mm at the end of one hour by Westergren's method.

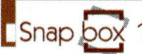 Snap box 1

Historical Updates: Edmund Faustyn Biernacki: Edmund Faustyn Biernacki (born on December 19, 1866 in Opoczno–died on December 29, 1911 in Lwów) was a Polish physician. He was the first one to note a relationship between the sedimentation rate of red blood cells in a human blood sample and the general condition of the organism. This method, known as the Biernacki Reaction, is used worldwide to assess erythrocyte sedimentation rate (ESR).

VIVA VOCE QUESTIONS

Q1. Define ESR. What are the factors which affect ESR?

Ans. The rate at which the red blood cells settle down is known as erythrocyte sedimentation rate. ESR depends on the shape, size and number of RBCs, temperature, tendency for rouleaux formation, plasma viscosity, length, diameter and position of ESR tubes and the anticoagulant used for the procedure.

Q2. Name the two methods used to assess the ESR.

Ans. Westergren's and Wintrobe's methods are used to assess the ESR.

Q3. What is the effect of temperature on ESR?

Ans. The increase in temperature decreases the viscosity of blood and hence increases the ESR.

Q4. Mention the clinical importance of performing the erythrocyte sedimentation rate.

Ans. The high values of ESR indicate the presence of acute inflammatory reaction in the body and it also serves as a prognostic indicator for various diseases.

Q5. Mention any two pathological causes for raised ESR.

Ans. Hereditary spherocytosis and tuberculosis.

Q6. Define haematocrit. Mention the different methods for measuring the haematocrit.

Ans. Haematocrit or packed cell volume (PCV) is defined as the percentage of the volume (or parts) of blood occupied by the red cells.

The different methods for measuring PCV includes: (a) Macrohaematocrit method, (b) Microhaematocrit method and (c) Automated method.

Q7. What is the clinical significance of assessing the packed cell volume?

Ans. The percentage of error associated with PCV method is less as compared to the haemoglobin estimation or red cell count. Hence, PCV is a more accurate test to determine the presence of anaemia or polycythemia. It is also used in the calculation of various red cell indices.

Q8. What are the advantages of microhaematocrit method?

Ans. The procedure is easy, cheap, less time consuming and requires very less quantity of blood when compared to the macrohaematocrit method. The procedure is very useful in mass screening for anaemia.

Q9. How do you calculate the 'true' haematocrit or true cell volume?

Ans. 'True' haematocrit or true cell volume is calculated by multiplying the haematocrit value obtained with 0.98.

Q10. Why is the haematocrit of venous blood more than that of arterial blood?

Asn. The red cells in venous blood contain higher concentration of chloride ions when compared to the red cells of arterial blood due to the mechanism of chloride shift. Since chloride ions are osmotically active particles, water enters into the red cells leading to increase in the size of these cells. Hence, the haematocrit of venous blood is more than that of the arterial blood.

Q11. What is the normal haematocrit in males and females?

Ans. The haematocrit is normally about 45% for men and 40% for women.

Q12. State the clinical significance of ESR and PCV.

Ans. The erythrocyte sedimentation rate (ESR) is increased in inflammation, anaemia, pregnancy, kidney diseases, autoimmune disorders such as rheumatoid arthritis and lupus erythematous, and cancers such as multiple myeloma and lymphoma. The ESR is decreased in polycythemia, hyperviscocity, sickle cell anaemia, leukaemia, hypoprotenemia and congestive heart failure. The packed cell volume is the volume percentage of red blood cell in blood. The low haematocrit values are observed in anaemia and high haematocrit values in polycythemia.

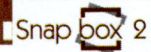 Snap box 2

Recent Updates

1. Dengue fever is an acute viral illness and may affect children and adults. It can also progress to a severe form know as dengue haemorrhagic fever (DHF). Disease is transmitted through the bite of the infected mosquitoes of the genus *Aedes*. The high haematocrit value in dengue fever increases risk of dengue shock syndrome. The haematocrit levels are kept under observations for a minimum of 24 hours period. A haematocrit level elevated more than 20% of the normal range suggests haemoconcentration, especially after treatment with intravenous fluids and these finding precedes shock.

2. Professional athletes' haematocrit levels are measured as part of tests for erythropoietin (EPO) use or blood doping. The level of haematocrit is compared with the long-term level for that athlete taking into consideration individual variations in haematocrit level, and against an absolute permitted maximum.

3. Anabolic androgenic steroid (AAS) use can also increase the amount of RBCs and thus affects the haematocrit particularly in persons addicted to the compounds boldenone and oxymetholone.

OBSERVATIONS: EXERCISE FOR STUDENTS

Results

Note

Results:

1. The ESR by the Wintrobe's method is .... mm at the end of first hour. (Normal values: Wintrobe's method: Males: 0 to 9 mm at end of first hour and Females: 0 to 20 mm at the end of first hour.

2. The ESR by the Westergren's method is .... mm at the end of one hour.

3. Normal values as per Westergren's method—(Males: 3 to 5 mm at the end of first hour and Females: 4 to 7 mm at the end of first hour)

4. Haematocrity value is .... %

   Normal Values: Wintrobes's Method: Adult men: Average 45% (range 40–50%) and Adult women: Average 42% (range 37–47%).

....

....

....

....

16

Determination of Osmotic Fragility of Red Blood Cells

Learning Objectives

The students should be able to:

1. Understand and explain the principal and procedure of determination of osmotic fragility of red blood cells.
2. List the factors affecting osmotic fragility.
3. Explain the mechanism and complication of haemolysis of RBC in the human body.
4. They should be able to explain the clinical importance of osmotic fragility of red blood cells in health and disease conditions.

Aim: To study the osmotic fragility of red blood cells.

Background and definition of osmotic fragility: The ease with which the RBCs are haemolysed in hypotonic solution is termed osmotic fragility of RBCs. The concentration of hypotonic solution in which the cells are getting haemolysed represents the osmotic fragility in percentage.

Principle

1. The red blood cells in isotonic solution remain suspended in it. [Isotonic solutions are those solutions having same tonicity as that of plasma (e.g. 0.9% sodium chloride; 5% glucose; 10% mannitol and 20% urea)]. They neither swell nor shrink in the solution because the osmotic pressure of the isotonic solution and the osmotic pressure within the RBCs are same.
2. While the red blood cell in hypotonic solution (e.g. <0.9% sodium chloride), absorb fluid from outside and swell and eventually burst.
3. Red blood cell when placed in hypertonic solution (e.g. >0.9% sodium chloride), the fluid within the red blood cell move out of cells and the cell shrinks.

Materials and chemicals: Lancet, cotton, spirit, a set of clean test tubes, test tube rack, distilled water, freshly prepared 1% NaCl solution, pipette (2 ml) and dropper.

Procedure

- Place the test tubes in the rack and assign numbers to the tube from 1 to 12.
- The hypotonic solutions of various strengths are to be prepared by mixing the required number of drops of 1% sodium chloride solution and distilled water in the test tubes 1 to 12, as given below:

Test tube no	1	2	3	4	5	6	7	8	9	10	11	12
No. of drops of 1% NaCl	22	16	15	14	13	12	11	10	9	8	7	0
No. of drops of distilled water	3	9	10	11	12	13	14	15	16	17	18	25
Strength of saline solution (%)	0.9	0.64	0.60	0.56	0.52	0.48	0.44	0.40	0.36	0.32	0.28	0

Note: That the first tube contains nearly isotonic saline and that the last tube contains distilled water (tonicity—nil).

- Add a drop of blood in each tube.
- Mix the blood with saline by inverting each tube carefully.
- After one hour, note your observations. Take care not to shake the tubes.
- Note the % of sodium chloride in the tube which shows the beginning of haemolysis and the % of sodium chloride in the first tube that shows complete haemolysis.
- The clear, straw-coloured, supernatant fluid indicates absence of haemolysis with unhaemolysed RBCs settled at the bottom.
- A tube with partial haemolysis will show a red coloured upper supernatant fluid proportionate to the extent of haemolysis and a layer of unhaemolysed RBCs at the bottom of the tube.
- Complete haemolysis is confirmed by a uniformly red coloured solution with no RBCs at the bottom.

Results: Record your observation and results as given below.

Beginning of haemolysis occurs in ......% saline.

Complete haemolysis of cells is seen in ......% saline.

The osmotic fragility of RBCs ranges from ......% to ......% saline.

Compare your results with the fragility range for normal RBCs and interpret.

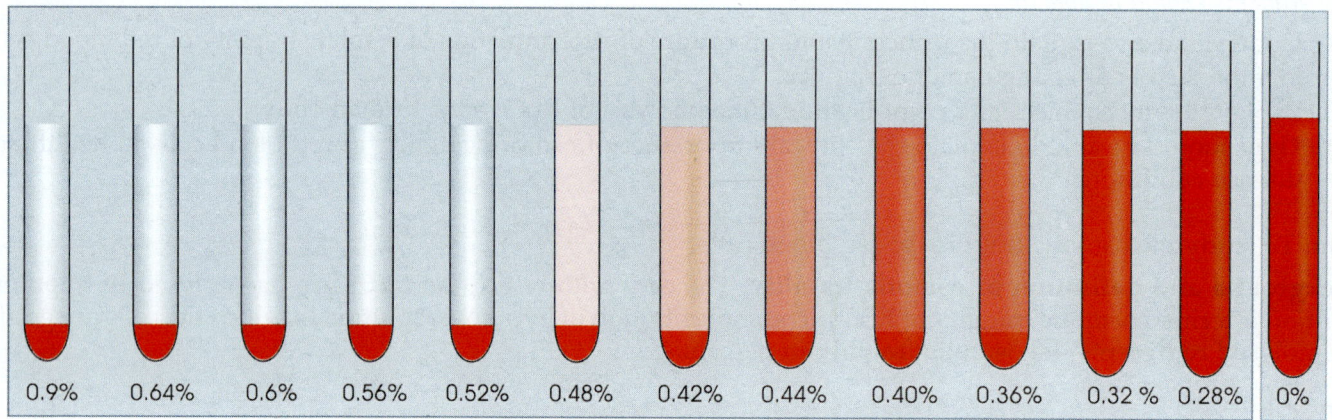

Concentration of sodium chloride in percentage

Fig. 16.1: Osmotic fragility of red blood cells (the onset of fragility occurs at 0.48% and is completed around 0.34%)

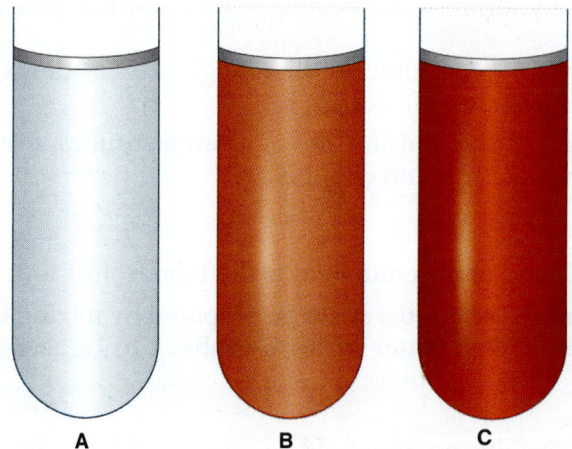

Fig. 16.2: A. No haemolysis, B. Partial or some haemolysis and C. Complete haemolysis

PRECAUTIONS

1. Prepare hypotonic solutions of various strengths by mixing the required number of drops of 1% sodium chloride solution and distilled water carefully.

2. As blood is added to the tube, ensure that the tube is not shaken for mixing because this may lead to mechanical haemolysis.

3. Wait for one hour to observe complete haemolysis.

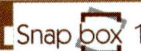
Snap box 1

Significance

1. The osmotic fragility of red blood cell starts at 0.48% sodium chloride and ends in 0.34% sodium chloride solution in normal healthy individuals.

2. In spherocytosis (spherical shaped RBC), autoimmune haemolytic anaemia, G6PD deficiency, etc. the RBC's osmotic fragility increases and it begins in 0.7% sodium chloride and ends in 0.45% sodium chloride solution.

3. RBC's osmotic fragility decreases in iron deficiency anaemia, sickle cell anaemia and thalassemia (they become slender). Osmotic fragility commences in 0.36% sodium chloride and ends in 0.24% sodium chloride solution.

OSPE NON-SKILLED QUESTIONS

Q1. What does osmotic fragility test signify?

Ans. The osmotic fragility test is a measure of the resistance of erythrocytes to haemolysis by osmotic stress. The test consists of exposing red cells to varying strengths of hypotonic saline solutions and measuring the degree of haemolysis by colorimeter at room temperature.

Q2. State the principle of osmotic fragility test.

Ans. The principle of the test is that the normal RBC is able to resist the influx of water to a limited extent. When the cells are placed in a hypotonic solution, the RBC absorbs water due to osmotic pressure and leads to swelling of RBC. In hypertonic solution the RBC shrinks.

OSPE FOR PRACTICE

1. Perform the osmotic fragility test and record your observations.

2. Add a drop of the given sample of blood to the test tube containing urea solution and record your observation.

3. Add a drop of the given sample of blood to the test tube containing 10% sucrose solution and record your observation.

4. Add a drop of the given sample of blood to the test tube containing 5% dextrose solution and record your observation.

VIVA VOCE QUESTIONS

Q1. What does osmotic fragility test signify?

Ans. The osmotic fragility test is a measure of the resistance of erythrocytes to haemolysis by osmotic stress. The test consists of exposing red cells to varying strengths of hypotonic saline solutions and measuring the degree of haemolysis by colorimeter at room temperature.

Q2. State the principle of osmotic fragility test.

Ans. The principle of the test is that the normal RBC is able to resist the influx of water to a limited extent. When the cells are placed in a hypotonic solution, the RBC absorbs water due to osmotic pressure and leads to swelling of RBC. In hypertonic solution, the RBC shrinks.

Q3. What is the normal range of osmotic fragility of red cells?

Ans. Haemolysis begins at 0.48% NaCl and ends at about 0.34% saline NaCl.

Q4. What would you observe if the red cells are suspended in a solution containing 10% glucose?

Ans. Since 10% glucose is a hypertonic solution, water moves out from the red cells into the surrounding medium resulting in shrinkage of the red cells.

Q5. **List a few conditions characterized by increased red cell fragility.**

Ans. The conditions such as hereditary spherocytosis, congenital/autoimmune haemolytic anaemia and G6PD deficiency are characterized by increased red cell fragility.

Q6. **List a few conditions characterized by decreased red cell fragility.**

Ans. Conditions such as iron deficiency anaemia, thalassemia, sickle cell anaemia and acholuric jaundice are characterized by decreased red cell fragility.

Q7. **Mention the clinical significance of osmotic fragility test.**

Ans. Osmotic fragility test is used as a screening tool for hereditary spherocytosis.

Q8. **Enlist factors affecting the osmotic fragility.**

Ans. The factor affecting the osmotic fragility test is the shape of the red cell, which, in turn, depends on the volume, surface area and functional state of the red blood cell membrane. The other factors which influence osmotic fragility are pH of the blood (decreased pH increases fragility) in saline, relative volume of blood and saline and temperature (increase in temperature decreases fragility of red blood cells).

Q9. **Describe the complication of haemolysis of red blood cell in human body.**

Ans. *The complications of haemolysis of red blood cell in human body are:*

1. The increased breakdown and metabolism of haemoglobin results in increased bilirubin level and may cause haemolytic jaundice and there is also increased fecal and urinary urobilinogen. Moreover, presence of free haemoglobin and free haeme in the circulation may lead to vascular dysfunction, injury, and inflammation.
2. Orthostasis and mild splenomegaly.
3. The free haemoglobin which passes via the tubules may get precipitated as acid haematin, thus blocking the tubules producing renal tubular damage and dysfunction and may eventually lead to anuria and renal failure.
4. Chronic haemolysis may lead to anaemia, reticulocytosis, low haptoglobin, high LDH, and high indirect bilirubin levels in circulation.

Q10. **What are the complications associated with chronic haemolysis?**

Ans.

1. The chronic haemolysis may lead to increased excretion of bilirubin into the biliary tract, thereby forming gallstones, release of free haemoglobin increases pressure over the pulmonary artery leading to pulmonary hypertension.
2. Increased pulmonary pressure in its artery leads to episodes of syncope, chest pain, and progressive breathlessness and condition eventually progressing to right ventricular heart failure.
3. The free haemoglobin which passes via the tubules may get precipitated as acid haematin, thus blocking the tubules producing renal tubular damage and dysfunction and may eventually lead to anuria and renal failure.
4. Chronic haemolysis may lead to anaemia, reticulocytosis, low haptoglobin, high LDH, and high indirect bilirubin levels in circulation.

Q11. **What is isoosmotic hyperhydration and what are its causes?**

Ans. Isoosmotic hyperhydration is the enhanced excessive blood plasma volume and interstitial volume. The increase in extracellular fluid volume may be due to administration of an excessive amount of isoosmolar solutions (Examples—fast parenteral administration of large amount of solution, viz. blood transfusion, plasma transfusion and blood substituents).

Q12. **What are signs and complication of isoosmotic hyperhydration?**

Ans. The general oedema is the most common sign observed in isoosmolar fluid's retention and increase in ECF volume. Its complication includes cardiac failure, nephrotic syndrome and liver cirrhosis.

Q13. **What is hyperosomotic hyperhydration? What physiological changes in circulation it may lead to?**

Ans. Hyperosomotic hyperhydration is a condition where both the volume and the osmolarity of the ECF are increased. This may lead to a shift of water from the intracellular space into the ECF. It persists till a new osmotic balance between ECF and ICF is established.

Q14. **What will hyperosomotic hyperhydration lead to?**

Ans. It may lead to intracellular dehydration.

Q15. What are the causes of hyperosomotic hyperhydration?

Ans. There are two likely causes for hyperosmotic hyperhydration: Increased intravenous administration of NaCl (in patients of renal insufficiency) and an excessive administration of infusions (infusion of hyperosmolar salts or hyperosmolar sugar solutions).

Q16. What are the etiological factors associated with hyperosmotic hyperhydration?

Ans. The etiological factors associated with hyperosmotic hyperhydration are adrenal tumours, acute renal failure, acute glomerulonephritis, administration of high doses of steroid hormones, etc.

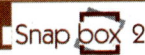 Snap box 2

The micro fluidic chip-based system which determines the osmotic fragility of RBCs is made from a Y-shaped polydimethylsiloxane (PDMS) micro channel and is sealed to a glass cover plate. The different degrees of haemolysis (no haemolysis, partial haemolysis, and complete haemolysis) are estimated with this micro fluidic chip-based system platform. This device is helpful in screening for diseases marked by RBC abnormalities, and also aids differential diagnosis with procedural simplicity, high speed accuracy and minimal requirement of blood samples.

OBSERVATIONS: EXERCISE FOR STUDENTS

Results

Note

Results: Record your observation and results as given below.

Beginning of haemolysis occurs in ....% saline.

Complete haemolysis of cells is seen in ....% saline.

The osmotic fragility of RBCs ranges from ....% to ....% saline.

Compare your results with the fragility range for normal RBCs and interpret.

....

....

....

....

....

....

....

....

....

....

....

....

....

....

Spotters 1
Instrument and Procedures

Q1. Identify the objects below and state their uses.

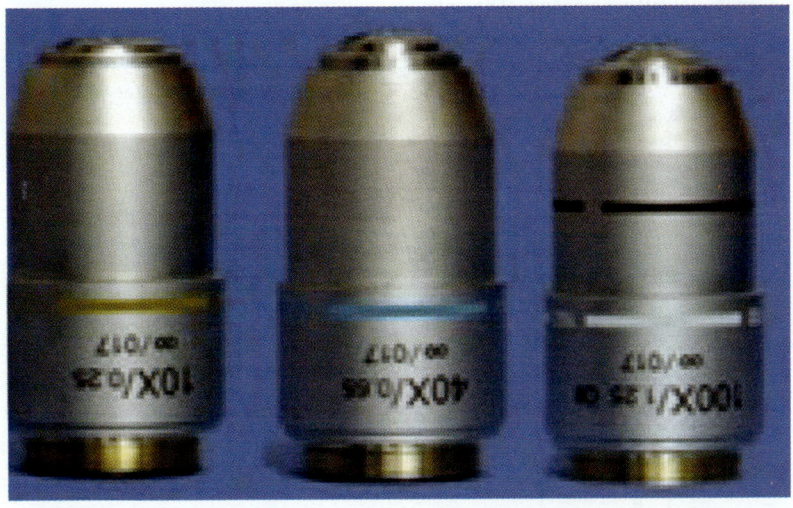

Ans. The three objective lenses commonly present on a microscope are having 10X (low power), 40X (high power) and 100X (oil immersion) powers. Together with a 10X eyepiece lens the total magnifications produced will be of 100X (10X times 10X), 400X and 1000X.

Q2. Identify the method of pricking of blood. What aseptic precaution should be taken before giving a prick?

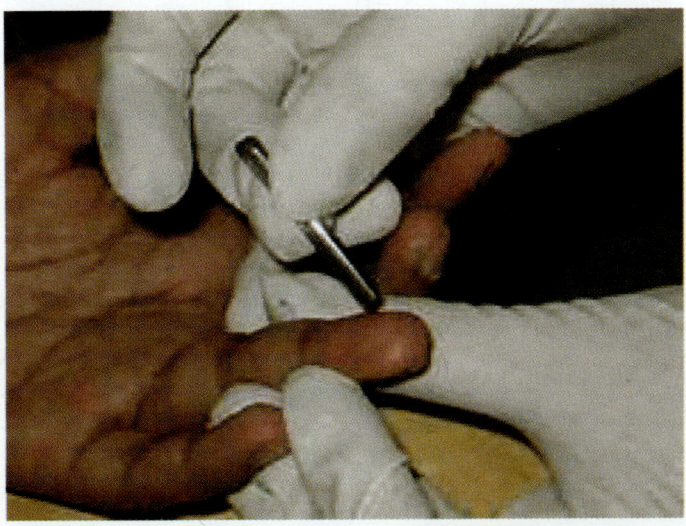

Ans. The photograph above shows method for collecting capillary blood from fingertip. The examiner is giving a bold prick using a lancet. The fingertip should be wiped with spirit using a sterile cotton gauze.

Q3. What are the advantages of capillary blood sampling over venous blood sampling?

Ans. *The advantages of capillary blood sampling over venous blood sampling are*:

- Capillary blood collection is simple and easy to obtain; while venous blood collection may be difficult to obtain in obese individuals and in infants.
- The capillary blood can be collected from varied locations while venous collection is via intravenous route.
- A person can self-perform the test.

Q4. What are the commonly used diluting fluids for WBC and RBC count?

Ans. *The commonly used diluting fluids are*:

1. **WBC diluting fluid (Turk's fluid):** It contains glacial acetic acid (3%) 3 ml, gentian violet (1%) 1 ml and distilled water to make 100 ml (solvent).
2. **RBC diluting fluid (Hayem's fluids):** Mercuric chloride 0.25 gm; sodium sulphate 2.50 gm; sodium chloride 0.50 gm and distilled water 100 ml.

Q5. Explain the method of cell counting.

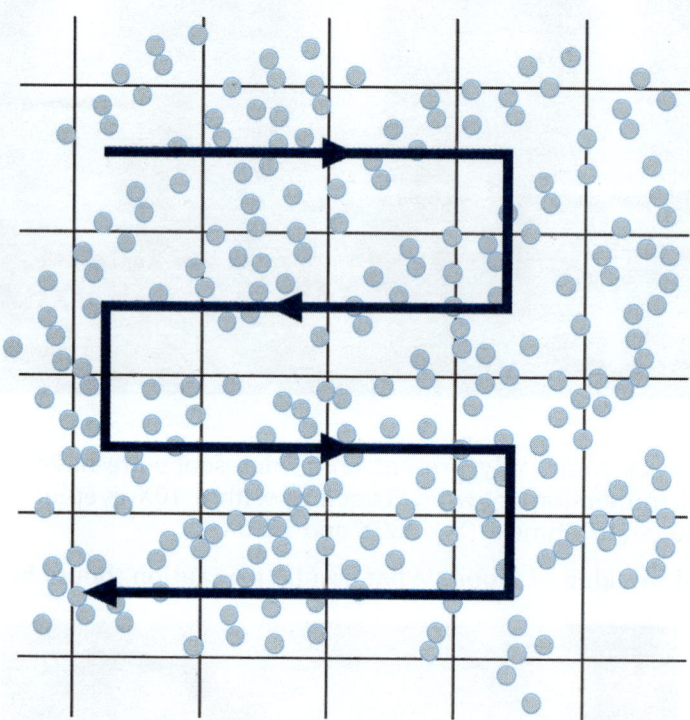

Ans. The cell count is to be conducted by counting the cells in the first square and further proceeding in Z pattern for further counting. Ensure counting cells lying over the square grid marking.

Q6. Identify the objects from right to left in the figure below.

Ans. The objects from right to left in the figure are dropper, stirring rod, haemoglobinometer tube, comparator box and haemoglobin pipette.

Q7. What are the features of RBC diluting pipette?

Ans. *The features of RBC diluting pipette are*:

a. The markings on the pipette include 0.5, 1 and 101.

b. The luminal diameter of the stem of RBC pipette is smaller when compared to that of WBC pipette.

c. The bulb contains a red bead.

d. The volume of the bulb of the RBC pipette is larger than that of the WBC pipette.

Q8. Identify the pipette below and compare them for their features.

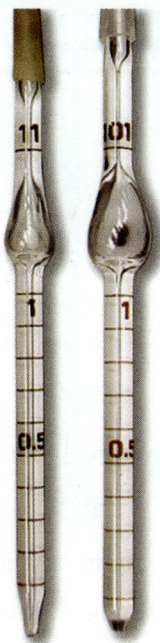

Ans. These are WBC and RBC pipette.

Differences between WBC and RBC pipette

	WBC pipette	*RBC pipette*
Graduation on	**Stem:** 0.5 and 1	**Stem:** 0.5
Pipette	**Above bulb:** 11	**Above bulb:** 101
Bulb size	Smaller	Larger
Bead of the bulb	White coloured bead	Red coloured bead
Mouthpiece	White in colour	Red in colour
Size of lumen of pipette	Larger	Smaller

Q9. Identify the procedural stage in the figure below.

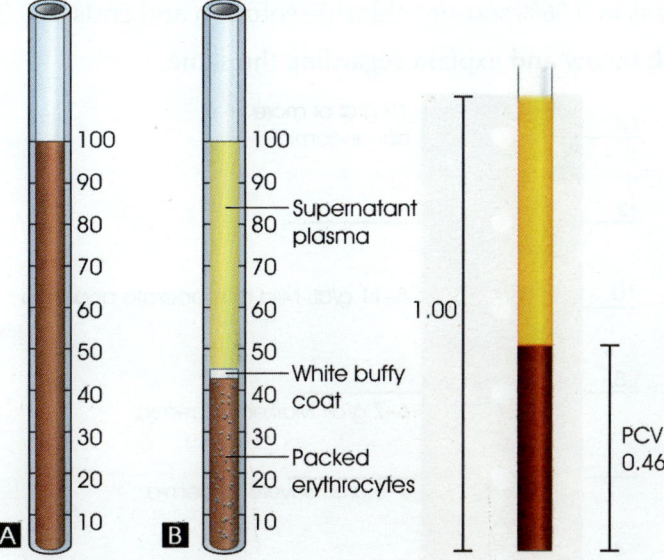

Ans. (A) Blood sample before centrifuging in the haematocrit; (B) The same after centrifuging in the haematocrit.

Q10. Identify the procedure and the instrument.

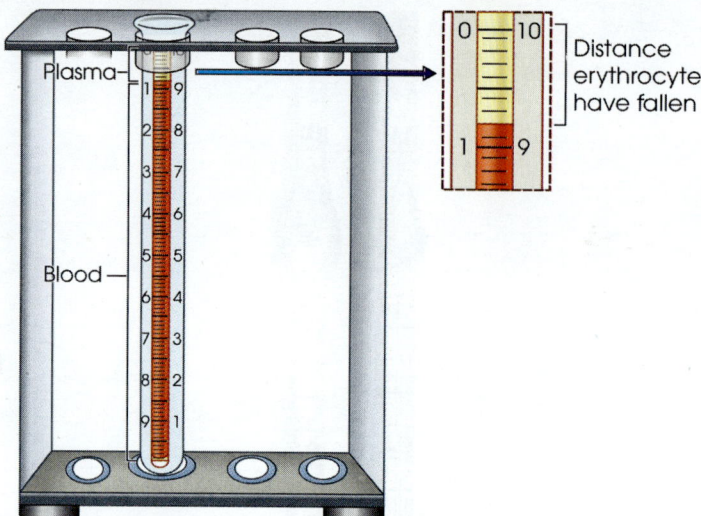

Ans. The procedure is determination of erythrocyte sedimentation rate. The instrument is Wintrobe's tube with stand.

Q11. What are the characteristic features of ideal blood smear?

Ans. *The characteristic features of ideal blood smear are:*
  1. An ideal smear covers around ¾ the entire slide area.
  2. Ideal smear is tongue shaped, slightly rounded or curved at the feathery edge tail region. It is thick at head end, and thin at tail end.
  3. The upper and lower edges of the smear are clear and visible.
  4. The smear is smooth without any streaks or vacuoles.
  5. It is single cell layer thick.

Q12. What is the osmotic fragility of red blood cell? Enlist the condition in which osmotic fragility increases and decreases.

Ans.

  1. In normal healthy individuals, the osmotic fragility of red blood cell begins in 0.48% sodium chloride solution and ends in 0.34% sodium chloride solution.
  2. RBCs osmotic fragility increase when they become spherical, e.g. in hereditary spherocytosis (independent of the cause). Osmotic fragility of red blood cell begins in 0.7% sodium chloride solution and ends in 0.45% sodium chloride solution.
  3. RBCs osmotic fragility are decreased when they become slender, e.g. in iron deficiency anaemia and thalassaemia. It begins in 0.36% sodium chloride solution and ends in 0.24% sodium chloride solution.

13. Identify the photograph below and explain regarding the same.

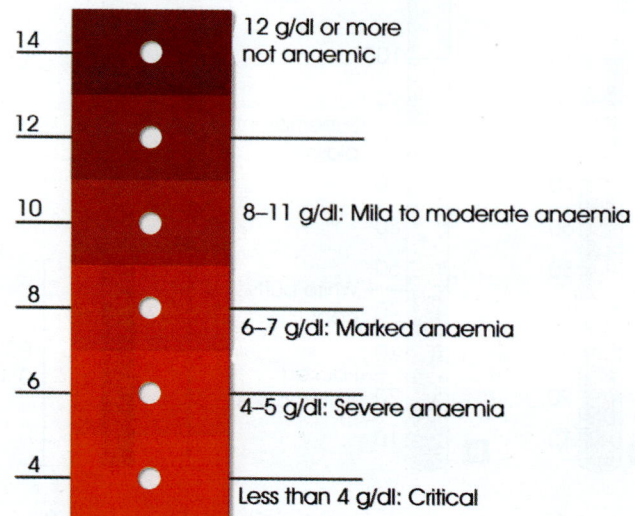

Ans. The photograph above is WHO Haemoglobin Colour Scale. The colour of a drop of blood is absorbed on a chromatography paper and the colour of the drop of blood is matched against a printed scale of colour corresponding to varied levels of haemoglobin ranging from 4 to 14 g/dl.

Q14. Identify cell below. Describe its characteristic features.

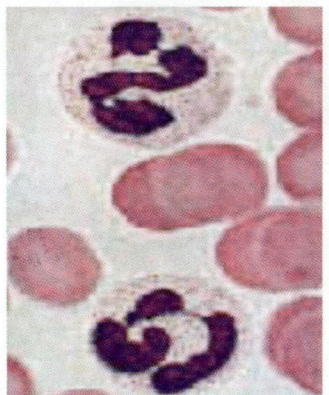

Ans. The cell is neutrophil.

The characteristic features are:
1. They are also known as polymorphonuclear leukocytes.
2. They are 10 to 14 micron in diameter.
3. The nucleus is multilobed (1–6 lobes), cytoplasm is bluish pink in colour with plenty of red brown or purple colour granules.

Q15. Identify cell below. Describe its characteristic features.

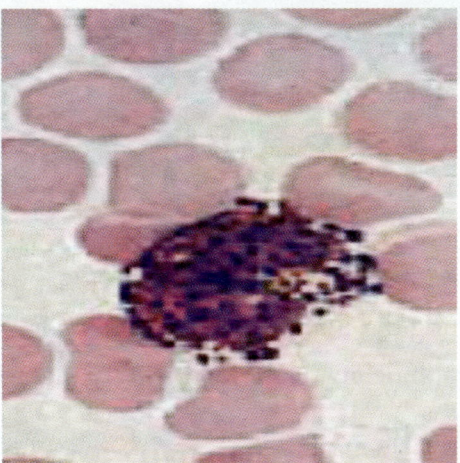

Ans. The cell is eosinophil.

The characteristic features are:
1. Eosinophil is 10–14 micron in diameter.
2. The nucleus is purple in colour and has bilobed and spectacle shaped or horseshoe shaped nucleus.
3. The cytoplasm is pink in colour having large coarse brick red-coloured granules.

Q16. Identify the diagram.

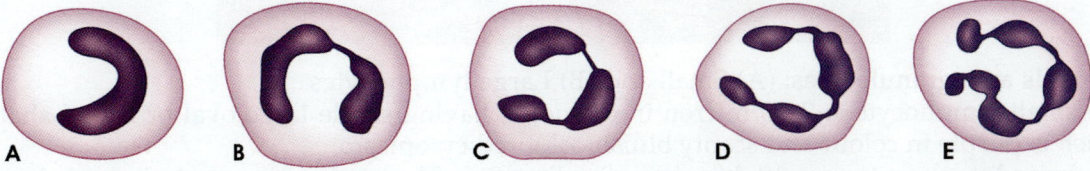

Ans. The diagrammatic representation of lobes of neutrophil is seen in A, B, C, D and E. The details are as follows: A. Stab or Schaf cell; B. Two lobes; C. Three lobes; D. Four lobes; E. Five lobes.

17. **Identify the objects from right to left in the figure below.**

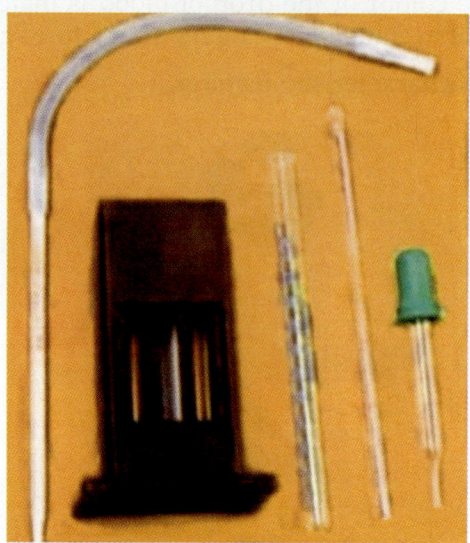

Ans. The objects from right to left in the figure are dropper, stirring rod, haemoglobinometer tube, comparator box and haemoglobin pipette.

Q18. Identify the procedure from the photograph.

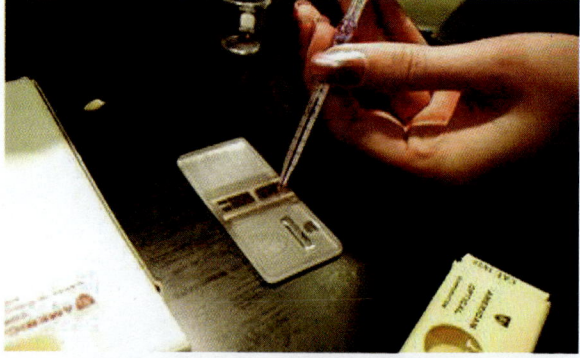

Ans. The photograph above is depicting the charging of the Neubauer chamber.

Q19. Identify the cells in the photograph below. Describe their characteristics.

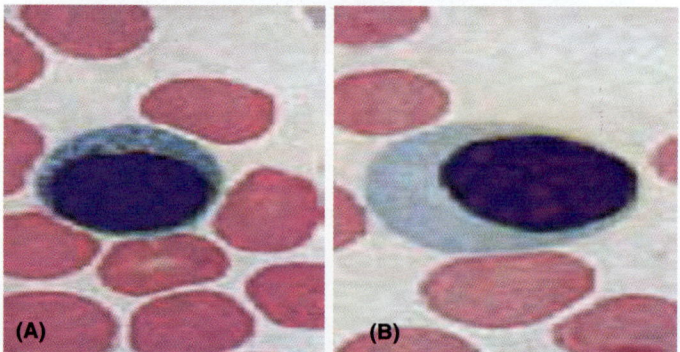

(A)   (B)

Ans. **These cells are agranulocytes:** (A) Small and (B) Large lymphocytes
  1. The small lymphocyte is 7–10 micron in diameter; having single large oval or round shaped nucleus which is purple in colour and scanty bluish coloured cytoplasm.
  2. The large lymphocytes are 10–14 micron in diameter. The nucleus is mostly indented, and occupies almost entire cell. Nucleus is oval or round shaped and is purple in colour. The cytoplasm is sky blue and cytoplasm to nucleus ratio is more than small lymphocyte.

Q20. Identify the cell below. Describe its characteristics.

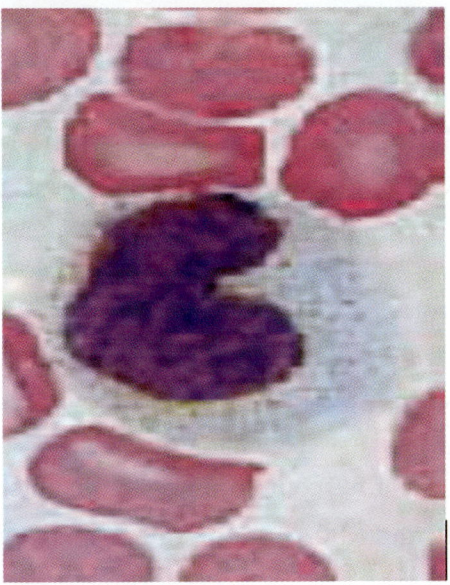

Ans. The cell is monocyte.

Its characteristic features are:

1. They are 14–18 micron in diameter.
2. Nucleus is large round, oval or kidney shape and deeply indented, it is pale purplish blue in colour and its location is usually eccentric.
3. The cytoplasm is abundant and greyish blue in colour.

Spotters 2
Calculations

Q1. **Calculate the mean corpuscular volume (MCV): RBC count is 5 millions/cu mm; and haematocrit is 40%.**

Ans. *The mean corpuscular volume (MCV):*

$$MCV = \frac{\text{Haematocrit (\%)} \times 10}{\text{RBC count (millions/mm}^3 \text{ blood)}}$$

PCV in 1000 ml or in 100 ml × 10 and RBC count in millions/cu mm

MCV = 40/5 × 10

MCV = 80 μm^3

Q2. **Calculate the mean corpuscular haemoglobin (MCH) from data below: RBC count is 5 millions/cu mm; and haemoglobin level is 15 gm/dl.**

Ans. *The mean corpuscular haemoglobin (MCH) is:*

$$MCH = \frac{\text{Haemoglobin in gm/dl} \times 10}{\text{RBC in millions/μL}}$$

Thus MCH = 15/5 × 10

Thus, MCH = 30 pg or micro microgram.

Q3. **Discuss from the schematic representation below regarding the distribution of body water in different compartments.**

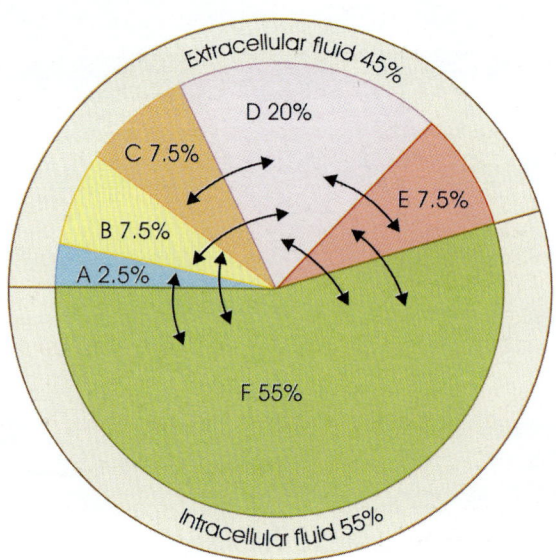

Ans. *The distribution of body water in different compartments as shown in the above schematic diagram includes:*

A = Transcellular water (2.5 percent).

B = Dense connective tissue and cartilage water (7.5 percent).

C = Plasma water (7.5%).

D = Interstitial and lymph water (20%).

E = In accessible bone water (7.5%).

F = Intracellular water (55%).

Q4. Calculate the MCHC value from given data: For example, haemoglobin level is 15 gm/dl and haematocrit reading is 45%.

Ans.

$$\text{MCHC} = \frac{\text{Haemoglobin in gm/dl} \times 100}{\text{PCV per 100 ml of blood}} \times 100$$

MCHC = 15/45 × 100

Thus MCHC = 33% (Approx)

Q5. Calculate colour index: Haemoglobin is 14.8 μ/dl and RBC count is 5 millions/μL of blood.

Ans. Colour index = Haemoglobin%/RBC%

> **Note:** For standard reference: Haemoglobin of 14.8 μ/dl is 100%; and RBC count of 5 million/μL of blood is 100%.

Thus colour index = 100%/100%

Colour index = 1

Q6. In an individual of 70 kg what will be the total body water?

Ans. The total body water is 60% of body weight.

Therefore, 60% of 70 kg = 42 L

Thus the total body water in individual within 70 kg is 42 L.

Q7. In an individual of 70 kg what will be his extracellular fluid volume and intracellular fluid volume?

Ans. The extracellular fluid volume is 20% of total body weight = 20% of 70 kg = 14 L.

Similarly intracellular fluid volume is 40% of total body weight = 40% of 70 kg = 28 L

Q8. Calculate the number of WBCs in 1 mm³ of undiluted blood when number of WBCs in 0.4 mm³ of diluted blood (*n* cells) is 150 cells.

Ans. The number of WBCs in 0.4 mm³ of diluted blood = *n* cells is 150

The dilution factor = 1:20 (0.5 parts of blood in 10 parts of Turk's fluid).

Therefore, the number of WBCs in 1 mm³ of undiluted blood

$$= \frac{n \times 20 \text{ (dilution factor)}}{0.4}$$

$$= \frac{150 \times 20 \text{ (dilution factor)}}{0.4}$$

= 150 × 50 cells

Therefore, the number of WBCs in 1 mm³ (1 cubic mm) of undiluted blood is 7500.

Q9. Calculate the number of platelets in 1 mm³ of undiluted blood when *N* which stands for total number of cells in 25 RBC square is 150.

Ans. Volume of fluid under which platelet cells are counted is 1 mm × 1 mm × 0.1 mm (= 1 μL)

Dilution factor as determined for dilution using RBC pipette is 200.

Let the count be *N* for total number of cells in 25 RBC square, i.e. it represents total number of cells in 1 mm³ of undiluted blood and its value is 150.

Thus number of platelets in 1 mm³ of undiluted blood = *N* × 200/0.1

= *N* × 2000

= 150 × 2000 = 300000

Thus number of platelets in 1 mm³ of undiluted blood = 300000 platelets.

Q10. Calculate the oxygen carrying capacity when Hb level is 15 gm%.

Ans. As 1 gm of haemoglobin carries 1.34 ml of oxygen, hence the oxygen carrying capacity = haemoglobin level × 1.34 ml

$$= 15 \times 1.34$$

$$= 20 \text{ ml/dl}$$

Q11. If number of reticulocytes as counted are 10 and total number of red blood cells counted is 500, calculate normal reticulocyte count.

Ans. The percentage of reticulocyte = Number of reticulocytes/total number of red blood cells counted × 100

$$= 10/500 \times 100$$

$$= 2\%$$

Normal reticulocyte count = 0–2% in children and adult.

Results: The reticulocyte count of given sample is 2%.

Q12. If you have to calculate the mean corpuscular thickness, which blood indices value are required and what is the formula for calculating mean corpuscular thickness?

Ans. The blood indices value required for calculation of mean corpuscular thickness (MCT) are mean corpuscular volume (MCV) and mean corpuscular diameter (MCD). The formula to calculate MCT is:

$$MCT = MCV \times \frac{1}{\pi \left(\text{mean diameter}/2\right)^2}$$

Q13. How can the blood volume be calculated? What is the average blood volume in humans?

Ans. The blood volume can be calculated if the haematocrit value and plasma volume are given using the formula as follows:

$$\text{Blood volume} = \frac{\text{Plasma volume}}{1 - \text{Haematocrit}}$$

Q14. Which is the more accurate equation used to calculate blood volume in males and females and state the equation?

Ans. The Nadlers equation is the most preferred equation in use to calculate the blood volume.

In males: Blood volume = $(0.3669 \times H^3) + (0.03219 \times W) + 0.6041$.

In females: Blood volume = $(0.3561 \times H^3)$

$$+ 0.03308 \times W + 0.1833$$

where H is body height in metres.

and W is body weight in kilograms.

Spotters 3
Applied Clinical Physiology

Q1. Enlist any three conditions in which specific gravity of blood is increased.

Ans. *The specific gravity of blood rises in the following conditions:*

1. When water is lost from the body, such as in excessive sweating, diarrhoea, cholera, etc.
2. By exudation of fluid into tissues or serous cavities due to inflammation or surgical operation.
3. When water intake is inadequate.

Q2. Enlist any three conditions in which specific gravity of blood is decreased.

Ans. *The specific gravity of blood decreases in the following conditions:*

1. When large quantity of water is taken.
2. In severe haemorrhage after which fluid is drawn in from the tissue spaces and the blood is diluted.
3. Injection of saline into the veins causing dilution of blood.

Q3. Peripheral smear shows spherocytosis. What is this abnormality?

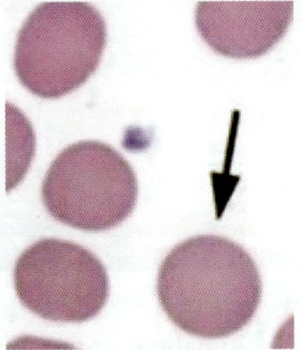

Ans. Spherocytosis: It is the deficiency of spectrin in red blood cell membrane due to a primary defect in ankyrin gene protein. This reduces red blood cell membrane stability/plasticity leading to premature lysis of the cells in spleen and the patient may present with anaemia, splenomegaly and jaundice.

Q4. Identify the defect in RBC in smear below. What are the clinical manifestations in this disease?

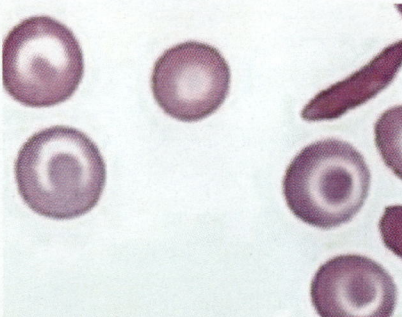

Ans. The cells are sickle-shaped and seen in patients of sickle cell anaemia. The clinical manifestations in this disease include symptoms of fatigue, breathlessness, jaundice, increased susceptibility to infections, painful joints, chest syndrome (pain in the chest wall), priapism (prolonged, painful erections), anaemia and "pain crises" which are also referred to as sickling crisis.

Q5. Enlist conditions in which blood volume is decreased.

Ans. *Blood volume is reduced in the following conditions:*
1. Loss of whole blood, e.g. haemorrhage due to traumatic injury, during operation, etc.
2. Decrease in number of RBC, e.g. anaemia.
3. Loss of plasma alone, e.g. burns.
4. Loss of blood water or anhydraemia—diarrhoea, dehydration, etc.
5. Acute exposure to cold causes moderate loss.
6. Posture: Blood volume is lower in the erect position than in the recumbent state.

Q6. Enlist causes for haemoglobinuria.

Ans. *Haemoglobinuria may be caused under the following conditions:*
1. In strenuous exercise.
2. Due to mismatched blood transfusion.
3. Black water fever due to virulent type of malaria and red water fever due to another type of parasite which invades the erythrocyte causing release of Hb in the plasma.
4. Paroxysmal nocturnal haemoglobinuria
5. Hypotonicity of plasma
6. Thermal or chemical injuries
7. Paroxysmal cold haemoglobinuria.

Q7. Identify the sign in the photograph below.

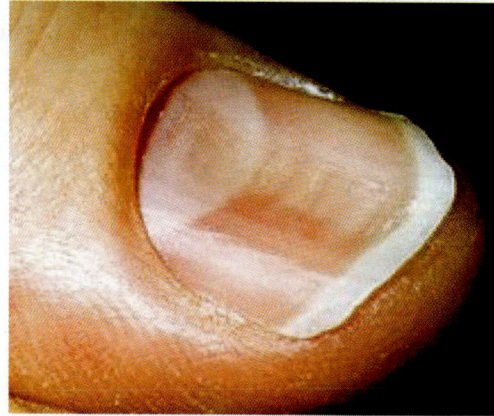

Ans. It is koilonychia and is a specific physical sign of severe iron deficiency anaemia.

Q8. Identify the sign in the photograph below in patient of purpura. What are the types of purpura?

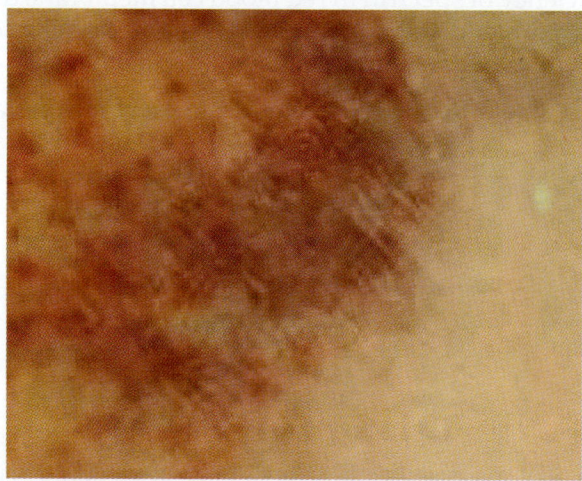

Ans. It is a skin rash usually characterized by small, purplish-red spots on skin in purpura. There are two types of purpura: Non-thrombocytopenic (normal platelet levels) and thrombocytopenic (lower platelet count). In this disease there is diminution of platelets in the blood.

Q9. **What is the most common cause of anaemia rashes as seen in photograph?**

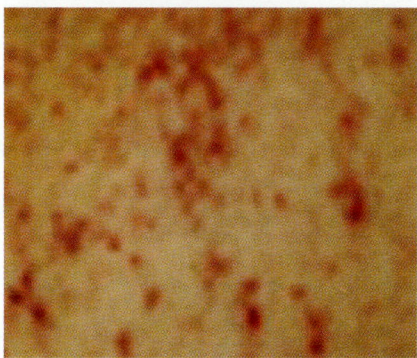

Ans. Aplastic anaemia is one of the most common causes of anaemia rashes.

Q10. **The peripheral blood smear shows neutrophils with hypersegmented lobes and macrocytosis of cell. Identify the clinical condition. What are its causes?**

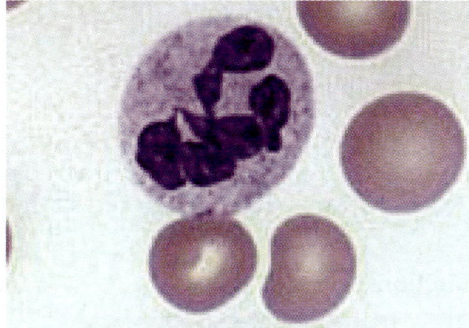

Ans. The clinical condition is megaloblastic anaemia. Its causes are vitamin B_{12} deficiency, pernicious anaemia and may also occur in patients of alcoholism, hypothyroidism, liver dysfunction, etc.

Q11. **What is the role of metals in erythropoiesis?**

Ans. *The role of metals in erythropoiesis is*:

   1. Iron: It is required for synthesis of haem.

   3. Copper and manganese: They help in the conversion of iron into haemoglobin by catalytic action.

   4. Cobalt: As a component of vitamin B_{12}, they help in maturation of red blood cells.

   5. Calcium: It helps in directly by conserving more iron and its subsequent assimilation.

   6. Bile salts: The presence of bile salts in the intestine is important for the proper absorption of these metals.

Q12. **Identify the stage of cell as per Arneth count. What is its normal staging?**

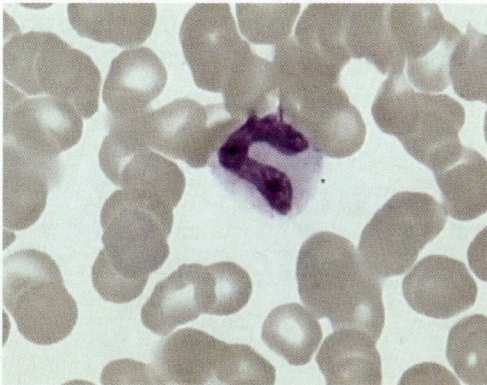

Ans. **Stage I**

   The stage classification of Arneth count is as follows:

   Stage I—N1 (nucleus is C or U-shaped, the two limbs connected by thick band of chromatin)—5–10%.

Stage II—N2 (Nucleus is bilobed and connected by thin band of chromatin—20–30%.

Stage III—N3 (Three lobes and connected by chromatin filament)—40–50%.

Stage IV—N4 (Four lobes and connected by thin band of chromatin)—10–15%.

Stage V—N5 (Five lobes with unclear outline)—3–5%.

Q13. The peripheral smear showing eosinophil cells in patient of hypereosinophilia. What is this condition?

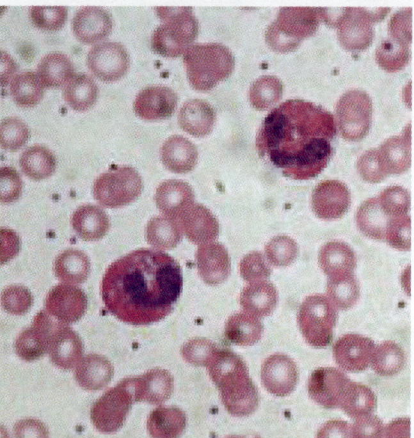

Ans. Hypereosinophilia is defined as moderate to severe eosinophilia (i.e. ≥1500/μL). The end-organ manifestations help to diagnose the cause. If the cause of the eosinophilia is unknown and no clinical manifestations are seen, then such patients are considered to having hypereosinophilia of unknown significance.

Q14. Identify the cell. What are its functions?

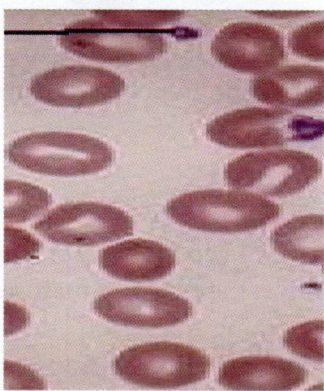

Ans. It is platelet. The functions of platelets are that they are important functionally for blood coagulation, haemostasis, clot retraction, they store 5HT and histamine (these are mediators of inflammation) and they engulf carbon particles, viruses and immune complexes.

15. Identify the cell.

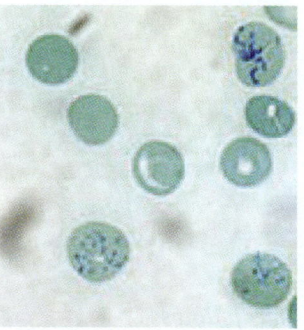

Ans. Reticulocytes as seen in peripheral smear.

Q16. What is dengue fever?

Ans. Dengue fever is an acute viral illness and may affect children and adults. It can also progress to a severe form known as dengue haemorrhagic fever (DHF). Disease is transmitted through the bite of the infected mosquitoes of the genus Aedes.

Q17. What is the normal platelet count? What is thrombocytopenia?

Ans. The normal platelet count is 150,000 to 450,000 platelets per microlitre of blood. Thrombocytopenia: It is a condition of lowered platelet count leading to mild to serious bleeding. The risk for serious bleeding occurs when platelet count becomes as low as 10,000 or 20,000 platelets per microlitre. Mild bleeding sometimes occurs when the platelet count is less than 50,000 platelets per microlitre.

Bibliography

1. John P. Greer, Daniel A. Arber, Bertil E. Glader, Alan F. List, Robert T. Means, Frixos Paraskevas, George M. Rodgers, John Foerster (All Editors). Wintrobes Clinical Haematology, Lipincott Williams and Wilkins, 13th Editions; 2013.
2. Lee, G. Richard, et. al. Wintrobe's Clinical Hematology, 9th ed. Lea and Feblger, Philadelphia, 1993.
3. Martin Howard Peter Hamilton. Haematology. Elsevier Publications. Fourth Edition: 2013: 10–133.
4. Nobel Prizes and Notable Discoveries. Erling Norrby. Publisher: WSPC Publishers. 2016: 1530.
5. Williams WJ. Examination of the blood. In: Williams WJ, Beutler E, Beutler E, Erslev AJ, Lichtman MA, eds. Hematology, 3d ed. New York: McGraw-Hill, 1983;9–14.
6. www.nobelprize.org. (The Nobel Prize in Physiology or Medicine).

Unit

2

Clinical Practicals with Spotters

1. General Clinical Examination
2. Examination of Arterial Pulse
3. Blood Pressure Recording
4. Cardiorespiratory Response to Exercise
5. Autonomic Function Test
6. Clinical Examination of Cardiovascular System
7. Electrocardiography: Recording of Normal Electrocardiogram
8. Experiment to Record Blood Flow in the Arm
9. Spirometry—Measurement of Lung Volume and Capacities and Recording Peak Expiratory Flow
10. Clinical Examination of the Respiratory System
11. Stethography Recording of Respiratory Movements
12. Determination of Physical Fitness of the Subject
13. Examination of Abdomen
14. Reproduction
15. Pregnancy Diagnostic Test
16. Examination of Central Nervous System
17. Examination of the Sensory System
18. Examination of the Motor System
19. Reflexes
20. Cranial Nerves
21. Cerebellar Function Tests
22. Perimetry
23. Electroencephalogram (EEG)
   Clinical Spotters

General Clinical Examination

PY 5.15*

INTRODUCTION

All students should note that your effective communication with patient and appropriate history taking is important as nearly 80% of diagnosis are made on history alone and 5 to 10% on examination and investigations. The doctors should be relaxed and smile to radiate confidence in patient reporting to them. A physical or clinical examination is the process by which a doctor investigates the body of patient for evidence of any disease. The patient symptoms are recorded on history taking. The detail personal history, family history and occupational history with physical examination help to arrive to accurate diagnosis. Routine physical examinations are performed on asymptomatic patients for purpose of screening for any evident disease. Rapport with patients plays a significant role in the doctor–patient relationship which provides benefits in other medical encounters while management of patient. A physical examination may include checking vital signs.

Vital Signs

Vital signs may reflect abnormalities in the nervous system.

1. Note his general appearance—whether conscious and alert or drowsy or in semicoma for coma.
2. Assess his mental state, his mood, behaviour and his intelligent quotient.
3. Assess the general buildup of patient in reference to his age and sex.
4. Record his height, weight and body mass index.
5. Record body temperature (Recorded by clinical thermometer). May be recorded in the mouth, axilla, ear or rectum. Normal mouth temperature is 35.8–37°C, axilla is 0.5°C lower than oral temperature, rectum is 0.5°C higher than oral temperature (close to core temperature). Ear temperature can be recorded which is close to rectal temperature.
6. Diurnal variations are there in temperature, lowest in the early morning and maximum between 6 and 10 pm.
7. **Pulse:** Count and record the pulse rate and note whether the rhythm is regular or irregular. The normal pulse rate is between 60 and 100 beats per minute.
8. **Blood pressure:** The students should learn to record the systolic and diastolic blood pressure. Normal blood pressure is 120 mm Hg (systolic) and 80 mm Hg (diastolic).
9. **Respiration:** Communicate with patient as you count the respiratory rate. The normal respiratory rate is 14–18 breath per minute. Respiratory rate and pattern of respiration is particularly helpful in evaluating patients with altered consciousness. The abnormal breathing patterns represent loss of higher control particularly of the primary medullary and pontine respiratory centres. The suppression of the medullary and pontine respiratory centres by metabolic or direct damage results in hypoventilation.
10. **Eyes:** For pallor and icterus. Examine palpebral conjunctivae for paleness. If pale, the individual is having anaemia also when in shock. Observe for yellowness of sclera, if icterus positive the individual might be suffering from jaundice (Fig. 1.1A and 1.1B).
11. **Cyanosis:** Observe for any bluish coloration of skin, buccal mucosa, along tongue, anterior vaginal wall, etc. Cyanosis is defined as a bluish discoloration, especially of the skin and mucous membranes, due to excessive

---

*Competency achievement as per competency based Undergraduate Curriculum for the Indian Medical Graduate, 2018, 1; Medical Council of India.

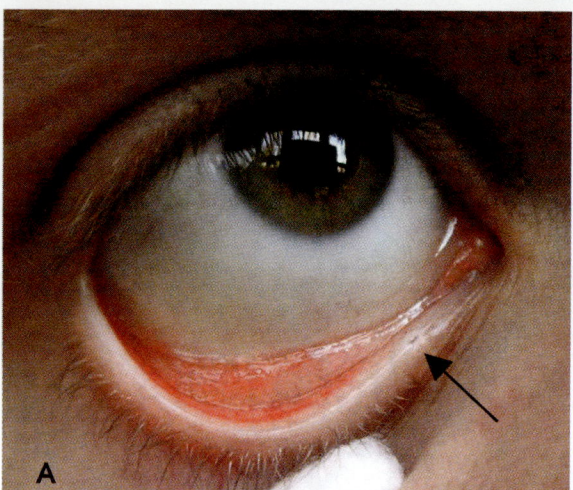
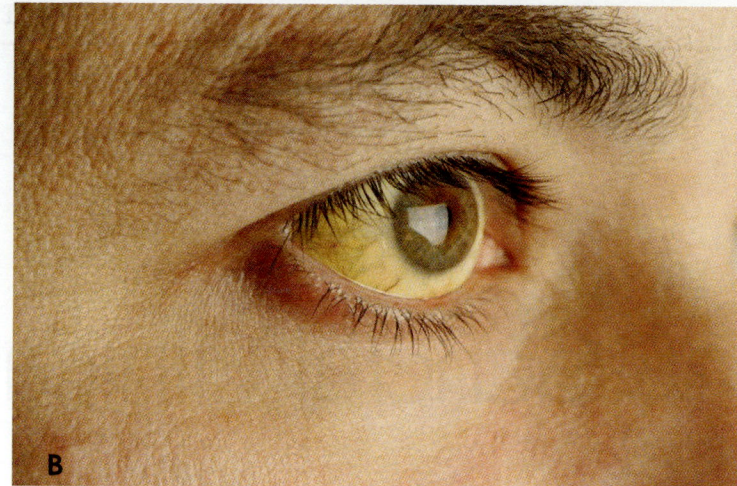

Figs 1.1A and B: A. Examination of conjunctiva, B. Examination of sclera

concentration of deoxyhaemoglobin in the blood caused by deoxygenation. Cyanosis is divided into two main types: Central (around the core, lips, and tongue) and peripheral (only the extremities or fingers). A few conditions leading to central cyanosis are pneumonia, broncholitis, pulmonary hypertension, chronic obstructive pulmonary disease (emphysema), intracranial haemorrhage, grand-mal seizure, congenital heart diseases, etc. Peripheral cyanosis is the blue tint discolouration in fingers or extremities due to inadequate circulation. The causes for peripheral cyanosis may be: All common causes of central cyanosis, heart failure, on exposure to cold, Raynaud phenomenon, deep vein thrombosis, etc.

12. **Clubbing:** Note for clubbing along nail bed and record it if present (Fig. 1.2).
13. ***The grades of clubbing are:***
   I. Fluctuation and softening of the nail bed.
   II. Loss of the normal <165° angle between the nail and the fold.

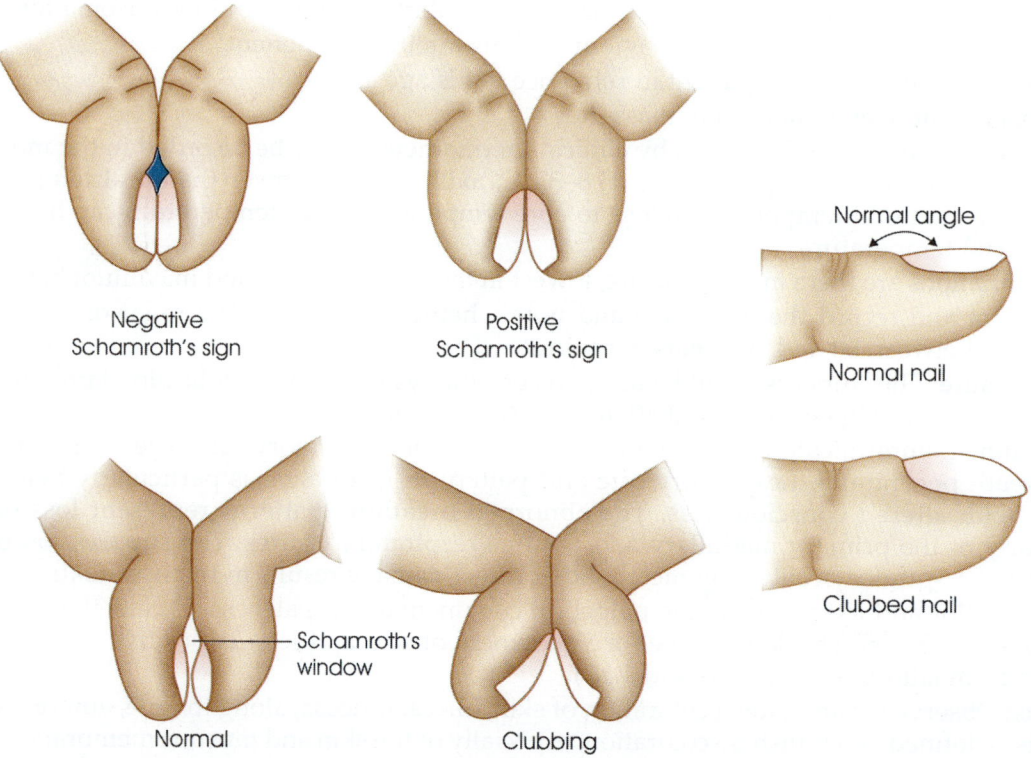

Fig. 1.2

III. Increased convexity of the nail fold.

IV. Thickening of the whole distal end part of the finger (resembling a drumstick)

V. Striation and shiny nail and skin.

Schamroth's test—in this test if the distal phalanges of corresponding fingers of opposite hands are directly opposed—a small diamond-shaped "window" is normally apparent between the nail beds. When the window is obliterated, the test is positive and clubbing is present.

14. **The neck is to be inspected and palpated**

The jugular venous pressure should be assessed (Figs 1.3 and 1.4) from the waveform of the internal jugular vein which lies adjacent to the medial border of the sternocleidomastoid muscle. Distension of the external jugular vein is a useful clue to an elevated JVP. The JVP is measured in cm vertically from the sternal angle to the top of the venous waveform. The normal upper limit is 4 cm. This is about 9 cm above the right atrium and corresponds to a pressure of 6 mmHg. Elevation of the JVP indicates a raised right atrial pressure. It is important to measure it in CVS disease and for severity of lung disease and in patients of suspected disturbance of fluid and electrolyte disturbance.

- Ensure that the neck muscles are relaxed by resting the back of the head on a pillow.
- Inspect by looking across the neck from the side of the patient.
- Identify the internal jugular pulsation, if necessary, by means of abdominojugular reflux.
- Measure the vertical height in centimetres between the top of the venous pulsation and the sternal angle to give the venous pressure.
- If necessary, readjust the position of the patient until the waveform is clearly visible.
- Identify the pattern of the pulsation and note any abnormality.
- Normally the jugular venous pressure falls on inspiration because of fall in intrathoracic pressure is transmitted to right atrium.

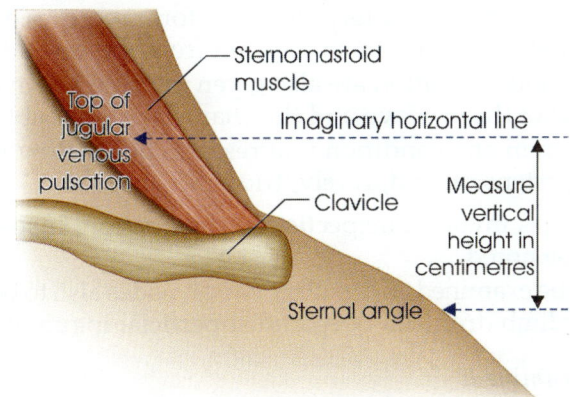

Fig. 1.3: Measuring the height of the JVP

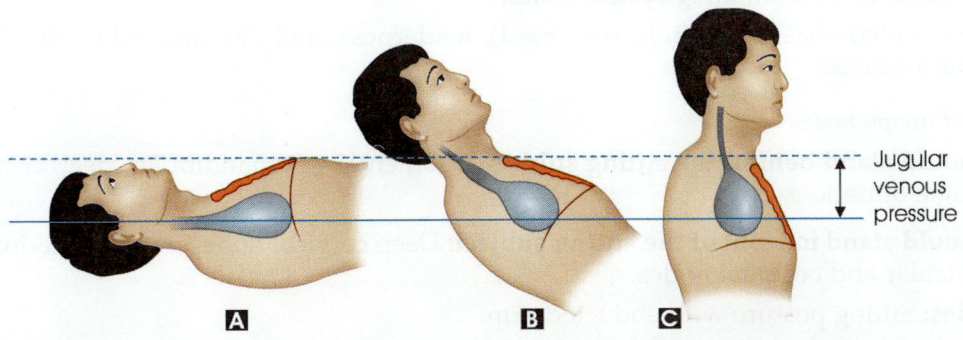

Fig. 1.4: Jugular venous pressure in a normal subject: (A) Supine: Jugular vein distended, pulsation not visible. (B) Reclining at 45 degrees: point of transition between distended and collapsed vein can usually be seen to pulsate just above the clavicle. (C) Upright: Upper part of vein collapsed and transition points obscured by sternum

Common Abnormalities

Raised jugular venous pressure: Heart failure is the commonest cause of a raised jugular venous pressure (Table 1.1). In milder degrees of heart failure abdominojugular reflux results in rise in pressure which is sustained while abdominal pressure is applied. In major pulmonary embolism the JVP may be so elevated that it is missed in a semirecumbent position. Marked elevation also occurs in SVC obstruction when the vessel is non-pulsatile. In pericardial constriction the JVP is elevated and there is a characteristic paradoxical rise on inspiration (Kussmaul's sign).

Table 1.1: Abnormalities of the jugular venous pulse

Condition	Abnormalities
Heart failure	Elevation, sustained abdominojugular reflux
Pulmonary embolism	Elevation
Pericardial effusion	Elevation, prominent 'y' descent
Pericardial constriction	Elevation, Kussmaul's sign
Superior vena caval obstruction	Elevation, loss of pulsation
Atrial fibrillation	Absent 'a' waves
Tricuspid stenosis	Giant 'a' waves
Tricuspid regurgitation	Giant 'v' wave
Complete heart block	'Cannon' waves

Serial estimations of the jugular venous pressure give valuable information regarding response to treatment, e.g. a reduction in the pressure as a result of effective diuretic therapy in the patient with heart failure.

15. **Waveform:** Identification of the jugular venous pulse waveform requires experience. The normal waveform comprises two peaks, which helps to distinguish the vein from the carotid artery.

    Abnormalities of jugular venous pulsation are also given in Table 1.1. In atrial fibrillation there is no atrial systole. This results in the loss of the 'a' wave and the characteristic double impulse.

    Prominent 'a' waves are seen in any condition that restricts blood flow from the right atrium to the right ventricle, e.g. pulmonary hypertension and, rarely, tricuspid stenosis.

16. Examination of the lymph nodes involves inspection and palpation. Inspection of the overlying skin to be done and associated pain to be noted.

    Lymph nodes of the neck to be examined and axillary lymph nodes also to be examined as they drain the arms. Lymph nodes from the lower limb drain via deep and superficial inguinal nodes and later can be palpated.

Other group of nodes to be examined:

Submental, submandibular, cervical, posterior auricular, occipital, supraclavicular, axillary, inguinal and popliteal nodes (Fig. 1.5).

Points to be noted while examining lymph nodes:

Site, size, number, consistency (soft, firm or hard), tenderness, mobility, matted or discrete, fixity to skin, generalized or localized.

Examination of lymph nodes:

Examiner should stand behind the sitting subject: Submental, submandibular, deep cervical nodes in the anterior triangle of neck.

Examiner should stand in front of the sitting subject: Deep cervical nodes in the posterior triangle of neck, posterior auricular and occipital nodes.

Axillary nodes: Sitting posture with abducted arm.

Inguinal nodes: Supine position with thigh flexed to 10°.

Popliteal nodes: Flex the knees and palpate deep into popliteal fossa.

17. Test for pitting oedema of the ankle if JVP is raised.

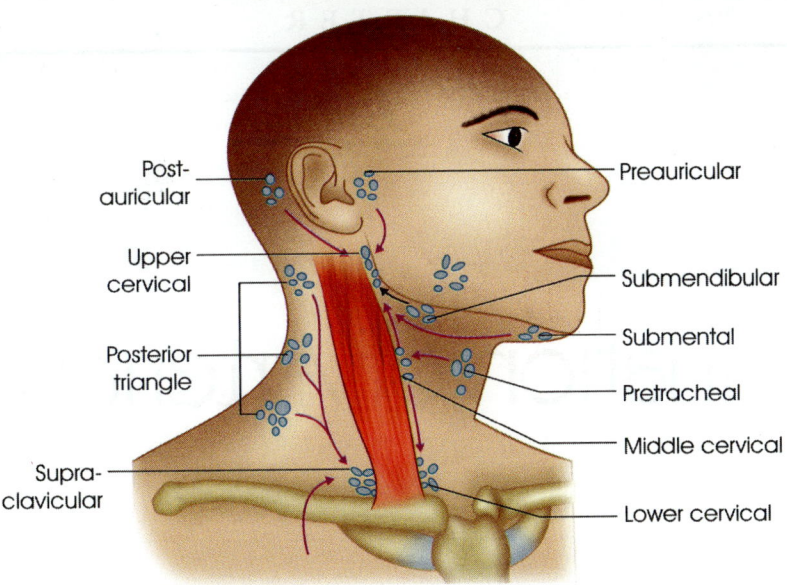

Fig. 1.5: The cervical lymph node groups

Observations

Name	Age	Sex
Height	Weight	BMI

General Appearance

Mental state: Consciousness and orientation

Build and nourishment

Afebrile/febrile

Skin, conjunctiva, mucosa any pale or blue colour or yellow colour

Clubbing

Pedal oedema

Lymphadenopathy

Vital Signs

Temperature	Pulse	BP	RR

Inference.

VIVA VOCE QUESTIONS

Q1. What is the cause of cyanosis?

Ans. Cyanosis occurs when there is increased amount of reduced haemoglobin in the blood.

Q2. Classify hypoxia.

Ans. Hypoxia is of four types—hypoxic hypoxia, anaemic hypoxia, stagnant hypoxia and histotoxic hypoxia.

Q3. Is there any physiological condition that causes hypoxia?

Ans. High altitude hypoxia.

Q4. What are the causes of anaemic hypoxia?

Ans. Anaemic hypoxia is present if haemoglobin content is low or the functional amount of haemoglobin is reduced as in carbon monoxide poisoning.

Examination of Arterial Pulse

PY 5.16*

Learning Objectives

After learning the practical the student should be able to:

1. Conduct clinical examination of radial pulse by palpation and examine arterial pulse at other sites. (Arterial pulse is the rhythmic expansion of the arterial wall due to the pressure wave produced by ventricular ejection.)
2. Discuss the physiological significance of various characteristics of pulse.

Aim of Practical

1. To examine the *radial pulse* in a human subject and record observations.
2. To palpate arterial pulse at other sites. *Carotid pulse, brachial pulse, femoral pulse, popliteal pulse* and *dorsalis pedis pulse.*

PROCEDURE

1. Radial Pulse

1. Ask the subject to sit comfortably on examination stool.
2. Ask the subject to keep his forearm semi-pronated and the wrist slightly flexed.
3. Palpate the radial pulse using his index, middle, and ring finger by placing the fingers along the radial side of the palmar aspect of the wrist, about 2 cm proximal to the thenar eminence (Fig. 2.1).

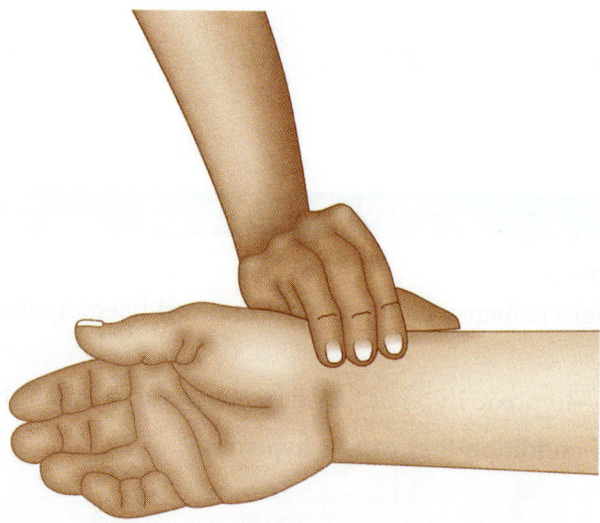

Fig. 2.1

*Competency achievement as per competency based Undergraduate Curriculum for the Indian Medical Graduate, 2018, 1; Medical Council of India.

2. Palpate Pulse at Other Sites

Carotid pulse, palpate carotid pulse (Fig. 2.2A) between thyroid cartilage and anterior border of sternocleidomastoid muscle. But **do not** examine simultaneously on both sides. Femoral pulse (Fig. 2.2B), brachial pulse (shown in the practical on BP).

Dorsalis pedis pulse is palpated by pressing against the tarsal bone just lateral to the extensor tendon of the big toe.

> **Note:** Radio-femoral delay, if any.

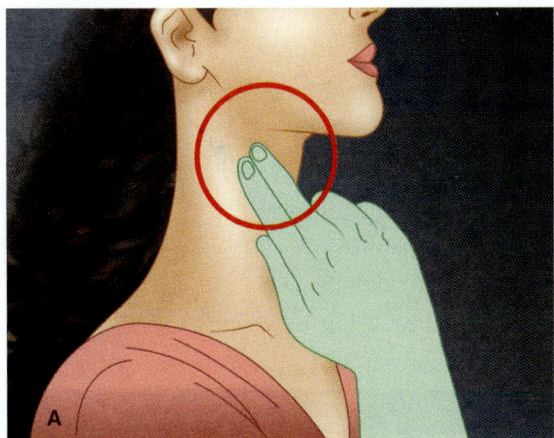 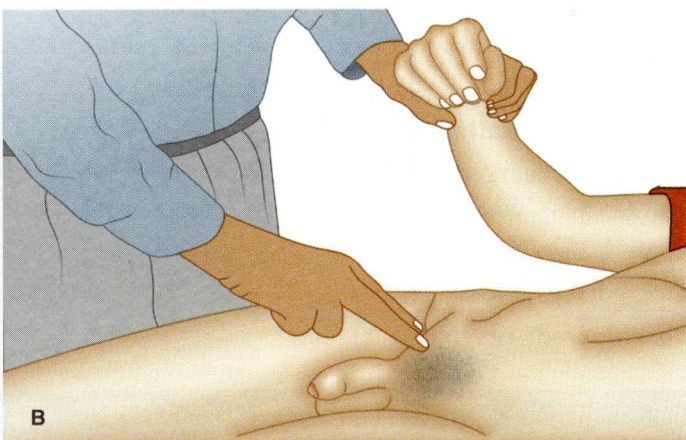

Fig. 2.2

OBSERVATIONS

Take a note of the following features of the radial pulse:

Rate: Examine the radial pulse by palpating radial artery and count the pulse rate of the subject for one minute. Take three readings, and take the mean of the values. The normal pulse rate ranges between 60 and 100/minute in an adult. It is an accurate indication of the heart rate in a normal person. Tachycardia is defined as a pulse rate more than 100/min and bradycardia as a rate less than 60/min.

Rhythm: Normally the pulse has a regular rhythm. Assess the interval between consecutive pulses. Confirm whether the rhythm is regular or irregular. In disease the rhythm may be regularly irregular, or irregularly irregular.

The heart rate increases during inspiration and slows during expiration. It is called respiratory sinus arrhythmia and it is most obvious in children, young adults and athletes.

Volume or amplitude: Volume indicates the upthrust imparted to a finger on palpating the pulse. Volume is assessed by the perception of expansion of the arterial wall. The pulse is weak or thready in heart failure, circulatory shock and aortic stenosis. The pulse is high volume and strong in pregnancy, thyrotoxicosis, aortic regurgitation, hyperthermia or after heavy exercise.

Character: It refers to an impression of the pulse waveform derived during palpation. Like volume, it needs to be examined at one of the large arteries. Alterations in the rate, rhythm and volume alter the normal character of the arterial pulse. Altered character of the pulse is seen in anacrotic pulse, dicrotic pulse, pulsus paradoxus, pulsus alternance, water-hammer pulse or collapsing pulse, pulsus bisiferens, etc.

Recordings of pulse can distinguish such alterations of pulse character.

Condition of the arterial wall: Obliterate the blood flow in the radial artery by pressing your index finger against bony prominence. Empty the radial artery peripherally using the ring finger. You have to feel for the condition of the vessel wall by rolling the segment of the radial artery on the underlying bone using your middle finger. Normally in young people it is not felt.

Compare the radial pulse on both sides: Atheromatous narrowing of axillary artery may cause reduced strength of one radial pulse compared to the other, as also in aortic dissection.

Examine other peripheral pulses: Carotid, brachial, femoral, popliteal, and dorsalis pedis at these arteries.

Radio-femoral delay: Examine for any delay between radial and femoral pulses.

In young patients with hypertension the radial femoral pulses on one side of body are palpated at the same time. The pulsation should occur simultaneously. Delay may suggest coarctation of the aorta where the aorta is constricted just beyond the subclavian artery. Blood flow to the arm is good but to the legs is poor so the pulse may be weak and delayed.

The dorsalis pedis pulse is palpated

Results

Pulse rate is/minute ....　1　　　　2　　　　3　　　　Average of 3

Rhythm: Regular/Irregular

Volume: Adequate/High/Low

Equal on two sides: Yes/No

Condition of the vessel wall: Soft/Hard/Rigid

Radial femoral delay: Yes/No

Carotid, palpated: Yes/No

Brachial, palpated: Yes/No

Popliteal, palpated: Yes/No

Dorsalis pedis palpated: Yes/No

OSPE

1. **Examine the pulse of the sitting individual for clinical examination.**
   - Ensure palm is warm before touching the patient. (Yes/No)
   - Palpate the radial artery with the tips of the index and middle fingers. (Yes/No)
   - Does not press too hard for fear of obliterating the pulse. (Yes/No)
   - Counts the pulse for a minute. (Yes/No)

2. **Identify the arterial pulse wave and interpret the same. The radial pulse can be recorded (Fig. 2.3) by instruments used in clinical practice may be Dudgeon's sphygmograph, for more accurate work optical recording instrument is used.**

Radial arterial pulse wave forms a contour wave generated by the heart when it contracts, and it travels along the arterial walls of the arterial tree.

Pulse waveform has two components: In Fig. 2.3 the upstroke is abrupt and without any secondary wave on it. Near the middle of the down stroke there is sharp depression called the dicrotic notch, followed by dicrotic wave.

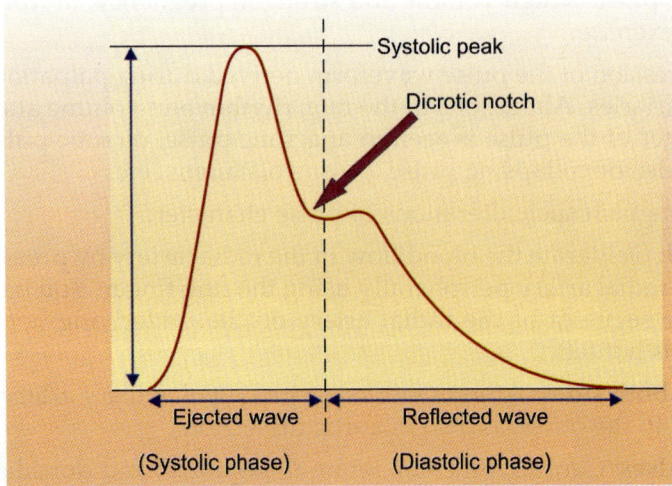

Fig. 2.3: Diagrammatic Representation of a radial arterial pulse wave

These two features are normally present in a normal **pulse tracing**. The waveform from beginning of the tracing up to the dicrotic notch is called primary wave or percussion wave and it corresponds to ventricular systole. Dicrotic notch is the sudden drop in pressure at the beginning of diastole. Sometimes secondary oscillations are found on down stroke both above and below the dicrotic wave known as the pre-dicrotic wave and post-dicrotic wave respectively are due to elastic oscillations of the aorta. The normal pulse is called catacrotic pulse. When a secondary wave is found on the upstroke the wave is called anacrotic wave and pulse called anacrotic pulse. When dicrotic wave becomes very prominent and can be felt easily with fingers the pulse is known as dicrotic pulse.

Water–hammer pulse: In Fig. 2.4 the rise and fall are steep and abrupt without any dicrotic notch or wave. This is found in aortic incompetence.

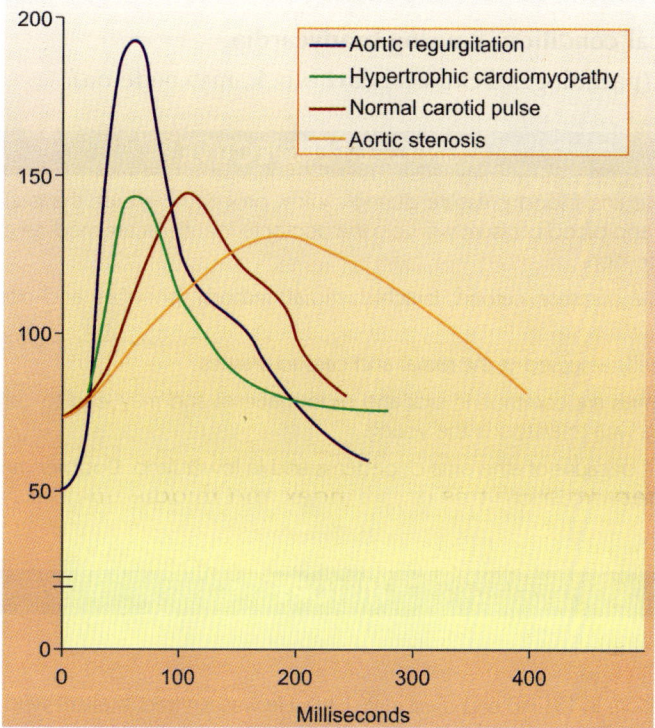

Fig. 2.4: The waveform of pulse is characterized by rate of rise of carotid upstroke. In aortic regurgitation the upstroke is rapid and followed by abrupt collapse. In aortic stenosis upstroke is slow with a plateau

Pulsus alternance: Pulse is alternately large and small. It is found in serious myocardial damage.

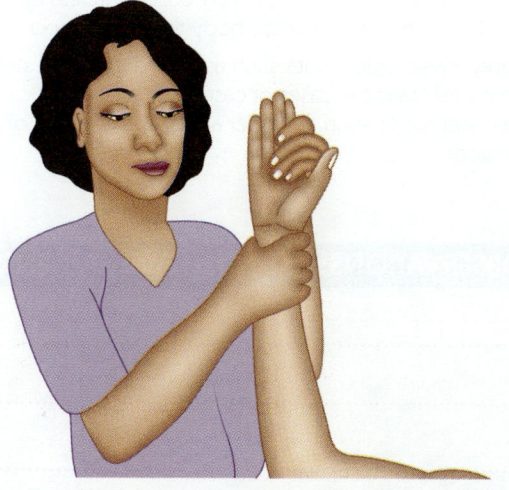

Fig. 2.5: Palpating pulse in aortic regurgitation

Pulses paradoxus: The volume and frequency is more during expiration than during inspiration, reverse of sinus arrhythmia.

VIVA VOCE QUESTIONS

Q1. What are the various reasons for irregular rhythm of pulse?

Ans. An irregular pulse may be due to sinus arrhythmia, premature beats, ectopic beats, atrial fibrillation, paroxysmal atrial tachycardia, atrial flutter, partial heart block, etc.

Q2. Enumerate some physiological conditions causing tachycardia.

Ans. Exercise, emotions, excitement, newborn (pathological causes, fever, anaemia, hyperthyroidism).

Q3. Name some physiological conditions causing bradycardia.

Ans. Sleep, old age, athletes (pathological causes heart block, myxoedema).

CLINICAL PERSPECTIVE

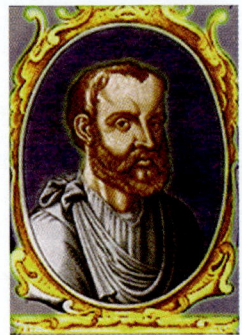

1. Monitoring a patient's vitals of pulse and blood pressure during clinical procedure ensure the patient's safety. Monitoring of vitals especially pulse and blood pressure will help the doctor to identify acute medical emergencies which could require immediate attention.

2. The arterial pulse can be felt in the common carotid, brachial, radial, femoral, popliteal and dorsalis pedis arteries.

3. The characteristics of pulse are ideally assessed at the radial and carotid arteries.

4. Bradyarrhythmias and tachyarrhythmias are common in sick and older patients and may lead to cardiovascular collapse despite similar rates being well-tolerated in the young.

5. Palpations of pulses can be difficult because of atheroma or oedema and in lower limb. Doppler measurements may be necessary to assess peripheral circulation.

HISTORY

Claudius Galen

Claudius Galen was a Greek physician born in 131 AD and died in 201 AD. He was a gifted intellect who studied at the famous medical school in Alexandria in Egypt. Galen was greatly influenced by the working methods of Hippocrates. He placed great importance on clinical observation through careful examination of patients and the recording of their symptoms. Galen advocated that pulse should be monitored meticulously and is important to detect it for abnormalities and it should be used as a tool to diagnose disease and suggest possible treatments.

Recent Update

The remote patient monitoring (RPM) enables monitoring of patients outside of conventional clinical settings; may be office, home, leisure places, etc. and this increases access to care and reduces health care delivery costs. Wireless Body Area Network (WBAN) integrates intelligent, miniaturized, low-power sensor nodes within, around or over a human body to monitor body functions.

Remote patient monitoring and patient care: Physiological data such as blood pressure, pulse, heart rate and ECG can be collected by sensors on peripheral devices. This helps in timely assistance in cases of casualty and emergencies and ensures positive patient outcomes. The newer applications also provide education, test and medication reminder alerts, and a means of communication between the patient and the provider. This is revolutionizing the future of history.

OBSERVATIONS: EXERCISE FOR STUDENTS

....

....

....

....

3

Blood Pressure Recording

PHY 5.12*

Learning Objective

After learning the practical student should be able to:

1. Define systolic, diastolic, mean blood pressure and pulse pressure.
2. Able to measure blood pressure by palpatory and auscultatory methods.
3. Understand the precautions to be taken while recording blood pressure.
4. Explain the importance of recording blood pressure in clinical practice.
5. Should understand physiological conditions affecting BP.
6. Should know the normal limits of systolic and diastolic blood pressures and define hypertension.
7. Should know the lifestyle modifications to control blood pressure.

Aim of Experiment

1. To determine the arterial blood pressure of a human subject by indirect methods. Note that direct method is used in animal and research and studies.
2. To study the effect of posture on blood pressure

Note: Arterial blood pressure is the lateral pressure exerted on the arterial wall by the column of blood while flowing through it.

PRINCIPLE

The principle of the experiment involves the balancing of air pressure against the pressure of the blood in the brachial artery, the air pressure being estimated by a mercury or an aneroid manometer.

APPARATUS

The sphygmomanometer is the instrument used for recording arterial blood pressure in humans. The mercury sphygmomanometer consists of a mercury manometer and inflatable cuff. The cuff is called a "Riva Rocci" cuff. It consists of an inflatable rubber bag covered by a non-distensible cotton fabric. The cuff is connected to the manometer to raise pressure to a desired pressure. To overcome tissue resistance the width of the cuff should be 20% more than the diameter of the arm. Width of cuffs for adults is 12 cm, length of inflatable rubber bag is 24 cm and for children the cuff sizes are smaller. Smaller cuffs used for children are of various sizes which cover most of upper arm leaving a gap of 1 cm or so below the axille and above anticubital fossa. Wider cuffs 15 cm have to be used to record the BP in obese individuals and for recordings in the lower limbs to overcome tissue resistance. Cuff is fitted with two rubber tubes, one connecting it to the mercury reservoir and the other to the hand bulb (Fig. 3.1).

The cloth covering keeps the rubber bag in position around the arm when arterial blood pressure is being measured. The manometer is a U-shaped tube. One limb being broader is the reservoir for mercury and the narrow limb is graduated from 0 to 300 mmHg, with the smallest division corresponding to a reading of 2 mmHg. A stopcock between the two limbs when closed prevents the mercury from entering the glass tube. The one-way valve fitted at the top of the mercury well prevents spilling of mercury when the lid is closed.

---

*Competency achievement as per competency based Undergraduate Curriculum for the Indian Medical Graduate, 2018, 1; Medical Council of India.

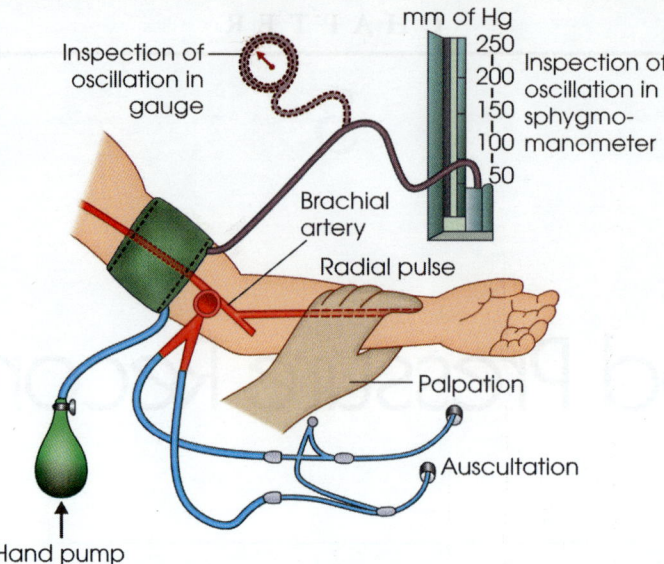

Fig. 3.1: Cuff and stethoscope position while recording blood pressure

Aneroid manometer: Used for measuring blood pressure does not contain mercury, the calibrated dial replaces the mercury manometer in aneroid manometer (Fig. 3.2).

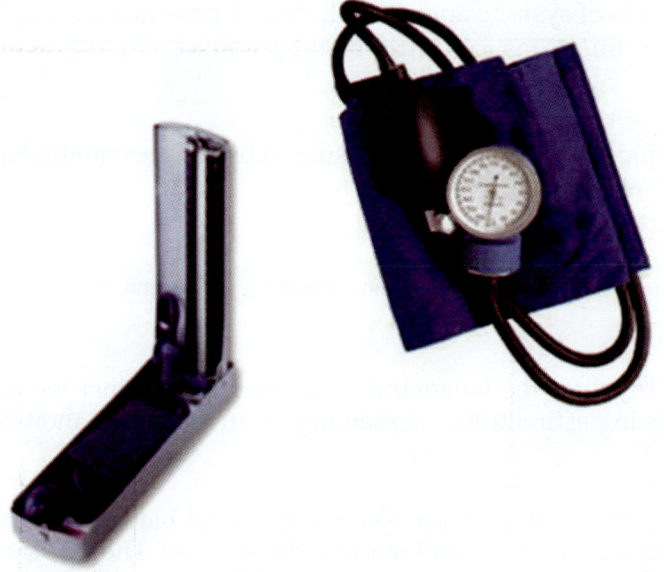

Fig. 3.2: Sphygmomanometer, mercurial, and aneroid type

Stethoscope: It is used to auscultate the Korotkoff sounds. It has a chestpiece which has the bell and diaphragm as two end pieces and there is ear frame of two curved metallic tubes joined together to a y-shaped spring. The y-shaped connector connects to chestpiece. Plastic knobs are attached to the curved metallic tube at their open end for comfortable feeling in the ear (Fig. 3.3).

PROCEDURE

Subject is made to sit down and the brachial artery is kept at the level of the heart to obtain a pressure that is uninfluenced by gravity and to reduce false baseline errors. The arm is exposed and cuff applied in such a way that the midpoint of the cuff overlies the brachial artery and the lower edge of the cuff is 1" above the cubital fossa. BP can be determined by 3 methods.

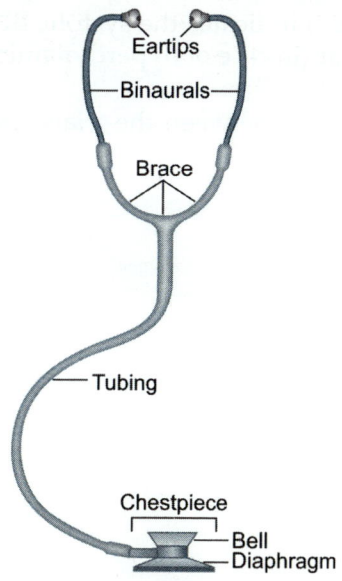

Fig. 3.3: Stethoscope

1. PALPATORY METHOD

Rubber bag is inflated until the air pressure within it overcomes the arterial pressure and obliterated the arterial lumen. This can be confirmed by feeling the radial pulse which will disappear, then pressure is raised beyond the point, by about 30 mmHg and then cautiously reduced again so that the pressure falls at the rate of 2–3 mmHg per second. Pulse starts reappearing at a point when pressure in the artery is equal to pressure of air in the cuff and blood escapes beyond the cuff into the peripheral section of the artery. In this method, the examiner takes the manometer reading as the radial pulse is first felt at the wrist, as the index of systolic pressure.

Disadvantages of the method:

1. The pressure recorded is about 2–5 mmHg less than that recorded by auscultation.
2. Only systolic blood pressure (and not diastolic) can be recorded by this method.

Advantage: The fallacy of auscultatory method in missing the auscultatory gap is avoided.

2. OSCILLATORY METHOD

The vibration produced by passing of blood through narrow channels (turbulent flow) produces oscillations of the mercury column indicating the pressure in the arteries. Point of appearance of oscillations indicates systolic pressure and point of minimum oscillation diastolic pressure. Not a reliable method. The method is no longer used.

3. AUSCULTATORY METHOD

Place the chestpiece of stethoscope over the arm medial to the tendon of biceps where pulsations of brachial artery are felt. Then inflate the cuff till the pressure is 30 mmHg more than the reading obtained by the palpatory method. Then gradually lower the pressure till a sharp light tapping sound, in rhythm with the heart beat, is heard. When the pressure in the cuff is further progressively lowered, the sound undergoes a series of changes in quality and intensity which were first obtained by Korotkoff, a Russian scientist, in 1905. He differentiated 5 phases of these sounds.

No sounds are heard if you place stethoscope in radial artery as such.	
Phase I	Sudden appearance of a clear but faint tapping sound growing louder during the succeeding 10 mmHg fall in pressure.
Phase II	The sound takes murmur-like quality during the next 15 mm fall in pressure.
Phase III	Sound changes a little in quality but become clearer and louder during the next 15 mm fall in pressure.
Phase IV	Muffled quality lasting throughout the next 5 to 6 mmHg fall.
Phase V	Complete disappearance of the sound.

The first appearance of the sound (phase I) indicates the systolic BP. For diastolic BP disappearance of sound (Phase V) is best. If sound does not disappear (in case of hyperdynamic circulation), muffling of sound (Phase IV) is taken as DBP.

The cuff pressure should be reduced to zero between the trials. Otherwise, inflated cuff will produce reflex spasm of the artery and false reading.

OBSERVATIONS

Blood pressure by palpatory method.

Reading:	1.	2.	3.	Average of 2

Blood pressure by auscultatory method.

Readings:	1.	2.	3.	Average of 2

Record BP in both the arms and compare.

The other arm

Readings:	1.	2.	3.	Average of 2

Result—concordant readings.   Same/different

Normal value:
Systolic 120 + 20 mmHg
Diastolic 80 + 10 mmHg

Effect of Posture on BP

Make the subject lie on bed for 5 minutes and record BP. Ask him to stand up and immediately record BP.

OBSERVATIONS

Blood pressure in supine position.

....

....

....

Blood pressure in standing position.

....

....

....

Compare the two values

Similarly make the subject to sit up from lying down position and compare BP recorded during the two positions.

Blood pressure in lying position

Blood pressure in sitting position

Effect of Exercise on Blood Pressure

Procedure

- Record resting blood pressure in sitting posture by palpatory and auscultatory method.
- The Riva Rocci cuff is disconnected from the BP apparatus.
- The cuff is still wrapped around the subject's arm.
- The subject is instructed to perform physical activities like on the spot jogging for five minutes or ten sit ups.
- Immediately after the exercise, BP is recorded by auscultatory method without any time delay.

Record your Observations

Blood pressure before exercise. ....

Palpatory method. ....

Auscultatory method. ....

Immediately after exercise. ....

Auscultatory method. ....

PRECAUTIONS

1. Subject to rest for 5 minutes before recording BP.
2. Brachial artery should be at the level of the heart.
3. The cuff should not be tied too tight or too loose.
4. The bladder of the cuff should be centered over brachial artery.
5. Take two or three readings each about two minutes apart and find average.
6. The cuff pressure should be lowered to zero between the trials to avoid reflex spasm.
7. The mercury column should be deflated slowly at a rate of 2–3 mm/sec otherwise the systolic blood pressure will be underestimated.
8. The subject should not have smoked for at least half an hour prior to recordings.
9. When you are taking your reading, keep still and silent. Moving and talking can affect your reading.
10. Mercury sphygmomanometers are considered the gold standard. They show blood pressure by affecting the height of a column of mercury, which does not require recalibration. Because of their accuracy, they are often used in clinical trials of drugs and in clinical evaluations of high-risk patients, including pregnant women. A wall mounted mercury sphygmomanometer is also known as a **Baumanometer.**

Aneroid sphygmomanometers (mechanical types with a dial) are in common use; they may require calibration checks, unlike mercury manometers. Aneroid sphygmomanometers are considered safer than mercury sphygmomanometers.

QUESTIONS

Q1. Define:
  a. Systolic BP
  b. Diastolic BP
  c. Pulse pressure
  d. Mean arterial pressure
  e. Basal blood pressure
  f. Causal blood pressure

Ans.

  a. **Systolic blood pressure:** It is the maximum pressure during systole. The normal value is 120 mmHg (100–120 mmHg).
  b. **Diastolic blood pressure:** It is the minimum pressure during the diastole. The normal value is 70–80 mmHg.
  c. **Pulse pressure:** The difference between the diastolic and systolic blood pressure is the pulse pressure. Normal range of pulse pressure averages around 40 mmHg.
  d. **Mean arterial blood pressure:** It is the average pressure exerted during the cardiac cycle. Mean blood pressure (MBP) is expressed as diastolic blood pressure +1/3rd of pulse pressure. The average mean blood pressure is 96 mmHg and ranges between 95 mmHg and 100 mmHg.

Q2. What is the effect of posture on BP?
Ans. When an individual stand up immediately from recumbent posture, there is pooling of blood in the legs the venous return to the heart is reduced, thereby reducing the cardiac output. Hence, the systolic blood pressure will fall, which may be recorded within 15 seconds usually difficult to record in normal subjects,

this will be brought back to normal by Baroreceptor reflex within 15 to 30 seconds, this is the function of autonomic nervous system (ANS).

Q3. What are normal limits of systolic and diastolic blood pressure?

Ans. Normal blood pressure—an optimal blood pressure level is reading under 120/80 mm Hg. Reading over 120/80 mm Hg and up to 139/89 mm Hg are in the normal to high range.

VIVA VOCE QUESTIONS

Q1. Define blood pressure, systolic blood pressure, diastolic blood pressure, mean blood pressure and pulse pressure.

Ans. Blood pressure is the lateral pressure exerted on the wall of the arterial vessels by the contained blood.

Systolic blood pressure: It is the maximum pressure exerted during the systole. The normal value is 120 mmHg (100–120).

Diastolic blood pressure: It is the minimum pressure exerted during the diastole. The normal value is 80 mmHg (60–80 mmHg).

Pulse pressure: The difference between systolic and diastolic blood pressure is called the pulse pressure. It averages around 40 mmHg.

Mean blood pressure: It is the average of systolic and diastolic blood pressure, for example, $(120 + 80)/2 = 100$ mmHg. But mean pressure can be more accurately determined by the following equation.

Mean pressure = Diastolic blood pressure + 1/3rd of pulse pressure.

It averages from 95 to 100 mmHg.

Q2. What is peripheral resistance? What are the factors affecting it?

Ans. It is the fractional resistance offered by the circulatory system to the flow of blood. The factors affecting peripheral resistance are: (a) Viscosity of the blood (b) size of the lumen of the blood vessels (c) velocity of blood flow.

Q3. What is orthostatic hypotension? What are its causes?
Postural hypotension is defined as a drop in stystolic blood pressure more than 20 mm Hg on standing.

Ans. It is postural hypotension when patients on sudden standing from sitting or lying down position experience dizziness, dim vision, decreased systemic blood pressure and loss of consciousness.

The causes are:
a. Autonomic insufficiency secondary to lower basal norepinephrine level, and in patients of diabetes mellitus and syphilis.
b. Those on sympatholytic drugs.
c. Primary hyperaldosteronism (These patients having abnormal barorceptor reflex).

Q4. What is the effect of exercise on blood pressure?

Ans. On exercising the systolic blood pressure rises because of increased cardiac output due to increased myocardial contractibility and increased venous return.

Depending on degree of exercise the diastolic blood pressure is affected. Diastolic blood pressure increases in mild exercise due to vasoconstriction and does not change or even may decrease in moderate exercise but may fall in intense exercise due to local vasodilatation because of accumulation of metabolites and decreased body temperature.

Q5. Explain the important short-term and long-term mechanism of regulation of blood pressure.

Ans.

A. *These mechanisms are:*
Neural (short-term mechanism) and Renal (Rennin Angiotensin Aldosterone: Long-term mechanism)
Neural mechanism (short-term regulation).

There are three different neural mechanisms:
1. Baroreceptor reflex (Marey's reflex)
2. Chemoreceptor reflex
3. Cushing's reflex

Baroreceptor reflex: These receptors are located in the carotid sinus and aortic arch, which respond to the stretch. They act by decreasing or increasing the **sympathetic** and **vagal tone** through **vasomotor centre** and **cardioinhibitory centre,** thus either BP is increased or decreased.

Chemoreceptor reflex: These receptors responsive to hypoxia, hypercapnia and acidosis are present in the carotid body and aortic body. They act through the respiratory center and come into action once the BP dips below 60 mm Hg. Low PO_2 and/or high PCO_2 levels in the arterial blood cause reflex increases in respiratory rate and mean arterial pressure.

Cushing's reflex: Also known as last ditch effort, this reflex comes into play when BP is below 40 mmHg and is due to ischemia of brain as also in increased intracranial pressure.

B. *Renal regulation (long-term regulation):*

Rennin angiotensin aldosterone: Long-term mechanism

Renin-angiotensin system: Renin is a glycoprotein produced by the juxtaglomerular cells of the kidney in an inactive form called prorenin. Whenever there is a fall in BP, the blood supply to kidney is reduced which stimulates the release of renin in circulation. (Renin is converted to active renin by action of kallikreins).

The renin acts on angiotensinogen to form angiotensin I.

This angiotensin I is converted to angiotensin II by converting enzyme and then into angiotensin III by angiotensinase.

The angiotensin II and III increase the peripheral resistance, increase blood volume by stimulating release of aldosterone, and thus raise blood pressure by vasoconstriction, aldosterone secretion which causes Na^+ reabsorption from tubules, ADH secretion and stimulation of thirst centre.

Q6. Define hypertension.

Ans. A. Hypertension is the persistent rise in systolic arterial pressure above 140 mmHg and/or diastolic arterial pressure above 90 mmHg

B. There are no recognized manifestations of hypertension.

Q7. What is the effect of posture on blood pressure?

Ans. In erect posture there is peripheral pooling of the blood in the dependent parts decreasing venous return to heart and thereby decrease in cardiac output and the blood pressure. Thus the systolic pressure would fall which may be recorded in 15 seconds but difficult to record. This decreases the discharge of baroreceptors, and by Baroreceptor reflex blood pressure is brought back to normal by sympathetic stimulation to increase arterial resistance and that usually result in slight increases in blood pressure with overcompensation.

In lying down position the systolic and diastolic blood pressure are lower than in sitting position.

Q8. What are the factors affecting blood pressure?

Ans. *The factors affecting blood pressure are:*

1. **Age:** Blood pressure increases with age.

   Newborn: The systolic blood pressure averages around 40 mmHg.

   Children: Systolic blood pressure is 90–110 mmHg and diastolic blood pressure is between 50 and 80 mmHg.

   Adult: Systolic blood pressure is between 100 and 140 mmHg and diastolic blood pressure is between 60 and 90 mmHg.

2. **Sex:** Blood pressure is less in females than males in the same age group prior to menopause.

3. **Food:** Blood pressure increases after food intake.

4. **Environmental temperature:** Blood pressure increases during winter when environmental temperature is low due to vasoconstriction. It decreases during summer when environmental temperature is high due to vasodilatation.

5. **Emotional status:** Anxiety and anger raises the blood pressure due to increase in sympathetic discharges. Depression may decrease blood pressure.

6. **Sleep and rest:** Sleep and resting condition decreases the blood pressures. Decrease normally occurs during sleep but in some hypertensives people called non-dipers, it does not decrease.

7. Exercise: It causes rise in systolic blood pressure but may be fall in diastolic blood pressure. The fall in diastolic blood pressure is due to accumulation of metabolites that decrease total peripheral resistance.

Q9. What lifestyle modification you will advice to a hypertensive patient?

Ans. These steps include maintaining a healthy weight; being physically active; following a healthy eating plan that emphasizes fruits, vegetables, and low fat dairy foods; choosing and preparing foods with less salt and sodium; and, if you drink alcoholic beverages, drinking in moderation is advised, avoid smoking.

OSCE

RECORD THE BLOOD PRESSURE OF THE SUBJECT

The following steps should be followed to record the blood pressure:

1. **Ensure** that you have the following necessary equipment: A sphygmomanometer, a stethoscope, hand cleansing gel. **(Equipment for measuring blood pressure)** (Yes/No).
2. **Rapport with the subject:** Ensure that you introduce yourself to the patient, explain the procedure answering any questions they may have, and ask for their consent. Make sure they are sitting comfortably, with their arm rested. (Yes/No).
3. **Positioning:** Level: Devices and columns at eye level, patient's arm held at heart level. (Yes/No).
4. **Placement:** Ensure correct placement of the cuff. Wrap the cuff around the patient's upper arm ensuring the lower edge of the cuff is placed one inch above the ante-cubital fossa. The bladder of the cuff should be centered over brachial artery (palpate medial to biceps tendon). Fasten the cuff evenly and snugly. (Yes/No).
   a. Palpating radial pulse and inflating the cuff until the pulse can no longer be felt. The reading at this point should be noted and the cuff deflated (Yes/No).
   b. Place the diaphragm of your stethoscope over the brachial artery and re-inflate the cuff to 20–30 mmHg higher than the estimated value taken before. Then deflate the cuff at 2–3 mmHg per second until you hear the first Korotkoff sound—this is the systolic blood pressure (Yes/No).
   c. Continue to deflate the cuff until the sounds disappear, this is the diastolic blood pressure. Record the true blood pressure (Yes/No).

MEASUREMENT OF BP BY DIGITAL RECORDING APPARATUS

The battery operated, palm top with LCD display screen digital blood pressure monitor is widely being used to monitor BP by patients or general public at home apart from its use by the practitioners. The cuff is wrapped around the upper arm. The pressure rises and then lowers and the arterial pressure and pulse reading appear on the screen. The pressure measuring ranges from 0 to 280 mmHg.

Simple Steps to an Accurate Reading

Before you Take your Blood Pressure Reading

1. Wear loose-fitting clothes like a short sleeved t-shirt so that you can push your sleeve up comfortably.
2. Before you take reading give five minutes rest. You should be sitting down in a quiet place, preferably at a desk or table, with your arm resting on a firm surface and your feet flat on the ground
3. Make sure your arm is supported and that the cuff around your arm is at the same level as your heart and is at the correct height. Your arm should be relaxed, not tensed.
4. When you are taking your reading, keep still and silent. Moving and talking can affect your reading.
5. Take two or three readings, each about two minutes apart, and then work out the average. Some people find that their first reading is much higher than the next readings. If this is true for you, keep taking readings until they level out and stop falling, then use this as your reading.

Clinical perspective: World Health Organization attributes hypertension or high blood pressure as the leading cause of cardiovascular mortality. An elevated arterial pressure is very important public health problem. It is a professional responsibility of a doctor to carefully examine vitals including blood pressure and informs the patient of their hypertensive state and to offer medical advice, including appropriate referral.

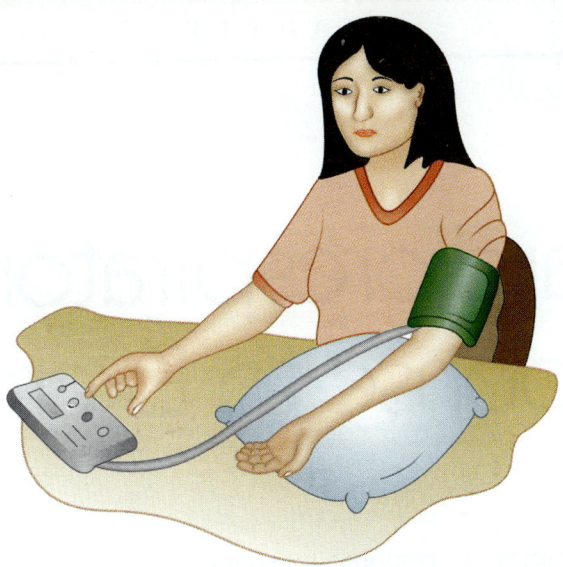

Fig. 3.4: Digital manometer. For recording blood pressure

HISTORY

The first time determination of arterial blood pressure was done by Rev Stephen Hales in the year 1733 in mare as experimental animal by inserting a brass cannula into the central end of femoral artery. He tied the cannula to a long glass which was having height of three meters. Rev Hales observed the oscillation and rise of blood column.

Riva Rocci invented the sphygmomanometer in the year 1886. Sphygmomanometer was thereafter used to record blood pressure in human beings.

OBSERVATIONS: EXERCISE FOR STUDENTS

....

....

....

....

....

....

....

....

....

....

....

....

....

....

Cardiorespiratory Response to Exercise

Experiment: To study the cardiorespiratory response to exercise.

Procedure

Record basal blood pressure in sitting position.

Record resting pulse rate and respiratory rate.

Instruct the subject to perform exercise, e.g. sit-ups, spot jogging, climbing stairs.

Record the observations as follows:

Basal	BP	Pulse rate	Respiratory rate
1.			
2.			
3.			
Immediately after exercise			
1. One minute after exercise			
2. Minutes after exercise			
3. Minute after exercise			
4. Minutes after exercise			
Till the values return to the basal level.			

....

....

....

VIVA VOCE QUESTIONS

Q1. What is the mechanism of increase in systolic BP in exercise?

Ans. There is increase in cardiac output because of increase in stroke volume and heart rate.

*Competency achievement as per competency based Undergraduate Curriculum for the Indian Medical Graduate, 2018, 1; Medical Council of India.

Q2. How much can be increased in cardiac output during exercise?

Ans. Cardiac output can increase to 24 liters per minute or even higher during exercise depending on the severity of exercise. It can still be greater in trained person.

Q3. How much heart rate can be increased during exercise?

Ans. Heart rate can reach up to 180 per minute in healthy adults.

Q4. What is the mechanism of increase in ventilation with exercise?

Ans. Neural impulses from the motor cortex to the medullary respiratory centre, afferents from muscles, tendons and joints or unknown mediators released from working muscles are believed to contribute.

Q5. What is the cause of limits of exercise performance?

Ans. Two main factors limit performance. The rate of oxygen utilization and oxygen supply to the muscles. Limitation could be caused by inability to increase cardiac output beyond a critical level, hence major factor could be pumping capacity of heart.

Q6. Describe the effects of different grades of isotonic exercise on cardiovascular function.

Ans. Figure shows the response of different grades of exercise on cardiovascular functions.

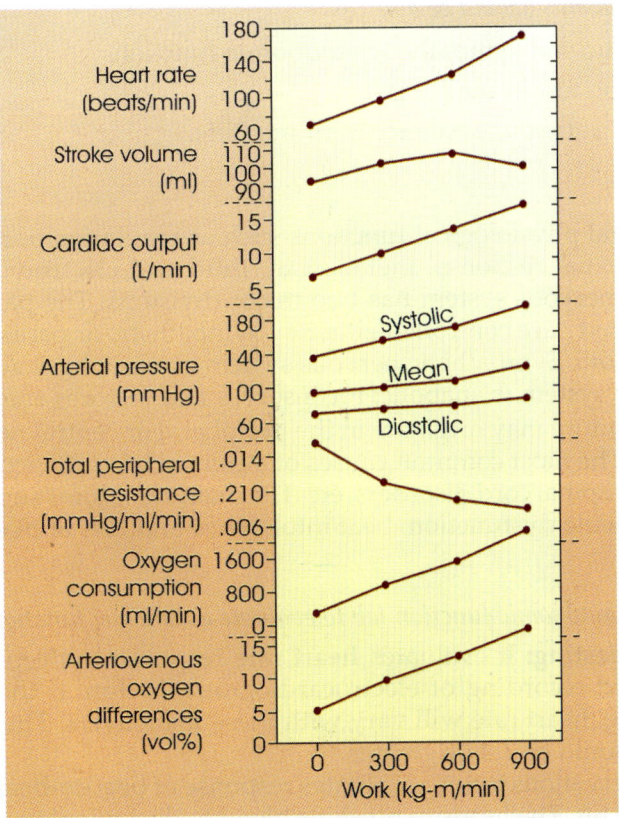

Fig. 4.1: Effects of different grades of isotonic exercise

Q7. What are cardiorespiratory changes on stoppage of severe exercise?

Ans. When exercise is stopped heart rate and cardiac output abruptly decrease, as sympathetic drive to the heart is removed. In contrast, TPR remains low for sometime after severe exercise is stopped, because of accumulation of vasodilator metabolites in the muscle during exercise peroid, arterial blood pressure falls below pre-exercise level for a brief peroid. BP is then stabilized at normal level by baroreceptor reflexes, ventilation returns to normal when the oxygen debt is recovered.

5

Autonomic Function Test

PHY 5.14*

Learning Objectives

After learning the practical the students should be able to:

1. Discuss the parasympathetic and sympathetic autonomic functions.
2. Perform autonomic function test in the subjects.
3. Discuss the significance of autonomic balance in human life.

Brief Review

Autonomic nervous controls vital physiological functions such as regulation of heart rate, cardiac output, blood pressure, body temperature, sexual response, metabolism, fluid and electrolyte balance, sweating, urination, defecation, etc. The autonomic nervous system has two major divisions: The parasympathetic and sympathetic systems. The organs in human body are controlled either by sympathetic or parasympathetic system though they might be receiving input from both. Sympathetic nervous system is catabolic; it activates fight-or-flight responses while parasympathetic nervous system is anabolic; it conserves and restores energy.

Autonomic insufficiency or failure may originate in the peripheral or central nervous system and could be also secondarily to other disorders. The most common causes of autonomic insufficiency are peripheral neuropathies, autoimmune neuropathy, aging, spinal cord disorders, etc. The main symptoms suggesting autonomic insufficiency are orthostatic hypotension, erectile dysfunction, heat intolerance and loss of bladder and bowel control.

Method

The following test is conducted in autonomic function lab to evaluate autonomic functions:

1. **Cardiovagal innervation testing:** It evaluates **heart rate** response to deep breathing and to the **Valsalva manoeuvers** using a traced recording of electrocardiogram rhythm. If the autonomic nervous system is physiologically functioning, heart rate will vary with these maneuvers. The ratio of longest to shortest R-R interval (Valsalva ratio) should be 1.4 or greater.
2. Vasomotor adrenergic innervations testing evaluates response of **beat-to-beat blood pressure** to the **Valsalva manoeuver** and to head-up tilt. The head-up tilt shifts blood to dependent parts, causing reflex responses. The Valsalva maneuver increases intrathoracic pressure and reduces venous return causing reflex vasoconstriction and causing blood pressure changes. The pattern of responses is an index of adrenergic function.

   Other adrenergic tests:

   Sustained hand grip: Sustained muscle contraction causes an increase in heart rate and systolic and diastolic blood pressure. This autonomic maneuver is performed using handgrip dynamometer and has been adapted as a clinical test of sympathetic autonomic function. The BP is measured using a sphygmomanometer cuff.
3. Quantitative sudomotor axon reflex test (QSART) evaluates integrity of postganglionic neurons using iontophoresis. Place electrodes filled with acetylcholine on the legs and wrist of volunteer subject to stimulate sweat glands. Measure the volume of sweat. The test can detect decreased, persistent (after stimulus discontinuation) or absent sweat production.

*Competency achievement as per competency based Undergraduate Curriculum for the Indian Medical Graduate, 2018, 1; Medical Council of India.

4. Thermoregulatory sweat test (TST) evaluates both preganglionic and postganglionic pathways. Dye is applied to the skin in a patient. He is asked to enter a heated closed compartment in order to produce maximal sweating. Sweating causes the dye to change colour, and areas of anhidrosis and hypohidrosis can be identified and is calculated as a percentage of body surface area.

5. Sympathetic skin response (SSR) provides an index of sweat production. It measures changes in skin resistance following random electrical stimulation over the palms and soles.

6. Quantitative direct and indirect axon reflex testing (QDIRT) also known as quantitative sudomotor axon reflex (QSART) evaluates the postganglionic sympathetic cholinergic sudomotor function by measuring axon-reflex mediated and direct sweat response in a dynamic manner. Stimulate sweat glands by acetylcholine iontophoresis and display sweat via an activator dye followed by taking digital photographs over time. Typically recording from the forearm and three lower extremity skin sites are used to evaluate the distribution of postganglionic deficits. The test has a high sensitivity and specificity.

Aim of Experiment

1. To study cardiovascular response to exposure of hand to cold
2. To demonstrate the effect of Valsalva manoeuver on heart rate.

Principle

The change in heart rate and the magnitude and duration of pressure response to a brief exposure of the hand to cold is a measure of vasomotor tone and autonomic activity in man.

Procedure

The subject is seated or made to lie down in quite surroundings. The blood pressure and heart rate is recorded and repeated at an interval of 2 minutes till three successive readings are identical.

One hand is immersed in cold water at 5°C. Immediately on immersing the hand blood pressure and heart rate are recorded. Water is stirred to maintain a uniform temperature. After two minutes the hand is removed and recordings of heart rate and blood pressure are repeated at intervals of one minute till the heart rate and blood pressure are back to the original levels.

Result

Tabulate the results

....

....

....

Draw two graphs

a. Showing the heart rate changes.
b. Showing the systolic and diastolic blood pressure, changes at various intervals.

VALSALVA MANOEUVER

Valsalva manoeuver is a procedure where the individual holds his breath for 15 seconds or more during forced expiration so as to sustain a pressure of 40 mmHg. During this procedure the increased intrathoracic pressure leads to a decrease in cardiac output and blood pressure. The resultant fall in blood pressure inhibits the response from baroreceptors, thus initiating a reflex tachycardia. Once the procedure is over, there is sudden increase in venous return to the heart. Increased venous return results in rise of blood pressure and increased impulses from baroreceptors that cause decrease in heart rate, so in a normal individual with an intact autonomic functions an increase in heart rate is expected during Valsalva manoeuver and a decrease in heart rate on termination of the manoeuver. The ratio between the maximum heart rate (during the manoeuver) and the minimum heart rate after termination of the manoeuver is called Valsalva ratio, normally the ratio is between 1.5 and 3.0. The value may be less than 1.5 in case of autonomic nervous system disorder. The test should not be performed in very old hypertensive persons.

Equipment Required

ECG machine, stethograph with transducers for recording, mercury manometer attached to mouthpiece.

Procedure

The subject is made to take a comfortable posture. ECG electrodes are placed and connected for recording on machine. Stethograph is placed around the chest and connected through volume transducers for recording. Subject is informed about the whole procedure.

Basal ECG and respiratory movements are recorded The subject is asked to breathe forcefully into a mouthpiece attached to mercury manometer so as to raise the mercury column up to 40 mmHg and to maintain it for 10–15 seconds. At the end of this asked to release the pressure and to continue normal breathing.

The ECG and respiratory recordings are continued throughout this procedure.

Calculation of Valsalva Ratio

This is the ratio of longest R-R interval to the shortest R-R interval during the manoeuver. To calculate it from the ECG strip find out the longest and shortest R-R interval and mathematically express these in terms of ratio.

Record the R-R interval and heart rate for 5 minutes after the manoeuver and find out the maximum R-R interval and convert it into heart rate. This will be the lowest heart rate after this manoeuver.

Plot the changes in 1. R-R interval and 2. heart rate against time during the whole procedure.

Recording of Data and Data analysis.

Parameter	R-R interval	Heart rate per minute
At rest:		
....		
During manoeuver:		
....		
Post-manoeuver		
....		
Valsalva ratio		
Conclusion		
The Valsalva ratio is /is not within normal ratio		
....		

VIVA VOCE QUESTIONS

Q1. Define Valsalva manoeuver.

Ans. When a person holds breath for (brief period) 15 seconds or more after forced expiration and closed glottis.

Q2. Explain the mechanism of changes in the heart rate during the manoeuver.

Ans. Valsalva manoeuver raises intra-thoracic pressure and so fall in venous return, fall in cardiac output and BP causing reflex tachycardia. This is valsalva manoeuver.

Q3. Enumerate clinical conditions where this test may be abnormal.

Ans. In long duration of diabetes mellitus due to impaired function of ANS.

Q4. Why there is an increase in blood pressure when hand is immersed in cold water?

Ans. It is the response of the body to stress of extreme cold temperature.

Q5. What is postural hypotension?

Ans. When an individual stands up immediately from recumbent posture, there is pooling of blood in the legs. The venous return to the heart is reduced, thereby reducing the cardiac output. Hence, the systolic blood pressure will fall, which may be recorded within 15 seconds (BP is usually difficult to record at this time in normal subjects). This will be brought back to normal by baroreceptor reflex within 15 to 30 seconds, This is a function of autonomic nervous system (ANS). Failure of appropriate response results in postural hypotension.

Q6. What is the mechanism of production of pain following immersion of hand in cold water?

Ans. Stimulation of pain receptors with intense cold that acts as a nocioceptive stimulus.

Q7. Describe the ganglionoic fibres of sympathetic and parasympathetic systems.

Ans. The preganglionic cell bodies of the sympathetic system are located between T1 and L2 or L3 in the intermediolateral horn of the spinal cord. The sympathetic ganglia consist of the vertebral (sympathetic chain) and paravertebral ganglia, including the superior and middle cervical, stellate, celiac, superior mesenteric, inferior mesenteric, and aorticorenal ganglia. The long fibers run from these ganglia to effector organs.

Preganglionic cell bodies of the parasympathetic system are positioned in the brain stem and sacral portion of the spinal cord. Preganglionic fibers traverse along the brain stem with the 3rd, 7th, 9th, and 10th (vagus) cranial nerves and from the spinal cord nerves from S_2 to S_4. The parasympathetic ganglia (e.g. ciliary, sphenopalatine, otic, pelvic, and vagal ganglia) are positioned within the effector organs, and postganglionic fibers are only 1 or 2 mm long.

Q8. Which are the neurotransmitters secreted in the ANS?

Ans. *The neurotransmitters secreted in the ANS are:*

1. **Acetylcholine:** The fibers secreting acetylcholine (cholinergic fibers) are all preganglionic fibers, all postganglionic parasympathetic fibers, and some postganglionic sympathetic fibers (those innervating sweat glands, piloerectors, and some muscle blood vessels).

2. **Norepinephrine:** The fibers that secrete norepinephrine (adrenergic fibers) are most of the postganglionic sympathetic fibers. Sweat glands on the palms and soles also respond to adrenergic stimulation to some degree.

Q9. Discuss the variability in heart rate and indication of autonomic status.

Ans. The higher variations in the heart rate lead to greater heart rate variability which indicates well-balanced sympathetic and parasympathetic autonomic function. While steadier heart rate leads to lower heart rate variability indicating altered autonomic function and implies the presence of physiological malfunction.

Q10. Describe sudomotor testing.

Ans. *The sudomotor testing includes:*

1. **Quantitative sudomotor axon-reflex test:** It evaluates integrity of postganglionic fibers. These fibers can be activated by iontophoresis using acetylcholine. The test is conducted on standard sites on the leg and wrist. The volume of sweat is measured. The test can detect absent or decrease in sweat production.

2. **Thermoregulatory sweat test:** It evaluates both preganglionic and postganglionic autonomic fibers. Dye is applied to the skin in a patient. He is asked to enter a heated closed compartment in order to produce maximal sweating. Sweating causes the dye to change colour, and areas of anhidrosis and hypohidrosis can be identified and calculated as a percentage of body surface area.

Q11. Describe cardiovagal testing.

Ans. Cardiovagal testing evaluates heart rate response (via ECG rhythm strip) to the Valsalva manoeuver and to deep breathing. The heart rate varies with these maneuvers if the ANS is intact. The normal responses to deep breathing and the Valsalva ratio vary with age.

Q12. How will you carry adrenergic testing?

Ans. Adrenergic testing is conducted by evaluating response of beat-to-beat BP to the head-up tilt test and with Valsalva manoeuver.

- **Head-up tilt test:** The blood shifts to dependent parts and produce reflex responses in heart rate and blood pressure. This test helps differentiate postural tachycardia syndrome from autonomic neuropathies.
- **Valsalva manoeuver:** This maneuver increases intrathoracic pressure and reduces venous return leading to reflex vasoconstriction and altered blood pressure.

OSPE SKILLED

Q1. Demonstrate quantitative sudomotor axon reflex test.

a. The quantitative sudomotor axon reflex test (QSART) evaluates integrity of postganglionic neurons using iontophoresis.

b. Place electrodes filled with acetylcholine on the legs and wrist of volunteer subject to stimulate sweat glands.

c. Measure the volume of sweat. The test can detect decreased, persistent (after stimulus discontinuation) or absent sweat production.

OBSERVATIONS: EXERCISE FOR STUDENTS

6

Clinical Examination of Cardiovascular System

PHY 5.15*

Learning Objectives

After learning the practical the student should be able to:
1. Discuss and explain the normal physiological functioning of heart.
2. Understand the importance of findings of inspection, palpation, percussion and auscultation of cardiovascular system and co-relate it with associated cardiovascular disorders.

Aim of the Experiment

Student should learn the method of conducting the examination of cardiovascular system and report if there is any abnormal finding.

Instruments: Stethoscope, sphygmomanometer, measuring tape, and torch.

Procedure

1. Ask the individual to sit upright on an examination table. Ensure adequate lighting is available in the room.
2. The patient is asked to remove the clothing over the chest.
3. Perform the general clinical examination in the patient/individual noting his pulse, body temperature, blood pressure, for the presence of pallor, cyanosis, clubbing, oedema, and lymphadenopathy.

The cardiovascular examination is carried out under the following headings:

- Inspection
- Palpation
- Percussion
- Auscultation.

Inspection

The cardiovascular examination should be carried out positioning the patient in the supine position tilted up at 45 degrees. The neck should be made prominent for visualization of pulsation.
1. Inspect the patient status for whether if they are comfortable at rest or obviously short of breath.
2. Identify the shape of the chest and observe its bilateral symmetry.
3. If any prominent veins visible on the chest wall. These are prominently seen in case of intra-thoracic growth, secondary to portal obstruction and obstruction to inferior vena cava.
4. Position of the trachea.
5. Presence of any precordial bulge or depression.
6. Position of apical pulsation, if visible.
7. Inspect the neck for increased jugular venous pressure (JVP) or abnormal waves. The JVP is increased in pregnancy (as a result of increased circulating blood volume), right heart failure, and atrial myxoma and in obstruction to superior vena cava. The jugular veins communicate directly with the right atrium. Therefore, the fluctuations in right atrial pressure during the cardiac cycle generate a pulse which is transmitted backwards into the jugular veins.

---

*Competency achievement as per competency based Undergraduate Curriculum for the Indian Medical Graduate, 2018, 1; Medical Council of India.

Palpation

1. The position of the trachea is to be confirmed by palpation for the trachea in the suprasternal notch and note if it is central or deviated to one side.
2. Confirm and note the position and character of the apex beat. Place the palm of the right hand over the apex, localize the apex beat by using the medial border of the palm and then feel it with the tips of the fingers (Fig. 6.1). The **apex beat** is defined as the lowermost and outermost definite palpable cardiac impulse usually felt in the fifth left intercostals space, 1 cm medial to the mid-clavicular line.
3. Place the hypothenar eminence of your right palm on the left mid and lower parasternal region of the patient/individual and confirm if parasternal heave is present.
4. Palpate the precordium for presence of a **thrill** (a palpable murmur which resembles the purring of a cat).

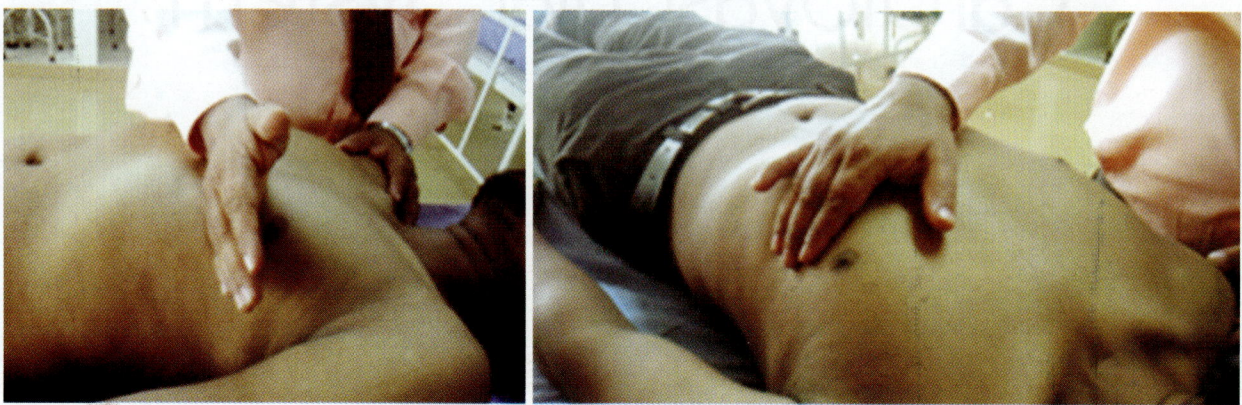

Fig. 6.1: Palpation of apex beat

Percussion

The rules of percussion are:

1. The stroke should be promptly made by movement at the wrist.
2. The long axis of the pleximeter finger should be parallel to the edge of the organ being percussed.
3. Percussion should be done from more resonant to a less resonant area.

Percuss lightly from the sides towards the heart in order to define the cardiac dullness, and to delineate the borders of the heart.

Auscultation

Auscultate the precordium in the following areas using a stethoscope (Fig. 6.2).

*   **Mitral area** corresponds to the region of the apex beat.
*   **Tricuspid area** is present to the left of the lower end of the sternum.
*   **Aortic area** is present to the right of the sternum, in the second intercostals space.
*   **Pulmonary area** is present to the left of the sternum in the second intercostals space.

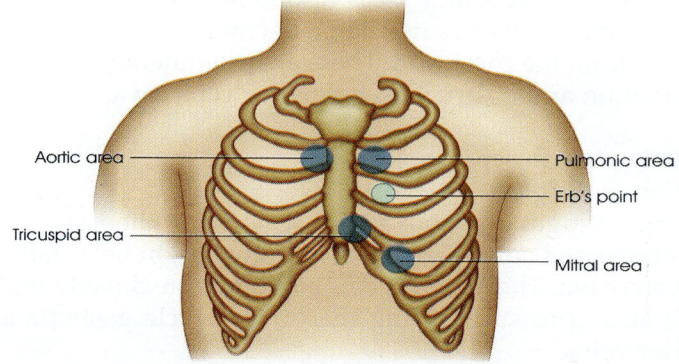

Fig. 6.2

In each of the above four areas note the character of the first and second heart sounds, this can be differentiated by their pitch and duration.

Palpate the left common carotid artery in the neck while auscultation for the heart sounds.

The students should note the reasons for the four heart sounds (S1, S2, S3 and S4).

Heart sound	Occurs during	Associated with
S1	Isovolumetric contraction	Closure of mitral and tricuspid valves
S2	Isovolumetric relaxation	Closure of aortic and pulmonary valves
S3	Early ventricular filling	Normal in children; in adults, associated with ventricular dilation (e.g. ventricular systolic failure)
S4	Atrial contraction	Associated with stiff, low compliant ventricle (e.g. ventricular hypertrophy)

OSPE NON-SKILLED CHART QUESTIONS

Q1. Enlist the clinical conditions in whom JVP is raised.

Ans. *The causes of raised JVP are*:
1. Pericardial effusion/pulmonary embolism/pericardial constriction
2. Quantity of fluid increased (iatrogenic fluid overload)
3. Right heart failure or congestive heart failure
4. Superior vena caval obstruction
5. Tricuspid regurgitation/tricuspid stenosis/tamponade (cardiac).

Q2. Discuss the procedure of palpation of apex beat.

Ans. **Apex beat:** The patient may be asked to lie down on examination couch and later asked to lie at left lateral decubitus position. Place the palm of the right hand over the apex, localize the apex beat by using the medial border of the palm and then feel it with the tips of the fingers. The apex beat is usually felt in the fifth left intercostals space, 1 cm medial to the mid-clavicular line.

Q3. Locate the position over chest where first and second heart sound are better heard.

Ans. The first heart sound is better heard in apex along the mitral and also at tricuspid area. The second heart sound is best heard in pulmonary and aortic area.

VIVA VOCE QUESTIONS

Q1. Name the pacemaker of the heart.

Ans. The SA node is the pacemaker of heart as physiologically it controls the heart rate.

Q2. Describe the heart valves.

Ans. *Heart contains four valves*:
- Two atrioventricular (AV) valves between atria and ventricles
- Aortic and pulmonary valves at junction of ventricles and great arteries.

Q3. Discuss the functions of heart.

Ans. The function of the heart is to generate blood pressure so as to produce a gradient that pushes blood through the vascular system. The heart works in conjunction with cardiovascular centers and peripheral blood vessels to achieve this goal. It regulates blood supply by the sympathetic and parasympathetic control by cardiovascular centre in CNS to alter the contraction rate and force to match blood delivery to meet the metabolic needs. The pulmonary circuit takes blood to and from the lungs and systemic circuit vessels transport blood to and from body tissues.

Q4. Define cardiac cycle.

Ans. Cardiac cycle is the sequence of events of pressure and volume changes, changes of the electrical potential and sound during the period between two successive ventricular contractions.

Q5. What are the causes for first and second heart sound?

Ans. The first heart sound is due to the closure of AV valves which occur at the beginning of ventricular systole. The second heart sound is due to the closure of the aortic and pulmonary valves at protodiastole phase of the cardiac cycle.

Q6. Enlist the factors which affect blood pressure.

Ans. *The factors which affect blood pressure are:*
- Cardiac output
- Total blood volume
- Blood viscosity
- Elasticity of arteries
- Resistance (vessel lumen size and smoothness).

Briefly: It is product of cardiac output and peripheral resistance.

Q7. What is baroreceptor reflex?

Ans. The arterial blood pressure is reflex controlled by pressure sensitive nerve endings known as *baroreceptors;* located in the carotid sinus and along aortic arch; which are sensitive to stretch of the arterial wall. Baroreceptors send afferent impulses through sinus and aortic nerves (Buffer nerves) to vasomotor areas of the central nervous system which monitor beat to beat changes in arterial pressure. The central nervous system as reflex response alters cardiac output by the sympathetic and parasympathetic divisions of autonomic nervous system which alter the cardiac output and vascular resistance by vasoconstriction or vasodilatation.

Q8. Discuss the long-term effect of exercise on heart.

Ans. *The long-term effects of exercise on heart are:*

Aerobic exercise strengthens the heart, the walls become thicker and stronger, the stroke volume increases and the heart becomes a more efficient pump. Training also results in new capillaries growing to improve the supply of blood to the muscles.

Q9. Describe the test for cardiovascular fitness.

Ans. *The test for cardiovascular fitness is:*

The best way of measuring cardiovascular fitness is to calculate a performer's VO_2 max. This measures the maximum amount of oxygen the body can take in. However, calculating VO_2 max requires very specialized equipment.

An alternative is the bleep test. Performers have to do 20 metre shuttle runs, keeping pace with a series of recorded bleeps which gradually get faster. The point at which the performer has to drop out is recorded.

The easiest test is the 12 minute run. Performers simply run for 12 minutes and the distance covered is recorded.

Testing Speed, Flexibility and Balance

Speed is easy to test. Simply record how fast a performer can sprint a short distance. 100 metre and 60 metre distances are often used.

Flexibility can be tested by measuring a performer's range of movement. A common test for flexibility is the **sit and reach test** (Fig. 6.3).

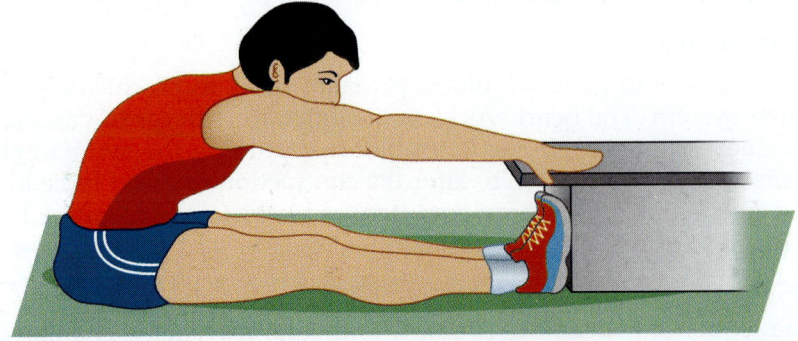

Fig. 6.3: Testing speed, flexibility and balance

How far the performer can reach relative to their feet is measured on a ruler.

Balance can be tested using the **stork stand test**. The performer stands on one leg, with their free foot on their standing knee. How long they can hold the position for is timed.

Agility can be tested by setting up an **agility run** and timing how long it takes for a performer to complete it (Fig. 6.4).

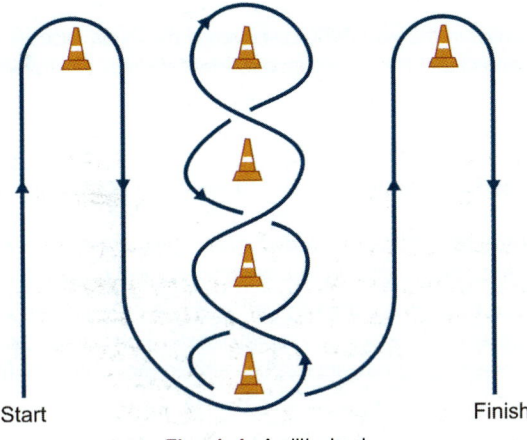

Start   Finish

Fig. 6.4: Agility test

When **retesting** performers to measure improvement, you must take care that the agility run is set up exactly the same as before.

Muscular endurance can be tested easily by seeing how many times a performer can repeat a movement requiring strength. **Sit-ups** and **press-ups** are often used (Fig. 6.5).

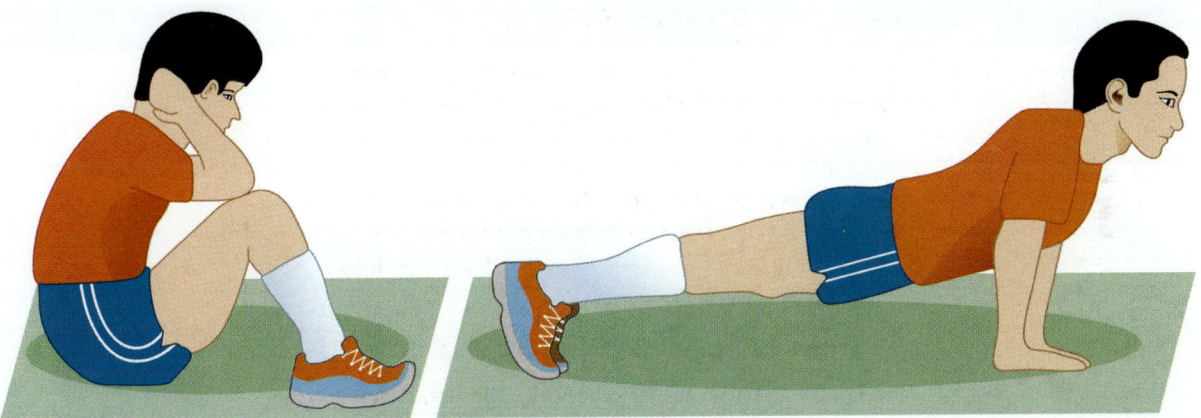

Fig. 6.5: Sit-ups and press-ups

I. HISTORICAL ASPECTS

Leonardo da Vinci (1452–1519)

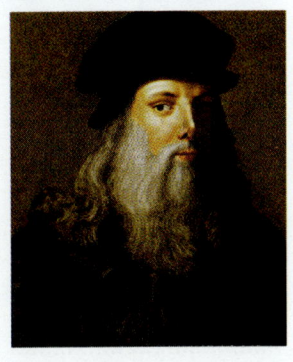

He investigated and studied the coronary arteries. William Harvey (1578–1657) Physician to King Charles I is credited with discovering circulatory mechanism of heart. Harvey understanding of the relationship between arteries and veins was existence of a unified circulatory system. Friedrich Hoffmann (1660–1742) was a Chief Professor of cardiology at the University of Halle and found that coronary heart disease emerged in the "reduced passage of the blood within the coronary arteries. He described the heart as a muscle, understood the role of the coronary vessels and was the first to mention the moderator band and the relation of the systole to the pulse. He also discovered the hemodynamic function of the sinuses of Valsalva in the closure mechanism of the aortic valve. Leonardo's notes and drawings on the heart are a fine example of his open mind and keen observation.

II. HISTORICAL ASPECT OF CORONARY DISEASES

William Osler (1849–1919) a cardiologist was first to explain angina and opined that it is a syndrome rather than a disease in itself.

In 1912, James B. Herrick (1861–1954), the American cardiologist discovered that the gradual narrowing of the coronary arteries could be the cause of angina. He is invented the term "heart attack".

John Gofman (1918–2007) in the year 1950, as a researcher along with his associates at University of California identified today's low-density lipoprotein (LDL) and high-density lipoprotein (HDL). He found out that patient who developed atherosclerosis had elevated levels of LDL and low levels of HDL.

Ancel Keys (1904–2004) an American Scientist in the year 1950 discovered that heart disease was rare in some Mediterranean populations who consumed a lower fat diet. He also observed that the Japanese had low-fat diets and low rates of heart disease as support to his theory of that fat was the cause of heart disease.

Recent Update

I. The aortic valve and the mitral valve are the most commonly replaced valves than pulmonary and tricuspid valve in adults. The commonest valve surgical procedure is valve replacement for aortic stenosis and mitral stenosis. Aortic regurgitation is another common valve problem that may require valve replacement. Aortic regurgitation can eventually lead to heart failure. **Mitral regurgitation** patients experience shortness of breath, irregular heartbeats and chest pain and also requires a valve replacement.

II. A cardiac stress test uses drugs or exercise to stimulate the heart and provoke a measurable response to the stress in order to gauge the heart's effectiveness. Angiogenesis represents a therapeutic target for cardiovascular disease. Defibrillation is used for treating fatal arrhythmias. Artificial pacemakers used to regulate the heartbeat can also incorporate a defibrillator.

Clinical Perspective

Heart is prone to several cardiovascular diseases and it becomes more prevalent with ageing. Myocardial infarction is a major cause of death. Obesity, hypertension, diabetes and high cholesterol can all increase the risk of developing heart disease. The students should gain sufficient knowledge of physiology and pathophysiology of heart and heart diseases for appropriate application in clinical practice. The precordial exam is also called the cardiac exam. It is carried out as part of a physical examination or when a patient presents with complaints of chest pain, associated breathlessness, palpitation, restlessness, sweating or any signs and symptoms suggestive of a cardiovascular pathology.

OBSERVATIONS: EXERCISE FOR STUDENTS

....

....

....

....

....

....

....

....

....

....

....

....

....

Electrocardiography: Recording of Normal Electrocardiogram

PY 5.5*

Learning Objectives

The recording of electrocardiogram enables to understand:

1. The anatomical orientation of the heart
2. The relative size of the chambers
3. Variety of disturbances of rhythm and conduction
4. The extent and location and progress of ischaemic disease to the myocardium.
5. The effects of altered electrolyte concentrations.

However, it gives no direct information about the mechanical performance of the heart as a pump.

Aim of the Experiment

1. To understand the unipolar and bipolar methods of recording the electrocardiogram (ECG).
2. To identify the various waves of the electrocardiogram (ECG) and explain the causes for the waves, calculate heart rate, note rhythm, and duration of each wave and PR and QT intervals.

Principle

As the cardiac impulse spreads through the heart electrical currents spread from the heart to the adjacent tissues surrounding the heart. A small portion of the current spreads to the surface of the body. If electrodes are placed on the skin on opposite side of the heart electrical potentials generated by the current can be recorded and the recording is called electrocardiogram.

The electrocardiograph is a high speed recording meter with a moving paper. An electrocardiogram (ECG) is the graphical record produced by an electrocardiograph machine. ECG picks up electrical impulses generated by depolarization and repolarization of cardiac muscle and translates into a waveform. The waveform is used to measure the rate and regularity of heartbeats, evaluate size and position of the chambers, identify underlying pathology in the heart. It can show the effects of drugs or devices.

The heart is actually suspended in a conductive medium. When one portion of it depolarizes and therefore becomes electronegative with respect to the remainder, electrical current flows from the depolarized to the polarized area in large circuitous routes (Fig. 7.1A). In the ventricles the cardiac impulse first arrives in the septum and spreads to the inside surface of ventricles. This provides electronegativity inside and electropositivity on the outer wall of the ventricles with current flowing through the fluids surrounding the ventricles. With algebraically averages of all lines of current flow, the average current flow occurs with negativity towards the base of the heart and positivity towards the apex. Later the current flows from the apex to the base (Fig. 7.1B).

A. Procedure

The routine recording is as follows:

Standard bipolar limb leads: Lead I, lead II and lead III. The electrocardiogram is recorded from two electrodes located on different sides of the heart on two limbs. Records the potential difference between the two leads (Fig. 7.2).

*Competency achievement as per competency based Undergraduate Curriculum for the Indian Medical Graduate, 2018, 1; Medical Council of India.

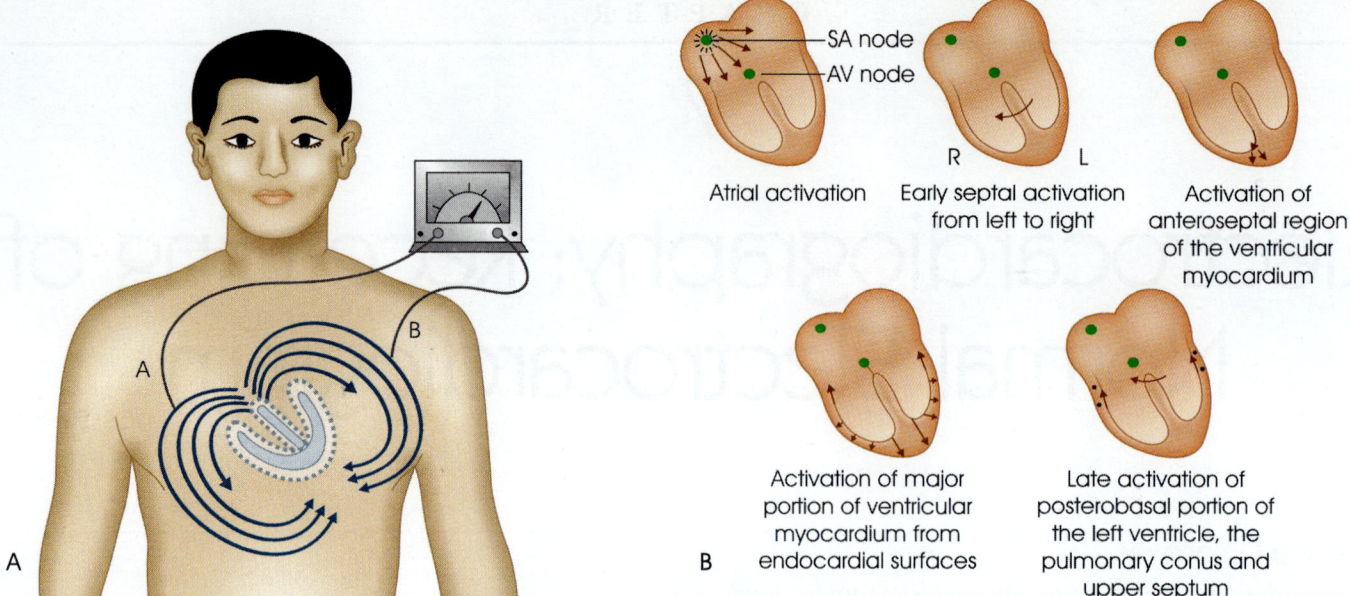

Figs 7.1A, B: The heart is suspended in the conductive medium, when one portion of ventricle depolarizes and therefore becomes electronegative with respect to the remainder, electrical current flows from the depolarized area to the polarized area in large circuits routes as in Fig. 7.1A. Pathway of cardiac impulse (Fig. 7.1B)

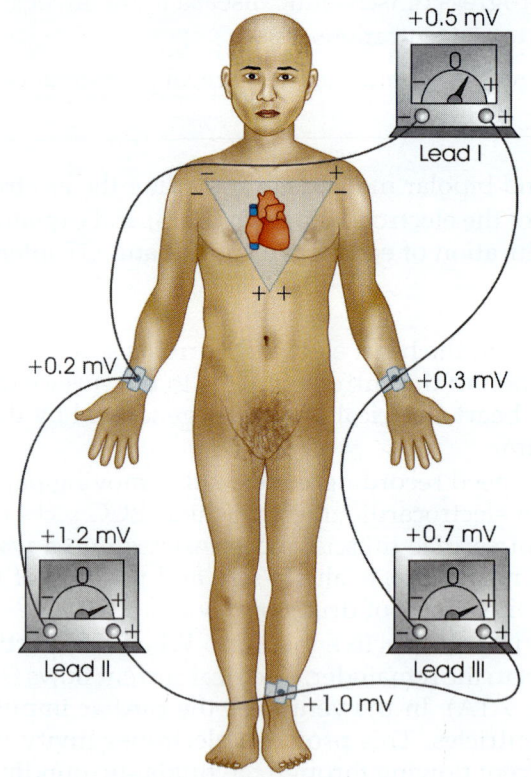

Fig. 7.2: Bipolar recording

Lead I: Negative terminal of the electrocardiograph is connected to the right arm and the positive terminal to the left arm. Therefore, when the point where the right arm connects to the chest is electronegative with respect to the point where the left arm connects the electrocardiograph it records positivity, i.e. the records above the isoelectric line in the electrocardiogram.

Lead II: The right arm is connected to the negative terminal and left leg to positive terminal. Therefore, when the right arm is negative in respect to left leg the recording is positive.

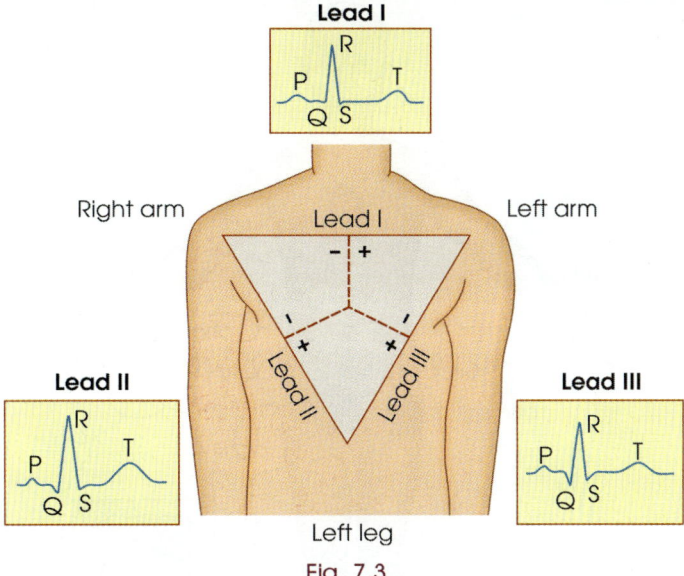

Fig. 7.3

Lead III: The negative terminal of machine is connected to the left arm and the positive terminal to the left leg. Therefore the electrograph records positivity when the left arm is negative with respect to the left leg.

Einthoven's triangle: A triangle drawn around the heart with two arms and left leg to form the apices of a triangle has been called the **Einthoven's triangle** (Fig. 7.3).

Einthoven's law: States that if electrical potentials of two of the three bipolar limb leads are known at any given instant the third can be determined mathematically by summing the two.

Lead I + lead III = Lead II polarity of lead II has been reversed to record major deflection as upright.

B. Unipolar Chest Leads

V1 to V6

In any unipolar recording one electrode is the exploring electrode, and the other electrode called the indifferent electrode assumed to be at zero potential as it is connected to all three limb positions (RA, LA and LL). The exploring electrode records the potential in chest leads over the six different points on the anterior surface of the chest over the position of the heart. It is connected to the positive pole, the other electrode the indifferent electrode is connected through equal resistances to the right arm, left arm and left leg at the same time and hence assumed to be at zero potential connected to the negative pole.

C. Unipolar Limb Leads. Augmented Unipolar Limb Leads

VR, VL, VF are unipolar limb leads where the active electrode is on right arm, left arm and left leg respectively and the indifferent electrode is at zero potential being connected to all three limb positions through resistances. The recordings obtained from unipolar limb leads are small, therefore, the augmented limb leads are generally used.

In augmented limb leads one limb position has active electrode and the indifferent electrode connects the other two limb positions. Leads aVR, aVL, and aVF are augmented limb leads (Named after their inventor Dr. Emanuel Goldberger and are collectively known as the Goldberger's leads). These leads record electrical activity between one limb and the other two limbs. The size of the potential is increased by 50 % without changing the configuration of the record. Hence the leads are called aVR, aVL, and aVF

As the exploring electrode is connected to the positive terminal of the machine and the other two limb terminals together through resistances are connected to the negative pole, in aVR exploring electrode at right arm is connected to positive terminal and LA and LL electrodes together are connected to negative terminal, in aVL, the left arm electrode is connected to positive terminal and the RA and LL together are connected to negative terminal, in aVF the electrode at left leg is connected to positive terminal and RA and LL together are connected to negative terminal.

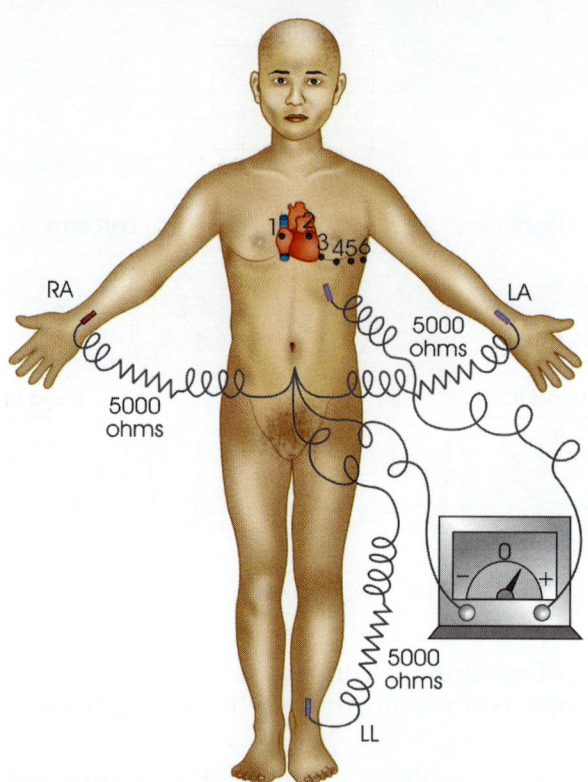

Fig. 7.4: Connections of the body with the electrocardiograph for recording chest leads. LA, left arm; RA, right arm; LL, left leg

Equipment

Electrocardiograph

Electrocardiograph picks up, amplifies and records the potentials of the heart from the body surface.

These amplified potentials move a heated stylus which records the ECG on a wax coated heat sensitive paper. The speed of the moving paper can be put at 25 or 50 mm/sec. The height of the vertical deflection of the stylus represents the voltage. The sensitivity may be adjusted to 1, 2 or 0.5 cm for 1 mV. Thus the machine is first standardized for recording.

ECG Paper

ECG machines when run at a standard rate of 25 mm per second the standard paper as used is with standard sized squares and each small square 1 mm represents 40 ms (0.04 seconds), and each large square of 5 mm represents 200 ms (0.2 seconds). On the y axis, each small square represents 0.1 mV in all routine recording.

ECG LEADS

There are 12 leads in the standard surface electrocardiogram, three bipolar and nine unipolar. There are six unipolar leads placed on the chest and are called the chest leads (Fig. 7.4). The three bipolar and three unipolar leads which are placed on the limbs are known as limb leads.

CHEST LEADS

Chest leads or precordial leads are unipolar leads that record the potential difference between an exploring electrode and a indifferent electrode. The six precordial leads V1–V6 are positive electrodes placed at six different positions as described later.

LIMB LEADS

The limb leads view the heart in a vertical plane.

BIPOLAR LIMB LEADS

1. **Lead I:** Records the difference in potential between right arm (RA) and left arm (LA).
2. **Lead II:** Records the difference in potential between right arm (RA) and left leg (LL).
3. **Lead III:** Records the difference in potential between left arm (LA) and left leg (LL).

UNIPOLAR AUGMENTED LIMB LEADS

aVR: Active (exploring) electrode on the right arm.

aVL: Active (exploring) electrode on the left arm.

aVF: Active (exploring) electrode on the left leg.

Leads aVR, aVL, and aVF are augmented limb leads (named after their inventor Dr. Emanuel Goldberger and are collectively known as the Goldberger's leads). Unipolar limb leads record the potential difference between one limb and an indifferent electrode. The recording obtained from earlier unipolar limb leads are small, therefore the augmented limb leads are generally used. These leads record electrical activity between one limb and the other two limbs. The size of the potential is increased by 50% without changing the configuration of the record.

PROCEDURE FOR RECORDING AN ECG

1. Ask the subject to lie supine on the hospital bed or examination couch.
2. Clean the skin and apply ECG jelly for better contact.
3. Place electrodes on the flexor aspect of the left and right wrists and the left and right legs above the ankle.

   The electrode on the right leg acts as the ground electrode:

   a. LL: Left leg, distally b) RL: Right leg, distally
   c. LA: Left arm, distally d) RA: Right arm, distally

4. Fasten the electrodes firmly to the skin by straps. The leads must be placed correctly.

5. The chest leads are placed as shown in Fig. 7.5.

   V1: Fourth intercostals space, to the right of the sternum
   V2: Fourth intercostals space, to the left of the sternum
   V3: Midway between V2 and V4
   V4: Fifth left intercostals space, along mid-clavicular line
   V5: At the horizontal level of V4, along anterior axillary line
   V6: At the horizontal level of V5 along mid-axillary line.

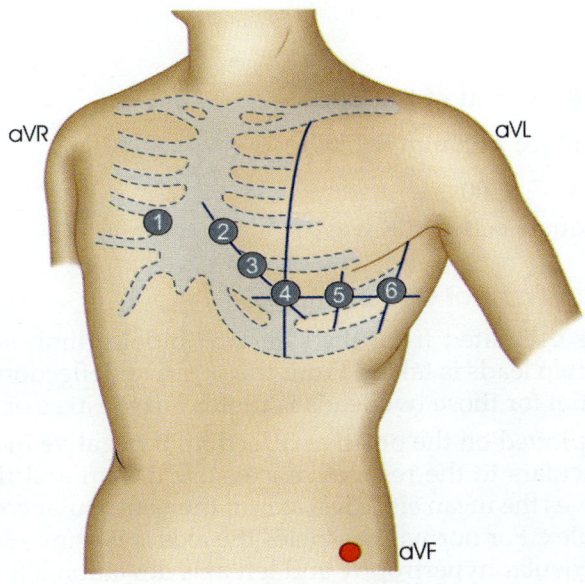

Fig. 7.5

6. Adjust the paper speed rate at 25 mm/sec. Center the writing pen.

7. Calibrate the voltage sensitivity such that 1 mV = 1 cm.

8. Connect the wires from the electrodes to the input socket of the ECG machine.

9. Record the ECG in each of the 12 leads as mentioned above, using the lead selector.

Observations

Paste your record. Compare with Fig. 7.6.

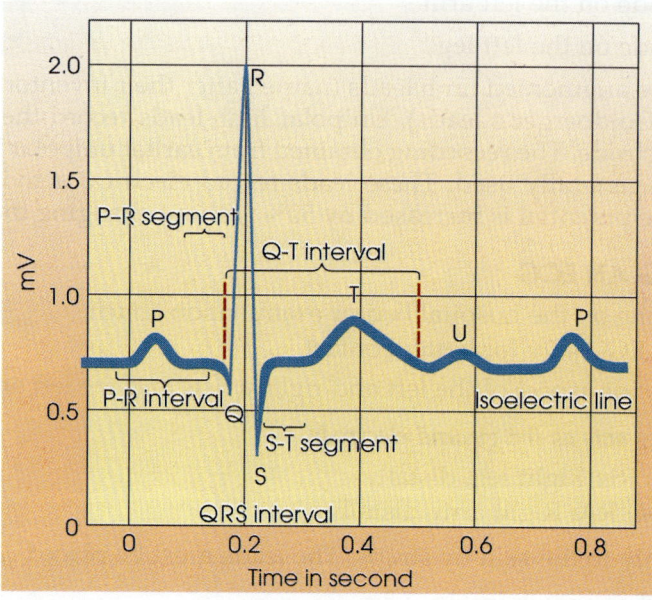

Fig. 7.6

Report on your ECG

P wave. Amplitude duration

QRS complex Amplitude duration

T wave upright/inverted duration

ST segment

PR interval

QT interval

Calculation of heart rate from RR interval of the ECG

At a paper speed of 25 mm/sec, 60 sec × 25 mm = 1500

$$\text{The heart rate/minute} = \frac{1500}{\text{No. of square between R waves}}$$

Determintation of Mean Electrical axis of QRS Complex

The electrical axis of the heart is estimated from the standard bipolar limb lead ECG. The net potential and polarity of the recordings in any two leads is taken. From the positive deflection negative potential is subtracted in each lead, then each net potential for those two leads is plotted in the axes of the leads.

If the potential is positive it is plotted on the positive direction, if negative in the negative direction. From the point on the two leads perpendiculars to the respective axes are drawn and the point where they intersect is joined to the central point. This gives the mean electrical axis of the ventricular complex (sum of the instantaneous axes) when plotted for QRS complex. For normal ventricles the axis is within. –30 degrees to +110 degrees. Right axis deviation suggests right ventricular hypertrophy and left axis deviation left ventricular hypertrophy. Taking your findings of ECG plot electrical axis of QRS complex as shown in Figs 7.7 and 7.8.

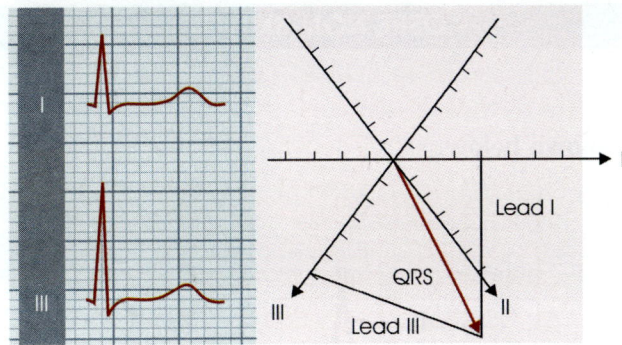

Fig. 7.7: Plotting of mean electrical axis of QRS complex

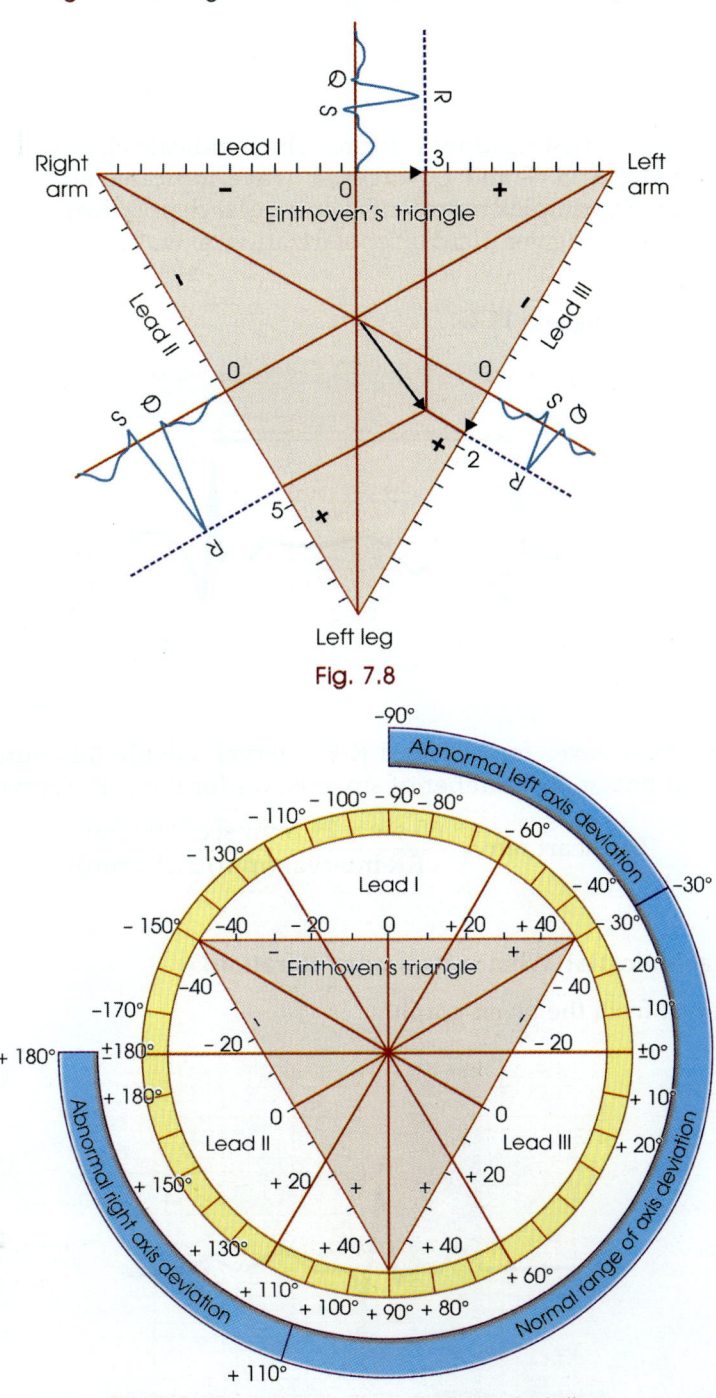

Fig. 7.8

Fig. 7.9: Normal and abnormal axis deviation

EXERCISE FOR STUDENTS

Q1. Interpret the Lead II ECG shown below.

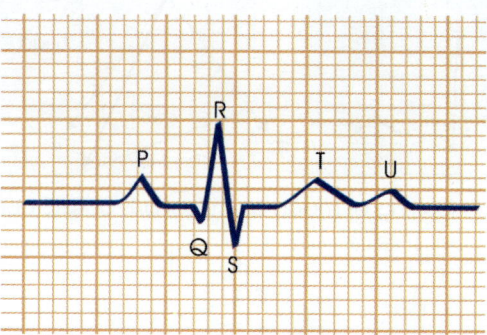

Ans. It is a normal ECG tracings consisting of waveforms which indicate electrical events during one heart beat. These waveforms are P, Q, R, S, T and U waves. P wave indicates atria depolarization. QRS complex follows the P wave. The QRS complex represents ventricular depolarization. T wave is normally a modest upwards waveform, representing ventricular repolarization. U wave indicates the recovery of the Purkinje conduction fibres.

Q2. Calculate the Heart Rate from given ECG.

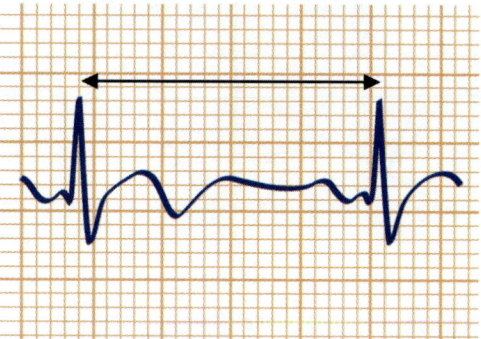

Ans. Count the number of small boxes for a typical R-R interval. Divide this number into 1500 to determine heart rate. In the second image, the number of small boxes for the R-R interval is 21.5.

$$\text{The heart rate} = \frac{60 \text{ sec} \times 25 \text{ mm/sec}}{\text{RR interval (mm)}} \frac{1500 \text{ (mm)}}{21.5 \text{ (mm)}}$$

The heart rate is 69.8

Q3. What does PR interval indicates? What is its normal duration?

Calculate the PR interval from the given graph.

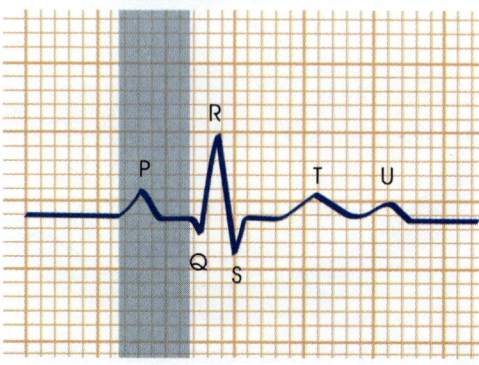

Ans. The PR interval indicates AV conduction time (recorded from the beginning of P wave). Normally this interval is 0.12 to 0.20 seconds. There are 5 small boxes from the beginning of P wave to the beginning of Q wave; 5 × 0.04 = 0.2 second.

The PR interval in the above ECG tracing is 0.2 second.

Q4. What does QRS indicate? Calculate the duration of the QRS wave.

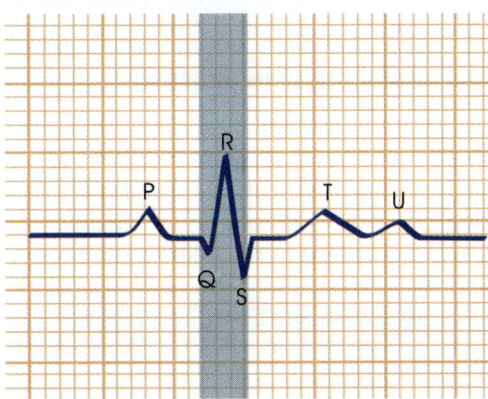

Ans. QRS complex indicates ventricular depolarization. The duration of QRS wave is 3 small squares; 3 × 0.04 = 0.12 sec

Q5. What does QT interval denote? What is its normal duration? Calculate the QT interval from the given graph.

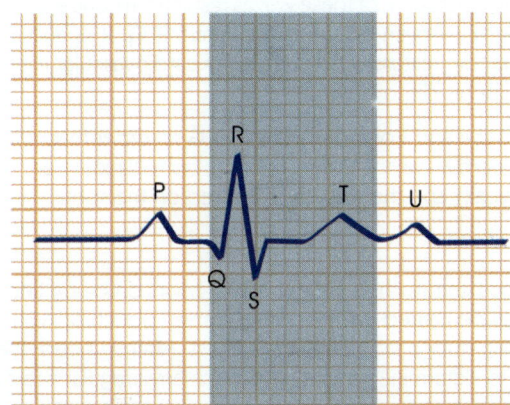

Ans. QT interval denotes ventricular depolarization and ventricular repolarization. The normally QT interval is 0.36 to 0.44 seconds (9–11 boxes). The QT interval is 10 small boxes: 10 × 0.04 = 0.40 sec.

Q6. What is the significance of ST segment morphology?

Ans. Minor ST deviations from isoelectric line may occur as normal variant. Pathological deviation = 2 mm or more of horizontal ST segment indicates myocardial ischemia, other important causes of ST depression are digoxin therapy and hypokalemia.

Q7. What is the significance of T wave morphology

Ans. The orientation of T wave is directionally similar to QRS complex. T wave inversion is normal in leads with dominantly negative QRS complex (aVR,V1) sometimes in lead III. Pathological T wave inversion occurs as a non-specific response to various stimuli (viral infections, hypothermia). More important causes of T wave inversion are ventricular hypertrophy, myocardial ischemia and mycardial infarction. Exaggerated peaking of T wave is the earliest change in ECG in ST elevation myocardial infarction. It also occurs in hyperkalemia.

VIVA VOCE QUESTIONS

Q1. What is electrocardiography?

Ans. Electrocardiography (ECG) is the recording of the electrical changes occurring during the process of depolarization and repolarisation of the heart.

Q2. What is the cause for P, ORS and T wave in ECG?

Ans. P wave is a positive wave, indicating the sum of all the electrical potentials produced during the depolarisation of both atria and the spreading of the electrical activity from SA node throughout the atrial musculature. P wave precedes atrial systole and initiates the atrial contraction. QRS wave is due to spreading of depolarization wave through the ventricular muscles, this initiates ventricular systole (depolarization). QRS wave precedes isovolumetric contraction. T wave precedes ventricular diastole and indicates the initiation of ventricular repolarisation.

Q3. What are the indications for echocardiography in patients?

Ans. Echocardiography is a non-invasive tool for imaging the heart of the surrounding intra-thoracic structures to diagnose various cardiac diseases to assess cardiac function.

It helps to evaluate size of cardiac chambers, study the thickness and movement of the wall, study the structure and movement of the valves, find out congenital cardiac anomalies, detect pericardial and pleural fluid, identify mass lesions within and adjacent to the heart and diagnose valvular and myocardial pathology.

HISTORICAL FACTS

Willem Einthoven

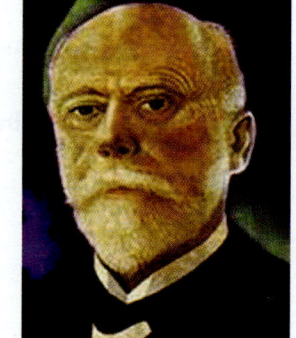

Einthoven, Willem (1860–1927) was a Dutch physiologist who discovered the procedure for recording the electrical activity of heart and it came to be known as electrocardiography. Einthoven invented a string galvanometer in 1903 (Fig below) and with it developed an improved method for measuring the electrical changes that take place in the body upon the contraction of the heart. Einthoven identified number of electrical waves associated with a beating heart. He opined that some of these waves result from contractions and electrical changes in the atria and ventricles of the heart. Einthoven assigned the letters P, Q, R, S and T to the various deflections and described the electrocardiographic features of a number of cardiovascular disorders. In 1924, he was awarded the Nobel Prize in Medicine for his discovery.

Present ECG recorders: Newer generation digital and Computer based ECG recorder machines are available today and are in routine use The direct pen recorder device is very suitable both clinically and experimentally because the nature of wave is recorded graphically and the wave is visualised on the spot.

RECENT UPDATES

Holter monitor device continuously records the heart rhythms usually for 24 hours on being tied and applied to the patient. This ambulatory electrocardiograph is battery operated and can be carried in a pocket or a small pouch or worn around the neck or waist. It is connected to electrodes (small conducting patches) which are stuck onto the patient's chest. After 24 hours, the monitor can be viewed by the physician so as to assess patient's symptoms and activities to determine if there have been any irregular heart beat.

Non-invasive imaging modalities (magnetic resonance perfusion imaging, stress echocardiography, CT coronary angiography) have higher rates of diagnostic accuracy and are now preferred in the assessment of patients with suspected coronary artery disease where available. The exercise ECG also provides prognostic information in patients of known coronary artery, myocardial infarction, indicated by ST depression.

Computerized analysis of ECG recordings are possible by modern ECG machines. Need of the hour is to develop tools for quantitative ECG analysis.

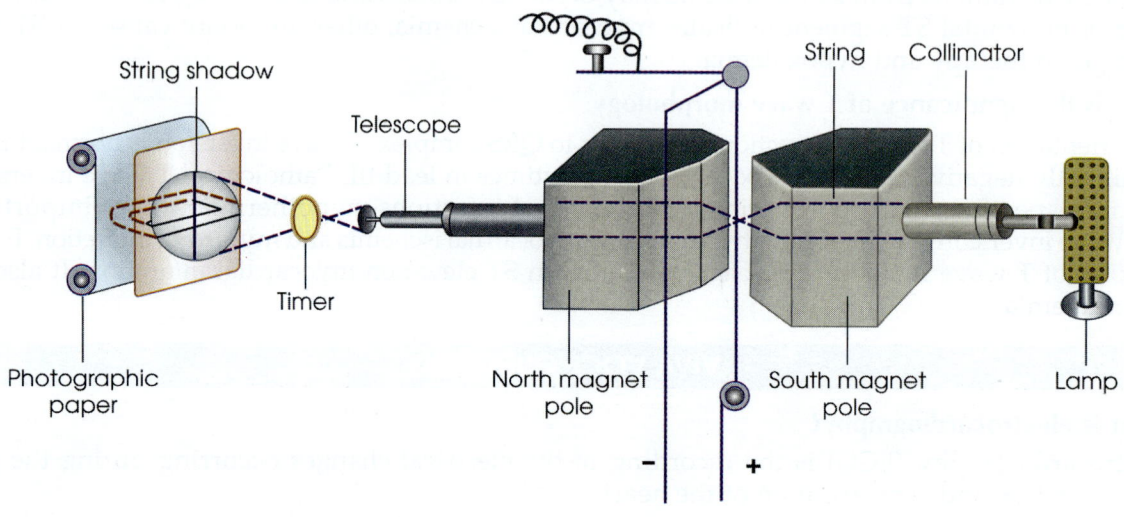

Clinical Perspective

Indications for Performing an ECG Include

1. Irregular heart rate or palpitations.
2. Chest pain.
3. Increased heart rates (>100 bpm).

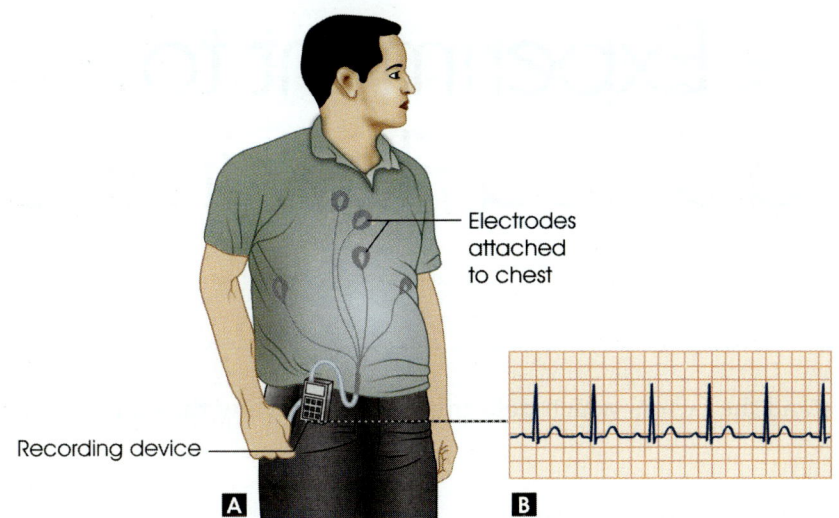

Electrodes attached to chest

Recording device

A   B

4. Decreased heart rates (<50 bpm).
5. To diagnose ventricular hypertrophy.
6. To evaluate conduction system blocks, myocardial infarction and drug effects, etc.
7. Chest trauma where cardiac injury is suspected, for example, blunt trauma to the chest (as might occur when a pedestrian is struck by car).
8. Pre-operative assessment of at-risk patients (for example, the elderly, patients of hypertension, diabetes mellitus, renal diseases, metabolic disorders, etc).

It is an invasive method to evaluate cardiac function.

OBSERVATIONS: EXERCISE FOR STUDENTS

....

....

....

....

....

....

....

....

....

....

....

8

Experiment to Record Blood Flow in the Arm

PY 5.16*

Learning Objective

Students should understand the factors which determine the blood flow through a part of the body.

Aim of the Experiment

Demonstration of recording blood flow in the arm.

Principal

If the venous return from the organ is stopped and arterial flow is allowed to continue the volume of the organ increases. The rate of change of volume is equal to the inflow of blood. The initial steady rate of change of volume before the venous pressure has risen much is taken to be equal to the normal rate of blood flow through the organ.

The part through which blood flow is to be determined is enclosed in plethysmograph. Part increases in volume and transducer system. The venous return is stopped by inflating the BP cuff placed proximal to the part and pressure is kept 50–60 mmHg applied for 30 sec. Increase in volume is recorded on a chart paper.

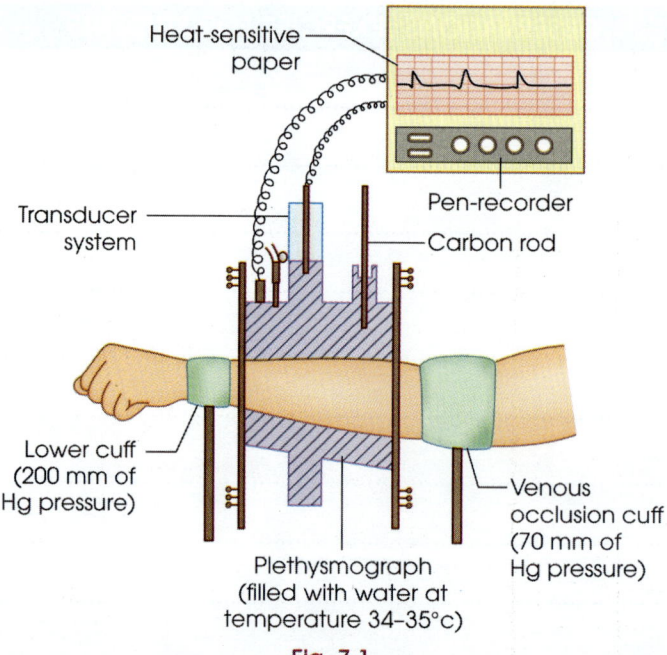

Fig. 7.1

---

*Competency achievement as per competency based Undergraduate Curriculum for the Indian Medical Graduate, 2018, 1; Medical Council of India.

Instrument

As shown in the figure is:

Water tight chamber, volume transducer, sphygmomanometer, recording equipment kymograph or recorder on a heat sensitive paper

Procedure

The arm is enclosed in the chamber filled with water at near the body temperature. The pressure in the proximal cuff enclosing the arm is raised to about 60–70 mm of Hg so that it is below the systolic blood pressure but obstructs the venous outflow from the part, the distal cuff also enclosing the arm distally is used to raise pressure to about 200 mmHg so that it is above the systolic pressure to prevent the outflow of the blood from the area of the arm enclosed into part distal to the enclosed area. The pulse wave may be seen on the record. The volume of the arm increases with blood flowing into this area and the change in volume of the arm increases the total volume in the chamber, this is recorded through the volume transducer system on an electronic recording system consisting of pen recorder on a heat sensitive paper. The blood flow can be calculated/estimated with this device.

The cuff pressure of 60 mm of Hg is sufficient to occlude the veins completely and being less than systolic pressure as well as diastolic pressure the arterial blood flow continues, the veins being capacitance vessels accommodate larger quantity of blood and the volume of the arm increases proportional to the arterial blood flow.

Precautions

If the flow is allowed to continue the venous pressure increases to a point where it equalizes and overcomes the cuff pressure. At this point there is some amount of venous outflow but less than arterial inflow, the volume of arm still would increase but this stage does not truly represent the blood flow as the venous occlusion becomes incomplete.

VIVA VOCE QUESTIONS

Q1. Define plethysmography.

Ans. Plethysmograph is an instrument for measuring changes in volume within an organ or whole body.

Q2. Describe the Principal of venous occlusion plethysmography.

Ans. When the venous drainage from the arm is briefly interrupted but arterial flow is unaltered and blood can enter the arm but cannot escape, volume of the closed system increases and increase is detected.

OSPE

Q1. What are the factors on which the blood flow through an organ or part of the body depends?

Ans. *The mean blood flow to an area depends on three factors:*

1. The total cross-sectional area of the vascular bed in that part.
2. The degree of vasodilatation or vasoconstriction of the vessels at that time.
3. Depends on the metabolism of the part.

Q2. Define cardiac output.

Ans. Output of each ventricle per minute is known as cardiac output.

Q3. How much is cardiac output in a resting adult person?

Ans. Cardiac output in an adult resting supine person is about 5 liters per minute. Stroke volume is about 70 ml per beat and with heart rate of 70 per minute the cardiac output would be equal to 70 × 70 = 4900 ml per minute = About 5 liters per minute.

Q4. What is meant by cardiac index?

Ans. Cardiac output divided by surface area is called cardiac index.

Q5. **Give normal value of cardiac index.**

Ans. Cardiac output divided by surface area of the person is called cardiac index. Hence in an individual with cardiac output of 5 L per minute with his surface area of 1.73 sqm it would be equal to 5 L per min/ 1.73 sqm = 3.2 liters per minute per square metre of body surface.

Q6. **What is the average normal blood flow to the coronary circulation under resting conditions?**

Ans. Coronary blood flow at rest in humans is about 250 ml/min 5% of the cardiac output.

HISTORICAL UPDATES

Changes in forearm volume are measured by a plethysmograph. Initially, air and then water-filled jackets were used, but these have been largely replaced by mercury-in-rubber (or silastic) strain gauges, which may themselves be ultimately replaced by indium-gallium gauges due to concerns over the potential toxicity of mercury. The strain gauges should be placed around the widest part of the forearm, and simply act as resistors. Changes in forearm volume result in a corresponding change in arm circumference and thus strain gauge length, which can be detected as an alteration in electrical resistance of the gauge, and thus potential difference. If the gauge length is made equal to the resting circumference of the limb, then changes in limb volume are directly proportional to the changes in resistance.

Venous occlusion plethysmography provides a measure of blood flow to that part of the forearm enclosed by the two cuffs. This is usually expressed as ml per 100 ml of forearm volume per minute, when electronic calibration is employed. Actual forearm volume can be estimated by calculation, assuming the forearm is a simple truncated cone, or by simple water displacement. When studies are conducted in a quiet, temperature-controlled room (22–26°C) with the subject resting in a comfortable supine position, measurement of FBF by strain gauge venous occlusion plethysmography compares favourably with values obtained by other established techniques. More recently, strain gauges employing a nonelastic loop attached to a passive inductive transducer, which acts as an electromagnetic sensor, have been developed and appear to be at least as accurate as mercury gauges.

ALTERNATIVE TO PLETHYSMOGRAPHY

Blood flow can also be measured using ultrasound. Usually this involves combining estimates of mean blood velocity with the cross sectional area of the vessel. Doppler ultrasound is used to estimate the mean blood velocity.

OBSERVATIONS: EXERCISE FOR STUDENTS

....

....

....

....

....

....

....

....

....

....

....

....

....

Spirometry—Measurement of Lung Volume and Capacities and Recording Peak Expiratory Flow PY 6.8* AND PY 6.10*

Learning Objectives

The students should be able to understand the procedure of spirometry for recording of vital capacity, timed vital capacity and other lung volumes and capacities. Spirometer is used to evaluate lung volumes and capacities which is helpful in diagnosis of respiratory disorders. It should be able to evaluate the type of respiratory disorder (obstructive or restrictive) from the findings. Though the prime aim of teaching this practical is to determine vital capacity and timed vital capacity, the normal lung volumes are also discussed for better understanding of the applied respiratory physiology. In patients of respiratory disease serial measurements of ventilator functions are important tool to assess the progress of the disease. Tests are also important for studying the efficacy of therapeutic measures as the change can be quantitatively measured.

Abnormal values are obtained not only in diseases of cardiorespiratory systems but also in neuromuscular, skeletal and metabolic disorders which decrease the overall efficiency of the body functions.

AIM of Experiment

1. Determination of tidal volume. Inspiratory capacity, expiratory reserve volume, vital capacity and timed vital capacity in the given subject. The graphical record which is obtained is called spirogram.
2. Determine the effect of posture on vital capacity.
3. Determination of peak expiratory flow rate.

Experiment I: Apparatus Required

Spirometer and a nose clip. Antiseptic solution.

SPIROMETER (Fig. 9.1)

The spirometer is a double-walled cylindrical chamber containing water between the two cylinders. An inverted cylinder of light metal dips into this water from above. The top of the inverted cylinder (bell) carries a hook to which is attached a chain which passes over a pulley. The other end of the chain carries a counter weight with a pen that moved up an down as the volume of air in the bell decreases or increases. These excursions of the pen on the kymograph paper are the permanent record of the respiratory excursions. The subject is connected to the spirometer through a mouthpiece. There is an inlet for filling oxygen into the chamber as well as another opening for putting water.

The paper on the kymograph drum is calibrated for time as well as volume. This is helpful in calculating timed vital capacity as well as mid-expiratory flow rates.

Method

Recording of Lung Volumes and Capacities

The subject is asked to sit comfortably.

1. After familiarizing the subject with the mouthpiece; close the nostril of the subject with nose clip.
2. Ask the subject to breathe from the atmosphere for 1–2 minutes.
3. Turn the three-way connector (not shown in Fig. 9.1) so that the subject can breathe the air under the spirometer bell.

---

*Competency achievement as per competency based Undergraduate Curriculum for the Indian Medical Graduate, 2018, 1; Medical Council of India.

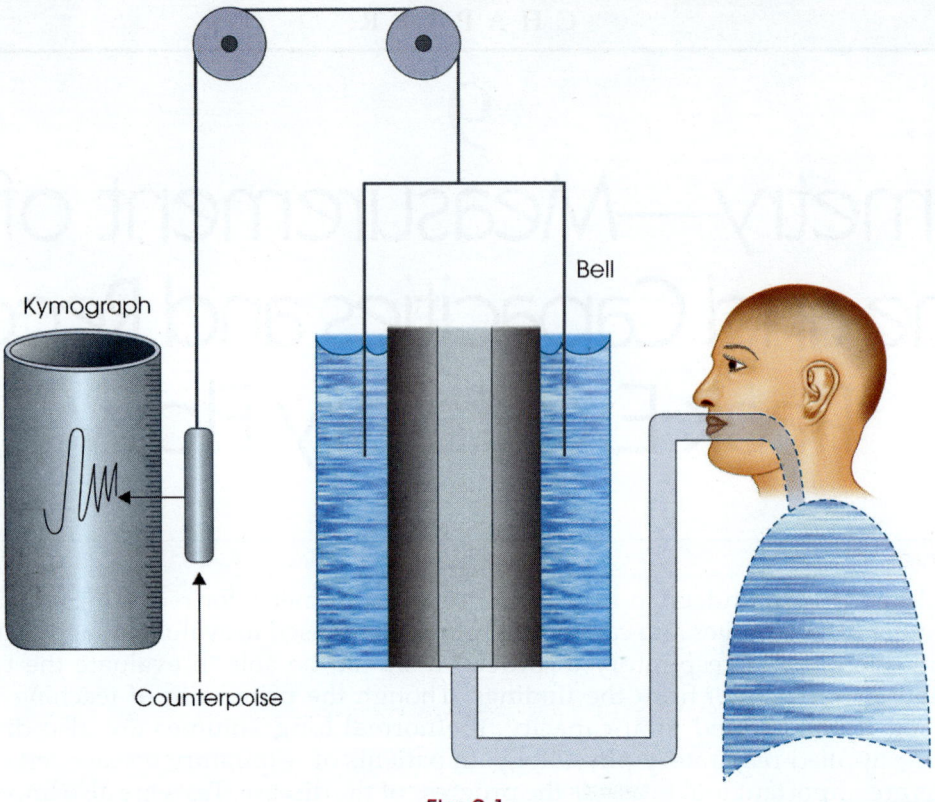

Fig. 9.1

4. Adjust the spirometer speed at 2 mm/second.

5. Record the normal breathing for a minute to calculate the tidal volume, the respiratory rate, and the resting pulmonary ventilation.

6. The subject should be asked to take a maximal inspiration after a normal expiration and the tracing for the same is recorded. Calculate the inspiratory capacity and the inspiratory reserve volume from the graph.

7. Ask the subject to make maximal expiration following normal inspiration. Use this to compute the expiratory reserve volume.

8. Ask the subject to make a maximal expiration after a maximal inspiration. This gives the vital capacity. Take 3 readings.

9. Next speed of the spirometer is set at the rate of 20 mm per second.

10. Ask the subject to take a maximal inspiration and then to make a maximal expiration quickly. Record this to compute timed vital capacity (forced expiratory volume: FEV).

11. Calculate the volume of air expired in 1st, 2nd and 3rd seconds. This will give the FEV_1, FEV_2, and FEV_3. Express these volumes as a percentage of the vital capacity.

Observations

Attach your graph paper and record.

Tidal volume   .... ml

Inspiratory capacity   .... ml

Inspiratory reserve volume   .... ml

Expiratory reserve volume   .... ml

Vital capacity   1.   2.

FEV1   .... ml   .... % of VC

Result any abnormal finding.

GRAPH

Q1. Study the graph and define the various lung volumes and capacity as shown in the graph.

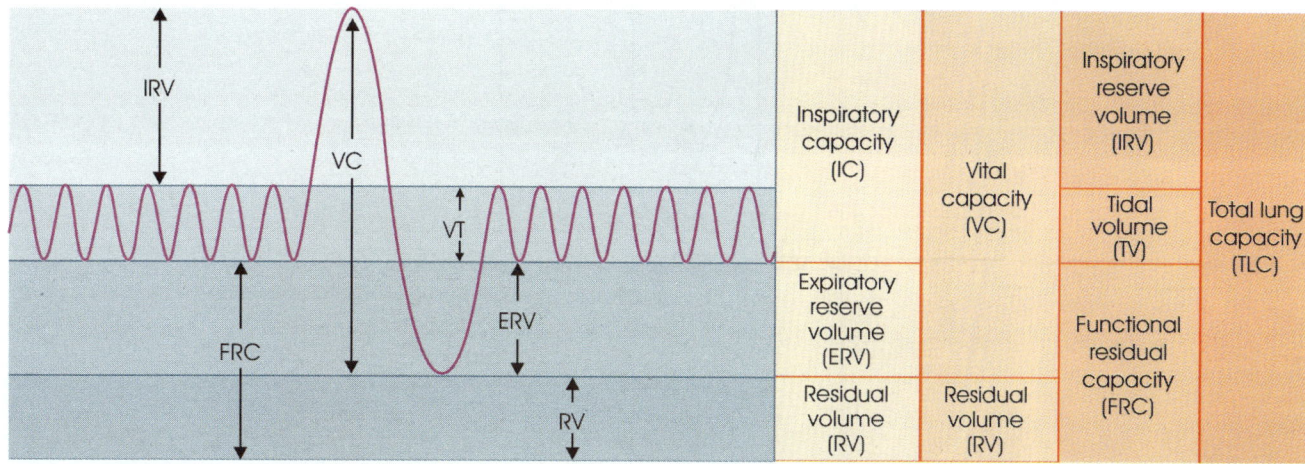

Ans. *The various lung volumes as shown in the graph are:*
- **Tidal volume (TV):** It is the amount of air inspired (or expired) during normal, relaxed breathing. It is about 500 ml.
- **Inspiratory reserve volume (IRV):** It is the maximum amount of air which can be inhaled after a normal tidal volume. It is about 1100 ml.
- **Expiratory reserve volume (ERV):** It is the maximum amount of air which can be exhaled after the expiration of a normal tidal volume. It is about 1200 ml.
- **Residual volume (RV):** It is the volume of air still remaining in the lungs after the expiratory reserve volume is exhaled. It is about 1200 ml.

Summing specific lung volumes produce the following lung capacities:
- **Total lung capacity (TLC):** It is the maximum volume of air present in the lungs (TLC = TV + IRV + ERV + RV). It is about 6000 ml.
- **The vital capacity (VC):** About 4,800 ml, it is the total amount of air that can be expired after fully inhaling (VC = TV + IRV + ERV = approximately 80 percent TLC). The value varies according to age, sex and body size.
- **Inspiratory capacity (IC):** It is the maximum amount of air that can be inspired (IC = TV + IRV). It is about 3600 ml.
- **The functional residual capacity (FRC):** It is the amount of air remaining in the lungs after a normal expiration (FRC = RV + ERV). It is about 2400 ml.

Q2. Describe the indicators of timed vital capacity.

Ans. The important indicators of timed vital capacity are FVC, FEV_1 and FEV 1%.

Forced Vital Capacity (FVC)

Forced vital capacity (FVC) is the volume of air that can forcibly be blown out after full inspiration. It is measured in liters.

Forced Expiratory Volume in 1 Second (FEV_1)

FEV_1 is the volume of air that can forcibly be blown out in one second, after full inspiration (Fig. 9.2).

FEV_1/FVC Ratio (FEV 1%)

FEV_1/FVC (FEV 1%) is the ratio of FEV_1 to FVC. In healthy adults it is approximately 75–80%. FEV_1 is diminished in cases of increased airway resistance to expiratory flow in obstructive diseases (asthma, COPD, chronic bronchitis, emphysema). In restrictive diseases (such as pulmonary fibrosis), the FEV_1 and FVC are both reduced proportionally and the value may be normal or even increased as a result of decreased lung compliance.

A derived value of FEV 1% is defined as FEV 1% of the patient divided by the average FEV 1% in the population for any person of similar age, sex and body composition.

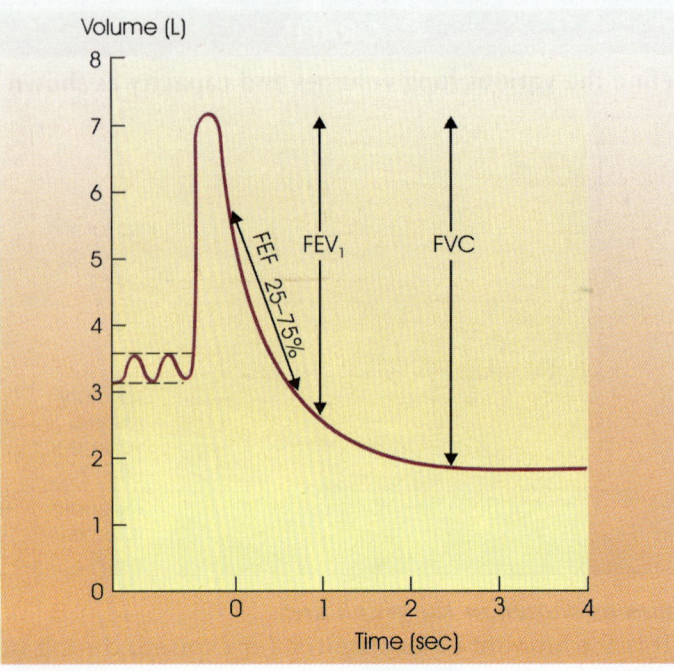

Fig. 9.2

Q1. Record your forced vital capacity (FVC).
A. Asked the subject to take deep breath, and then exhale into the sensor as hard as possible. (Yes/No)
B. The soft nose clips used to pinch the noise to prevent air escaping through the nose. (Yes/No)
C. Observing manoeuvre of subject ensuring that makes full and forceful exhalation. (Yes/No)
D. Noted the reading of the spirometer. (Yes/No)

Q1. Define vital capacity.
Ans. Vital capacity is the maximum amount of air a person can expel from the lungs after a maximum inhalation. It is equal to the sum of inspiratory reserve volume, tidal volume, and expiratory reserve volume.

Q2. What is the range for normal adult vital capacity?
Ans. A normal adult has a vital capacity between 3 and 5 litres.

Q3. Which device is used for measuring lung volume and capacity?
Ans. The lung volume and capacity can be measured using a device known as a spirometer.

Q4. Define functional residual capacity (FRC).
Ans. Functional residual capacity (FRC) is the volume of air that remains in the lungs during quite breathing. FRC = ERV + RV.

Q5. Which are the conditions in which restrictive lung disease occur?
Ans. The conditions in which restrictive lung disease occur are fibrosing alveolitis, severe scoliosis, ankylosing spondylitis, and even in weakness of the respiratory muscles (e.g. myasthenia gravis, Guillain-Barré syndrome and phrenic nerve palsy).

Clinical Perspective

Spirometry is indicated in for diagnosis and management of asthma, detection of respiratory disease in patients presenting with symptoms of breathlessness, measuring bronchial responsiveness in patients suspected of having asthma, diagnosis and differentiation between obstructive lung disease and restrictive lung disease, assessment of impairment from occupational asthma and conducting pre-operative risk assessment before anesthesia or cardiothoracic surgery.

TO STUDY THE EFFECT OF POSTURE ON VITAL CAPACITY

Aim: To study effect of posture on vital capacity.

Apparatus: Spirometer, nose clip, mouthpiece, antiseptic solution.

Spirometer: It is a double-walled cylindrical chamber containing water between two cylinders. An inverted cylinder of light metal dips into this water from above (Bell). Bell carries a hook to which a metal chain is attached, which passes over a pulley. Bell is counterbalanced by a weight. Pulley over which chain passes is converted into a scale graduated in litres. Movements of bell are recorded by a pointer passing over graduated scale (Fig. 9.3).

Procedure

Spirometer is filled with water.

Subject—made to stand facing spirometer.

Bring the bell to its lowest position by gently pushing it down; adjust pointer needle at zero.

After breathing normally for a minute, inspire deeply and fully.

Then after closing the nostrils with thumb and finger or with nose clip and mouthpiece held firmly between the lips exhale the air with maximum effort forcefully.

Note the reading on the spirometer scale.

Take 3 reading in standing posture and again 3 readings in sitting and 3 readings in lying position.

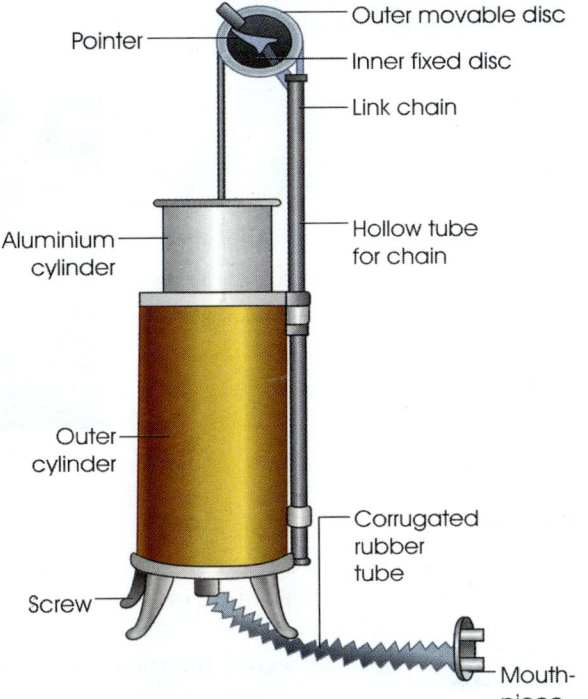

Fig. 9.3

Observations

Vital capacity:

Posture	1.	2.		
Standing	....	....	....	....
Sitting	....	....	....	....
Lying down	....	....	....	....

Result: Vital capacity is higher on standing

Q1. Give reasons why vital capacity is more in standing postion.

Ans. 1. Decrease in the thoracic blood volume enlarging the air space.
2. The abdominal viscera fall away from the diaphragm due to the effect of gravity bringing downward movement to the maximum. This ensure maximum space for air entry.

PEAK FLOW METER   (PY 5–10)

The peak expiratory flow (PEF), also called peak expiratory flow rate (PEFR), is a person's maximum speed of expiration, as measured with a peak flow meter, a small, hand-held device used to monitor a person's ability to breathe out air. It measures the airflow through the airways and thus the degree of obstruction in the airways. Peak expiratory flow is typically measured in units of liters per minuts (L/min)

To Measure Peak Expiratory Flow Rate

Principal:

Peak flow meter measures the maximum flow rate which is achieved during a single forced expiration. It does not measure the volume of air exhaled.

Reading on the apparatus is the PEFR in litres/min.

Aim of the Test

To determine the peak expiratory flow rate of the subject

Equipment:

Peak flow meter (Fig. 9.4).

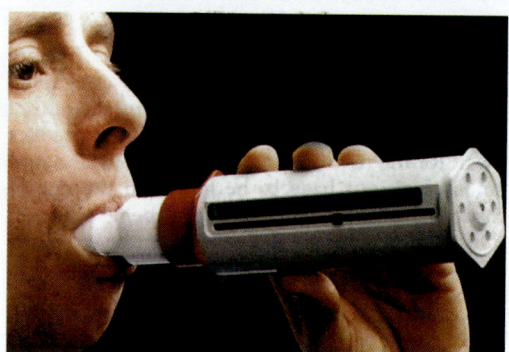

Fig. 9.4: Peak flow meter

Procedure

Ask the subject to take a deep breath and then to blow hard into the mouth piece of the flow meter forcefully with his nostrils closed. The reading on the dial apparatus is the PEFR in litres/min. Repeat the procedure thrice at an interval of 1–2 minutes.

Take 5 reading and record the mean of the 3 highest readings.

Observations:

1. ....
2. ....
3. ....
4. ....
5. ....

The maximal reading is taken as the result.

Result

....

....

....

....

Normal range is 300–500 litres/minute in an average adult.

Clinical Perspective

1. Measurement of PEFR requires training to correctly use a meter and the normal expected value depends on the patient's sex, age, and height. It is classically reduced in obstructive lung disorders such as **asthma**.
2. Peak flow readings are higher when patients are well, and lower when the airways are constricted. From changes in recorded values, patients and doctors may determine the severity of asthma symptoms, and treatment.
3. Due to the wide range of 'normal' values and the high degree of variability, peak flow is not the recommended test to **identify asthma**. However, it can be useful in some.
4. People with **asthma** may benefit from regular peek flow monitoring. When monitoring is recommended, it is usually done in addition to reviewing asthma symptoms and frequency of reliever medication use.
5. It is important to use the same peak flow meter every time
6. Flow is being monitored regularly, the results may be recorded on a peak flow chart.

PEAK FLOW RATE (PFR)

Although spirometer tests have the advantage that a permanent record is obtained, their big disadvantage is that the apparatus is not very portable. a simple and portable device, the wright peak flow meter is very useful in mass surveys of lung function and as a screening test in suspected obstructive airways disease.

This device make use of a single forced expiration. This differs from other tests of this kind in that, instead of measuring the volume expired in a given time, it measures the maximum flow rate or peak flow.

HISTORY

John Hutchinson

John Hutchinson (1811–1861 A.D), a surgeon, had begun his work with spirometers. He invented the spirometer to measure vital capacity and he believed it to be a powerful indicator of longevity. His spirometer consisted of a calibrated bell inverted in water, which captured exhaled air from the lungs. Hutchinson recorded the vital capacities of over 4000 persons with his spirometer. Hutchinson's water spirometer is still used today with a few alterations, which include the reduction of the mass of the bell and the addition of graphic and timing devices.

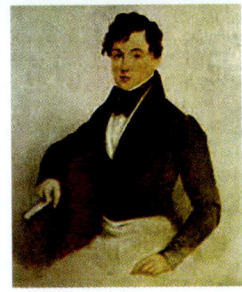

Recent Updates

The spirometry test is performed using a computerized device called a computerized spirometer.

Procedure

The patient is asked to take the deepest breath, and then exhale into the sensor completely. During the test, soft nose clips may be used to prevent air escaping through the nose. Sterilized filter mouthpieces must be used to prevent the spread of any infection. The computerized readings are obtained for lung capacity.

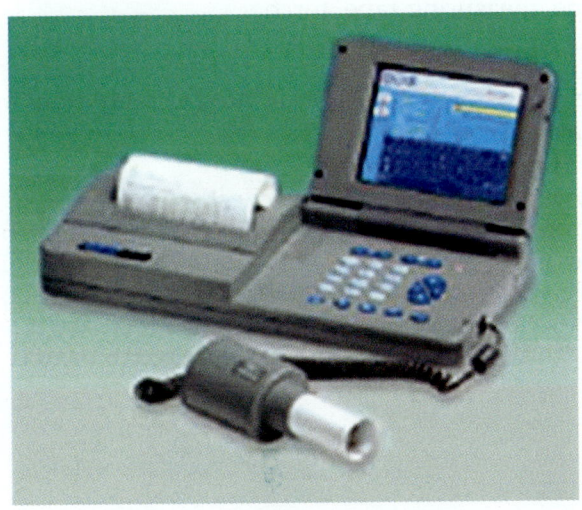

Fig. 9.5

Limitations of Test

The maneuver is dependent on patient cooperation and effort, and is normally repeated at least three times to ensure reproducibility. As results are dependent on patient cooperation, FVC can only be underestimated, never overestimated.

OBSERVATIONS: EXERCISE FOR STUDENTS

....
....
....
....

Clinical Examination of the Respiratory System

PY 6.9*

Learning Objective

The students should be able to understand the importance of findings of inspection, palpation, percussion and auscultation of respiratory system and co-relate it with associated respiratory disorders.

This examination is performed on every patient that is admitted to hospital and regularly in clinics and general practice.

Instruments required: Stethoscope, measuring tape, torch.

Method

Position of the patient: The subject in whom respiratory system is being examined is asked to sit comfortably on chair or may lie supine on examination couch:

1. Ensure adequate lighting is available in the room.
2. The subject is asked to remove the clothing over the chest.
3. Perform the general clinical examination in the individual noting his pulse, body temperature, blood pressure, count respiratory rate (as described below), assess jugular venous pressure, inspect hands for any pallor, cyanosis, clubbing if any, inspect for oedema, or any lymphadenopathy, ptosis and miosis.
4. The respiratory examination is carried out in four different stages:
   a. Inspection
   b. Palpation
   c. Percussion
   d. Auscultation.

Inspection

Inspect the chest from the front, back, along the mid-axillary line and over the shoulders and note for:

A. **Shape and deformity of the chest:** The normal chest is bilaterally symmetrical and elliptical in cross section. Observe for any kyphosis (abnormal anterior-posterior curvature of the spine), Scoliosis (abnormal lateral curvature of the spine), pectus excavatum (sternum sunken into the chest), pectus carinatum (sternum protruding from the chest) or barrel shape of chest.

B. **Respiratory rate:** Count the respiratory rate and look for regularity of the rhythm. Holding the patient hand and continuing conversation with patient enquiring their health profile the respiratory moments can be observed and respiratory rate counted. This will not make the patient aware and conscious, otherwise voluntary efforts by patient in nervousness may alter the rate.

C. **Type of respiration:** Note whether the respiration is abdomino-thoracic (seen in men and young children) or thoraco-abdominal (seen in women).

D. **Chest expansion:** Note the degree of the chest expansion and whether it is similar on both sides of the chest.

E. **Position of trachea:** Normally the trachea is central or slightly deviated to the right.

---

*Competency achievement as per competency based Undergraduate Curriculum for the Indian Medical Graduate, 2018, 1; Medical Council of India.

Palpation

1. Palpate and confirm the position of the trachea and the apex beat.
2. Measure the chest expansion using a measuring tape. (Normally the chest get expanded by 5 cm or more during inspiration).
3. Compare the chest expansion on both sides. Place the palm of both hands on either side of the chest of the subject and touch the tips of the two thumbs in the midline in front as well as at the back of the chest. The subject should be asked to take a deep breath and the distance of displacement of the thumbs from the midline is noted and this indicates the extent of expansion.
4. Vocal fremitus—it refers to vibrations setup by the voice which is conducted from the larynx through the trachea, bronchi and lung tissue to the chest wall. This is detected by placing the hand of the examiner on the chest. The patients/individuals are asked to repeat "ninety nine" continuously. Place the ulnar border of your palm on corresponding areas on both sides of the subject's chest and compare the vibration set up by the voice. Vocal fremitus is decreased in pleural effusion and increased in consolidation.

Percussion

It is done to compare the degree of resonance over corresponding areas on either sides of the chest. The degree of resonance may differ in different parts of the chest wall. It is most resonant below the scapulae posteriorly and clavicles anteriorly.

Percussion is Performed as Follows (Fig. 10.1)

Place the middle finger of the left hand (Pleximeter) firmly on the part to be percussed and strike the back of its middle phalanx perpendicularly with the tip of the middle finger of your right hand. The percussing finger needs to be bent so that its terminal phalanx is at right angles and it strikes the pleximeter finger exactly perpendicular.

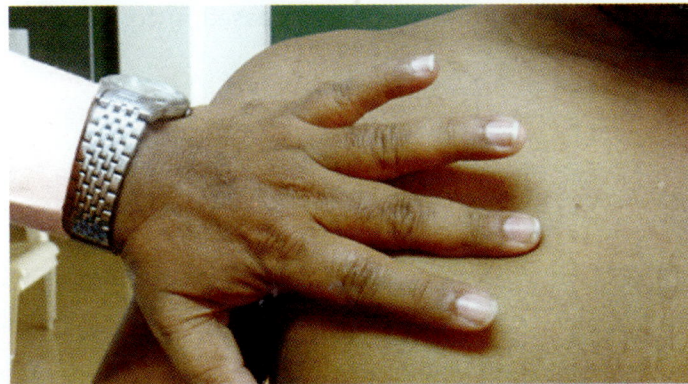 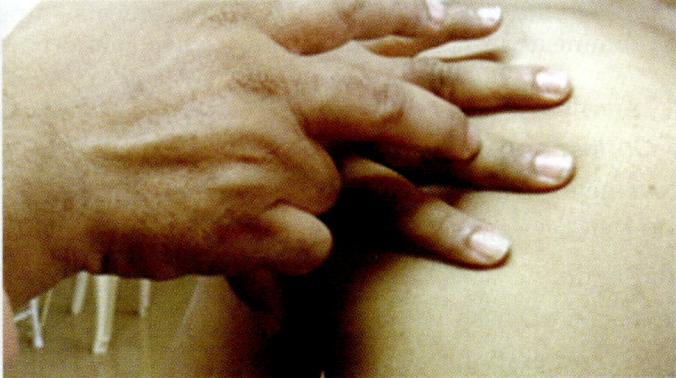

Fig. 10.1

Photograph—Demonstration of Percussion

Rules for Percussion

1. The stroke should be promptly made by movement at the wrist.
2. The long axis of the pleximeter finger should be parallel to the edge of the organ being percussed.
3. Percussion should be done from more resonant to a less resonant area.

The students should do percussion all areas of the chest keeping the pleximeter finger in the intercostals spaces. Ask the subject to keep his hand over the head while percussing the sides of the chest. Ask the subject to cross his arms in front as you percuss the back of the chest. Lung resonance is impaired in consolidation and fibrosis of the lung. The resonance is stony dull in pleural effusion. Lung resonance is increased in pneumothorax.

Auscultation

Auscultation is being performed all over the chest and the auscultatory findings of two sides are compared.

The following points are to be noted:

Character of the breath sounds: (Figure 10.2) There are two typical types of breath sounds **vesicular and bronchial.** Vesicular breath sounds are produced by the passage of air in and out of normal lung tissue and are heard all over

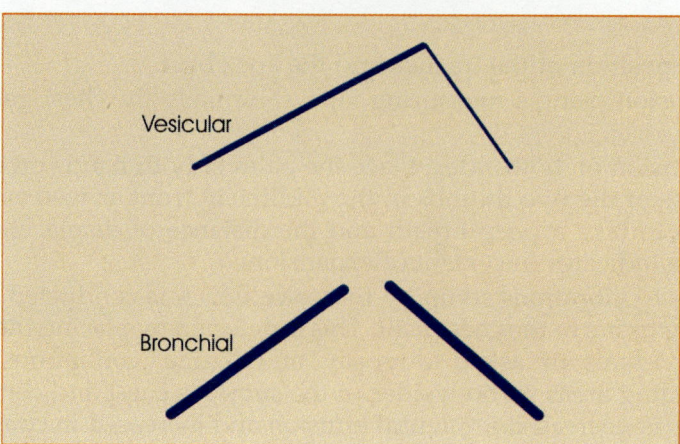

Fig. 10.2

the chest under normal conditions. The **vesicular breathing** is low pitched and rustling in character. The inspiratory sound is intense and audible during the whole of inspiration. The expiratory sound follows the inspiration without a distinct pause. The inspiratory sound is heard for a time twice as long as the expiratory sound. **Bronchial breath** sounds are produced by the passage of air through the trachea and large bronchi. This inspiratory sound is moderately intense and becomes inaudible before the end of inspiration. The expiratory sound is more intense and the duration extends through the greater part of expiration.

Vocal Resonance

Auscultate the chest each time the subject repeats "ninety nine". (Vocal resonance is increased in consolidation and diminished in pleural thickening, effusion and pneumothora).

Observations

1. On Inspection

Movements of chest

Shape and symmetry of chest

RR, Rhythm

Expansion of chest

Type of respiration

2. On Palpation

Position of trachea

Position of apex beat

Expansion of chest

Vocal fremitus

3. On percussion

Type of percussion note and intensity

4. On auscultation

Breath sounds and character

Vocal resonance

Abnormal sound found in disease states:

Wheeze: These are continuous musical sound on expiration or inspiration. A wheeze results of narrowed airways. It is commonly heard in patients of asthma and emphysema.

Rhonchi: They are characterized by low pitched, musical bubbly sounds heard on inspiration and expiration. Rhonchi are heard due to the presence of viscous fluid in the airways.

Crackles: This is an intermittent, non-musical and brief sounds heard during inspiration only. These are the result of sudden opening of alveoli due to increased air pressure during inspiration. This is seen in patients of congestive cardiac failure.

Stridor is a high-pitched musical breath sound resulting from turbulent air flow in the larynx or lower in the bronchial tree. The common causes are typically obstructive such as foreign body in airway.

VIVA VOCE QUESTIONS

Q1. What is normal respiratory rate?

Ans. Normal rate in a relaxed adult is 12–18 breaths per minute.

Q2. What is tachypnoea?

Ans. Increased rate of respiration in tachypnoea.

Q3. What is dyspnoea?

Ans. It is a symptom of breathlessness experienced by the patient.

Q4. Name the muscles of inspiration.

Ans. Diaphragm, external intercostal muscles. Accessory inspiratory muscles are scalene and sternocleidomastoid.

Q5. Name the muscles of expiration.

Ans. Internal intercostal muscles and anterior abdominal wall muscles.

Q6. In a man of 150 pound weight has tidal volume of 500 ml and respiratory rate of 12 per minute. Calculate alveolar ventilation.

Ans. Dead space air is expected to be 150 ml (normally equal to body weight in pounds). Hence the alveolar ventilation is 500 – 150 ml = 350 ml multiplied by RR = 350 ml × 12 RR = 4200 ml per minute.

Q7. Is the alveolar ventilation more when there is deep breathing than in shallow breathing at the same respiratory minute volume?

Ans. In deep breathing alveolar ventilation is more than in shallow breathing at the same respiratory minute volume (RMV).

Q8. Name one condition in which vocal fremitus is increased and decreased.

Ans. Increased in consolidation. Decreased in pleural effusion.

Q9. What are wheeze and crackles?

Ans. Continous musical sound on inspration or expiration is wheeze; intermittent non-musical brief sound during inspiration is crackles.

Q10. What are normal breath sounds?

Ans. Vesicular and bronchial.

Q11. Explain the physiological basis of compliance.

Ans. The slope of the pressure-volume curve, the volume change per unit pressure is known as compliance. The compliance in case of the human lung is 0.15 L/cm H_2O.

Compliance is reduced in pulmonary edema and interstititial pulmonary fibrosis

In chronic obstructive pulmonary disease (COPD, e.g. emphysema) the alveolar walls progressively degenerate that increases the compliance.

Q12. Define anatomical dead space.

Ans. It is the volume of the conducting airways where no gas exchange takes place. It is approximately 150 ml in an adult approximately equal to body weight in pounds.

Q13. Define forced expiratory volume (FEV$_1$)?

Ans. It is the volume of air exhaled in one second by a forceful expiration following a full inspiration (FEV$_1$). The total volume of the air exhaled after a complete and full inspiration represents the vital capacity. However, this value may be slightly smaller than the vital capacity measured with slow (normal speed) expiration. Therefore, this value is called forced vital capacity (FVC). The normal ratio of the FEV$_1$ with that of forced vital capacity is 80%.

Q14. Define forced expiratory flow (FEF25–75).

Ans. This measurement represents the expiratory flow rate over the middle half of the FVC (between 25 and 75%); obtained by identifying the 25% and 75% volume points of FVC, measuring the time between these points and therewith calculating the flow rate.

Q15. Discuss the criterion of classifying lung diseases as restrictive or obstructive disorder.

Ans. The lung diseases can be classified as restrictive or obstructive. In restrictive lung diseases the vital capacity is reduced to below normal levels; however, the rate at which the vital capacity is forcefully exhaled is normal. In obstructive lung disease the vital capacity is normal because there is no lung tissue damage and its compliance is unchanged but the increased airway resistance makes expiration more difficult and takes longer time. Obstructive disorders are therefore diagnosed by tests that measure the rate of forced expiration. A significant decrease in FEV 1% and FEF 25–75% suggests an obstructive lung disease.

Q16. Define physiological dead space.

Ans. Physiological dead space (total dead space) is sum of the anatomical dead space and any alveolar dead space. In healthy state physiological and anatomical dead spaces are equal. In disease condition if some alveoli receive ventilation but no exchange takes place between the gas in the alveoli and the blood and some of alveoli may be overventilated, these form the alveolar dead space which adds to physiological dead space.

Q17. What is normal ventilation perfusion ratio in the whole lung and what are the differences in the ratio in various parts of lung?

Ans. Normal ventilation/perfusion ratio of whole lung at rest is 0.8 (4.2 l/min ventilation divided by 5.5 l/min blood flow). In upright position ventilation/perfusion ratio are high in upper portion of lungs.

OSCE NON-SKILLED QUESTIONS

Q1. Describe the various types of shapes of the chest.

Ans. The variation in chest shape types are kyphosis (abnormal anterior-posterior curvature of the spine), scoliosis (abnormal lateral curvature of the spine), pectus excavatum (sternum sunken into the chest), pectus carinatum (sternum protruding from the chest) and barrel shape of chest.

Q2. Describe the method for counting the respiratory rate.

Ans. The respiratory rate is an observational evaluation and should be meticulously calculated by carefully observing the moments of the chest.

Can be counted by placing hand over the abdomen.

> **Clinical Perspective**
>
> In clinical practice the respiratory examination is performed as part of a physical examination or when a patient presents with respiratory complaints such as shortness of breath, cough, chest pain, difficulty in breathing or a history that suggestive of pathology of the lung. The respiratory examination aims to pick up on any respiratory (breathing) pathology that may be causing a patient's symptoms, e.g. shortness of breath, cough, wheeze, etc. Common conditions include chest infections, asthma and chronic obstructive pulmonary disease (COPD).
>
> This examination is performed on every patient that is admitted to hospital and regularly in clinics and general practice.

HISTORICAL ASPECTS

Michael Servetus (1553)

The first description of the function of pulmonary circulation was made by Ibn al-Nafis in the year 1242 in Egypt but later more relevant details regarding it was stated by Michael Servetus (1553) and William Harvey (1616). Servetus was a medical student from 1536–38 at the University of Paris. He followed the well-known anatomist Hans Gunther as assistant in dissection practical studies. Gunther wrote that "Michael Villonovanus" had perfect knowledge of Galens work. Servetus later came to differ from Galen in the understanding of pulmonary circulation. Galen had supposed that the aeration of the blood takes place in the heart and lungs as a fairly minor function. Servetus concluded from his experimentation that the transformation of the blood, accomplished by the release of waste gases and the infusion of air, occurred in the lungs.

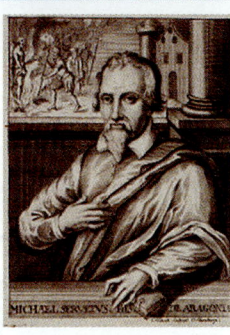

Recent Updates

Ventral respiratory group of neurons control inspiratory and expiratory muscles during exercise. Pre-Bötzinger complex is supposed location of central respiratory rhythm pattern generation circuitry. The pre-Bötzinger complex contains pacemaker cells which initiate spontaneous breathing. It is currently not known that how this system regulates its output to effect motor neuron bursting, which in turn is responsible for inspiratory muscle innervations. More research is required into the function of the pre-Bötzinger complex.

OBSERVATIONS: EXERCISE FOR STUDENTS

....
....
....
....
....
....
....
....
....
....
....
....
....
....
....
....
....

Stethography Recording of Respiratory Movements

PY 3.15*

Learning Objective

After learning the practical students should be able to:

Explain the physiological basis of changes observed in the respiratory movements after voluntary hyperventilation, with deglutition, exercise and of breaking point after breath holding.

Aim of Experiment

Record the normal respiratory movements in an individual and study the changes with voluntary hyperventilation, deglutition and exercise.

Measure the breath holding time.

Stethography is the process of recording of respiratory movements. The instrument used for recording of respiratory movements is called stethograph and the record obtained is called stethogram.

APPARATUS

1. **Kymograph:** It is a recording drum.
2. **Stethograph:** It consists of a corrugated rubber tube, with a metallic chain with a hook at its end, attached to the closed end of the stethograph, which is for tying the instrument around the human chest. There is a side tube to transmit pressure variations for recording.

Marey's tambour: The tambour is a flat saucer-shaped apparatus with its top occluded by a rubber membrane diaphragm. To the bottom is fixed a metal tube which connects with the stethograph through a pressure tubing. A pointer sits on the rubber diaphragm to record its excursions.

PROCEDURE

1. Ask the volunteer subject to sit comfortably on a stool with back towards the recording apparatus.
2. Tie the stethograph around the chest of the subject at the level of the fourth intercostals space and connect the tambour to it (Fig. 11.1).
3. Bring the writing lever/pen in contact with the paper of the kymograph and set drum movement at slow speed (2.5 mm/sec).
4. Record normal respiration for about 5 cm.
5. Ask the subject to drink water and record the effect of deglutition on the respiratory movement. Take a normal tracing after that.
6. After a normal tracing ask the subject to hold his breath as long as possible after (a) quiet inspiration (b) after normal expiration and (c) following deep inspiration (d) following deep expiration and record the effects.
7. Record normal respiration and ask the subject to take deep breaths and as rapidly as possible (hyperventilation) for one and a half minute. Immediately after hyperventilation note the effects.
8. Again record normal respiration. Disconnect stethograph from Marey's tambour and then ask the subject to exercise (spot jogging) for one minute. Immediately after exercise, connect the stethograph to the kymograph and record the effect of exercise on respiratory movements.

---

*Competency achievement as per competency based Undergraduate Curriculum for the Indian Medical Graduate, 2018, 1; Medical Council of India.

Precautions

1. The subject should be sitting comfortably in upright position.
2. Tie the stethograph at the level of 4th intercostals space as the expansion of the chest is maximum at this level.
3. Normal tracings should be taken before and after the recordings for each maneuver

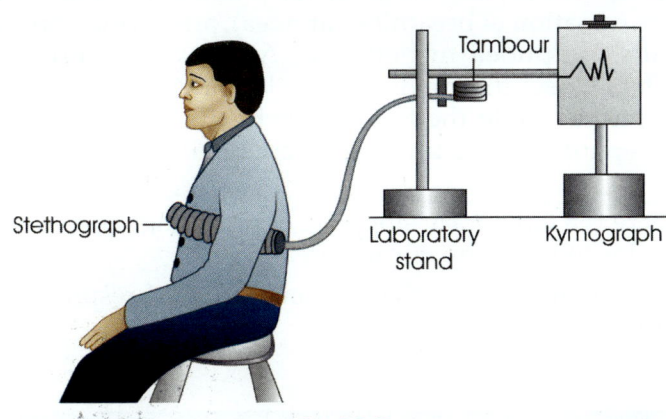

Fig. 11.1

Photograph—Respiratory Movements Being Recorded in a Subject

Observation

During inspiration the chest expands and the stethograph is stretched. The pressure inside the stethograph decreases, this fall in pressure is transmitted to the Marey's tambour. The rubber diaphragm is therefore pulled down causing a downward movement of the writing lever. During expiration recoil of the stethograph causes the reverse changes and therefore an upward movement of the writing lever. Thus down stroke in the tracing represents inspiration and upstroke, expiration.

1. During deglutition there is a temporary stoppage of breathing. This is called deglutition apnoea and is followed by normal breathing.
2. During voluntary hyperventilation, there is an increase in the rate and depth of respiration. This may be followed by a temporary cessation of breathing (apnoea) and then with a few breaths with decreasing duration of apnoea the normal breathing returns.
3. Breath holding time is recorded as a straight line. Note breath holding time up to breaking point. Repeat the procedure at the end of normal expiration. Maximum inspiration and maximum expiration and record the Breath holding time for each.
4. During exercise there is an increase in the rate and depth of respiration and after stopping exercise breathing gradually returns to normal.

Results

Breath holding at the end of	Time (sec)			Best value
	1st	2nd	3 rd	
Quiet inspiration				
Quiet expiration				
Deep inspiration				
Deep expiration				

Note your graphic observations:
Write the title of the experiment and label the various events recorded. Attach the graph.

OSPE NON-SKILLED

Q1. **Describe the changes seen in respiratory movements in voluntary hyperventilation, deglutition and exercise.**

Ans. *The changes seen in respiratory movements in voluntary hyperventilation, deglutition and exercise are:*

During voluntary hyperventilation, there is an increase in the rate and depth of respiration. This may be followed by a temporary cessation of breathing (apnoea), after which breathing returns to normal, there may be shorter peroids of apnoea in between. Apnoea is produced due to fall in PCO_2 with hyperventilation though PO_2 rises during hyperventilation. After apnoea there may be few breaths with decreasing periods of apnoea due to the fact that as breathing tends to resume due to fall of PO_2 but again due to low PCO_2 apnoea occurs till after a few breaths, normal breathing returns due to PCO_2 reaching normal level.

During deglutition there is a temporary stoppage of breathing. This is called deglutition apnoea and is a reflex phenomenon and is followed by normal breathing.

During exercise there is an increase in the rate and depth of respiration and after exercise breathing gradually returns to normal.

VIVA VOCE QUESTIONS

Q1. **Enlist the procedures for breathing movements and patterns.**

Ans. The breathing movements and patterns can be found out by stethography, magnetometers, respiratory inductive plethysmography, and optoelectronic plethysmography.

Q2. **What is deglutition apnoea?**

Ans. Stoppage of respiration with deglutition a reflex phenomenon.

Q3. **What is the effect of exercise on respiration?**

Ans. There is increase in rate and depth of respiration.

Q4. **What is the normal breath-holding time in adults?**

Ans. Breath-holding time after deep inspration is about 40–70 sec or more in an adult person.

Q5. **What is the physiological basis for breaking point?**

Ans. Breaking point is because of hypoxia and hypercapnea during breath holding.

Q6. **Mention the changes in respiration following hyperventilation.**

Ans. May show apnoea and after shorter peroids of apnoea in between breaths normal breathing returns.

Q7. **What is periodic breathing ? Give a few examples.**

Ans. Peroidic breathing is also called Cheyne-Stokes respiration, occurs in various diseases, most commonly in heart failure and uremia. Also occurs in brain disease, also in some normal individuals during sleep.

Q8. **What are the causes for abnormal patterns of breathing?**

Ans. The abnormal patterns of breathing are caused by injury to respiratory centres in pons and medulla, with use of narcotic medications, metabolic derangements and respiratory muscle weakness. The inspection of the pattern of breathing will often yield clues of the disease process.

CLINICAL PERSPECTIVE

A study of diaphragmatic and costal movements is important in the assessment of breathing capacity. Fluoroscopy can give a general idea of excursions of the diaphragm but by means of roentgen kymography it is possible to obtain an objective record of the respiratory movements of both the diaphragm and the ribs.

The physical assessment of breathing is mainly important for physical therapy evaluations. The impact of posture, age, and sex on breathing movements complicates these assessments.

HISTORICAL UPDATES

Leonardo da Vinci in 15th century explained the expansible nature of lung and opines that "The substance of the lung is dilatable and extensible like the tinder made from a fungus. But it is spongy and if you press it, yields to the force which compresses it, and if the force is removed, it increases again to its original size."

The record of respiratory movement was feasible after discovery of kymograph. A kymograph was invented by German Physiologist Carl Ludwig in year 1840. It is a device that gives a graphical representation of spatial position over time in which a spatial axis represents time. It was first use as a means to intrusively monitor blood pressure, and has found several applications in the field of medicine such as recording respiratory movements by process of stethography.

RECENT UPDATES

3-dimensional motion system are nowadays employed for recording breathing movements. It consists of 8 infrared cameras that track the movement trajectories of 14-mm passive markers attached to the thorax (chest wall), and abdominal wall. Cameras sample at a rate of 50 Hz. The motion analysis use optical and electromagnetic devices which permits accurate measurement of the kinematics of the chest and abdominal wall in various positions.

OBSERVATIONS: EXERCISE FOR STUDENTS

12

Determination of Physical Fitness of the Subject

PY 3.16*

Determination **of physical fitness** of the subject implies the ability to make adequate 'Physiological Adjustments' to the stresses imposed by a specific task. Good cardiorespiratory function as reflected by the ability to deliver oxygen to the tissues to maintain continuous activity is perhaps the single most important physiological factor in this respect.

There are a number of tests to measure physical fitness of the individual out of which the maximum oxygen intake test is considered to be the best single method for measuring the cardiorespiratory response to exercise. Treadmill exercise or exercise on bicycle ergometer is used to find out the maximum oxygen consumption while the expired air is collected in Douglas bag.

Tests have been designed so that maximum $VO_{2\,max}$ may be predicted by recording only the heart rate during and immediately after exercise. Pulse rate which is easy to measure coincides significantly with oxygen consumption during exercise. Response of the heart rate to increasing work rates is similar to the response of the body to requirement of oxygen. Maximum heart rate and maximum oxygen consumption are reached at approximately at the same time. The correlation has been employed successfully in a number of fitness tests.

Reasons for fitness tests are:
1. Providing basis for exercise prescription.
2. Evaluation of cardiorespiratory function.
3. Screening of coronary heart disease.

In the following experiment **heart rate during recovery** following a standard exercise will be used as a criterion of fitness of the individual. Test will be:
1. Simple step test for 3 minutes
2. Step design at Harvard.

Learning Objectives

1. Administer 3-minute step test and determine $VO_{2\,max}$ and provide percentile ranking of the subject from the table provided.
2. Calculate MET value from VO_2 max obtained from simple 3-minute step test.
3. Administer Harvard step test and determine physical fitness.

Procedure

Step test is used in assessing physical fitness.

Simple three minutes step test (McArnold, et al. 1981)

It is based on noting the heart rate recovery pattern over a fixed interval of time. In the first minute of exercise there is rapid increase in the heart rate which then levels off and remains fairly stable throughout the stepping period. The *recovery heart rate pattern* gives valuable information concerning the cardiorespiratory response to exercise. In the first minute the heart rate decreases rapidly. Thereafter the decline is more gradual and within two to three minutes depending on grade of exercise heart rate returns to the resting level.

*Competency achievement as per competency based Undergraduate Curriculum for the Indian Medical Graduate, 2018, 1; Medical Council of India.

EQUIPMENT REQUIRED

A stopwatch

Platform of required height

Metronome.

Conduction of the Test

The subject is asked to perform a four-step cadence up-up down-down (height of step 16 ½) women are asked to perform at a rate of 22 complete step ups per minute which can be regulated at 88 beats/min, using a metronome. For males this cadence is set at 24 steps/min or 96 beats on the metronome. Exercise is performed for 3 minutes. After the subject had completed the exercise, the subject is asked to remain standing and the heart rate is counted over a period of 15 sec, between 5–20 seconds after the cessation of exercise. It is converted into beats per minute (15 seconds heart rate × 4) and compared to percentile ranking as in Table 12.1.

Men: Max VO_2 in ml/kg/min = 111.33 – (0.42 × step test pulse rate, beats/min).

Women: Max VO_2 in ml/kg/min = 65.81 – (0.184 × step test pulse rate beats/min).

To simplify these conversions Table 12.1 gives the predicted maximal oxygen uptake, determined from this recovery rate. This predicted max VO_2 is within ±16% of max VO_2 of the person tested.

Table 12.1: Recovery heart rate (count between 5th, and 20th second X 4 = pulse rate) after simple 3-minute test and $VO_{2\ max}$. Read percentile for particular recovery pulse

Percentile ranking	Recovery HR (female)	Predicted max. VO_2 female (ml/kg/min)	Recovery HR (male)	Predicted max. VO_2 (ml/kg/min)
100	128	42.2	120	60.9
95	140	40.0	124	59.3
90	148	38.5	128	57.6
85	152	37.7	136	54.2
80	156	37.0	140	52.5
75	158	36.6	144	50.9
70	160	36.3	148	49.2
65	162	35.9	149	48.8
60	163	35.7	152	47.5
55	164	35.5	154	46.7
50	166	35.1	156	45.8
45	168	34.8	160	44.1
40	170	34.4	162	43.3
35	171	34.2	164	42.5
30	172	34.0	166	41.6
25	176	33.3	168	40.8
20	180	32.0	172	39.1
15	182	32.2	176	37.4
10	184	31.8	178	26.6
5	196	29.6	184	34.1

MET

MET is a unit for measurement of energy expenditure. One MET is equivalent to the resting oxygen consumption for an average man and women and it is approximately 230 and 200 ml per minute respectively. Work at two METs requires twice the resting metabolism or about 500 ml of oxygen per minute for a man and three MET is three times.

For more accurate classification the MET can be expressed in terms of oxygen consumption per unit of body weight with 1 MET equal to approximately 3.6 ml/kg/min. A young healthy subject can perform exercise work load of 8010 METS.

New York Heart Association has created functional classification method in conjunction with the exercise work load performed by a given patient. In this way each individual's/patient's functional capacity can be assessed. Healthy subjects more than 8 METS

Patients

Class I	6–8 METS
Class II	4–6 METS
Class III	2–3 METS
Class IV	1 MET

Harvard Step Test

Test was designed by Brouha, et al. (1943) in the Harvard Fatigue Laboratory during World War II. Test is simple to conduct and requires minimal equipment. There have been many variations of the test.

The test exposes the subject to a standard exercise test that one can perform in a "steady state" for more than a few minutes, it takes into account two factors: (1) The length of time the exercise can be sustained and (2) deceleration of the heart rate after exercise.

It consists of measuring the endurance in stepping up and down on a bench of standard height and the pulse response to this exercise.

Resource Required

Gym bench

Stopwatch

Assistant

Procedure

The subject should be in good physical condition. Ask to sit quietly for 5 minutes at least. Should be lightly clothed and wear rubber shoes or no shoes at all.

In the original test a 20 "step is used but to adjust to Indian standards it is lowered to 41 cm (16 ½").

The subject steps onto and down from a 41 cm platform 30 times a minute. At the signal 'start' the subject places one foot on the platform steps up, places other foot on the platform, straightens this legs and backbone and again steps down bringing the same foot that he placed up first. At a 2 sec interval the signal up is given. The subject should lead with the same foot each time and not alternate the foot. The observer has to call the rhythm by adjusting the metronome, and asking the subject to perform at the above rate. Subject performs the exercise as long as he can but not in excess of five minutes.

After the cessation of exercise record heart rate for 30 sec between one minute and one minute and thirty seconds.

Precautions

If the subject is dyspnoeic, or feels pain in the chest or in legs, or gets exhausted during the exercise period ask to discontinue the exercise immediately.

Observations

1. **Duration of exercise:** It is for five minutes or less ....
2. **Pulse rate:** Counted from 1 minute to 1½ minute after exercise. The count gives half minute value ....

Begin counting the time when the subject starts exercising and exercise him at a rate of 30 times a minute for five minutes continuously unless he stops before that from exhaustion. If he falls behind stop him after he has been unable to keep the pace for 20 seconds. In case he completes note the duration of the effort to the nearest second. In case he completes five minutes, he is asked to stop.

When the subject stops start counting the time and have him sit quietly on a chair. After exactly 1 minute count the number of heart beats for exactly 30 seconds.

Record the duration of effort and the number of heart beats in 30 seconds beginning after one minute after he stops.

The score depends on the above two values, the duration of exercise and pulse rate after the exercise. The score is obtained from the formula:

Index of fitness = (100 × test duration in seconds) divided by (5.5 × pulse count between 1 and 1.5 minutes).

Calculation

Fitness index: If the total test time was 300 sec (completed in 5 minutes) and the number of beats between 1 and 1.5 minutes was 90, taking the beats in 30 sec interval, not rate (beats per min). During this interval score would be:

Fitness index = (100 × 300) divided by (5.5 × pulse count between 1–1.5 sec) = 300 × 100 divided by 90 × 5.5 = 60

Long form of test can also be conducted. It requires measuring the pulse again from 2–2.5 minutes after finishing exercise and finally from 3–3.5 minutes after finishing exercise.

And then fitness index is calculated = 100 × duration of the test divided by 2 × sum of heart beats counted (in 1–1.5 sec + in 2–2.5 sec + in 3–3.5 sec).

The score ranges from 5 to 130. Interpretation is as:

Below 50 = Poor

50–80 = Average

Above 80 = Good

Validity: Correlation to direct V max O_2 has been reported between 0.6 and 0.8 in studies.

Advantages: The test requires minimal equipment and cost and can be self-administered.

Disadvantages: Biochemical characteristics vary between individuals, e.g. when the step height is standard, taller individuals are at advantage as it takes them less energy to step up into the step. Body weight is also a factor. Testing large group is also time consuming.

Observations

1. Simple 3-minute step test

Heart rate during recovery = (pulse rate from 5–20 sec × 4)

Fitness

MET value

2. Harvard step test

Duration

Pulse from 1 to 1 and ½ minute in recovery

Score from Table 12.2

Fitness grade.

Conclusions

1. The physical fitness of a person can be assessed using a simple test
2. Step test can be used on a large population in order to screen people before undertaking detailed tests.

Table 12.2: Scoring table for Havard step test

Instructions: (1) Find the appropriate line for duration of effort, (2) then find the appropriate column for the pulse counts, (3) read off the score where the line and column intersect and (4) interpret according to the scale given below:

Duration or effort	Heart beats for 1 minute to 1.5 minutes in recover										
	40–44	45–49	50–54	55–59	60–64	65–69	70–74	75–79	80–84	85–89	90–95
0–29′	5	5	5	5	5	5	5	5	5	5	5
0′ 30′–0″ 59″	20	15	15	15	15	10	10	10	10	10	10
1′ 0″–1′ 29″	30	30	25	25	20	20	20	20	15	15	15
1′ 30–1′ 59″	45	40	40	36	30	30	25	25	25	20	20
2′ 0″–2′ 29″	60	50	45	45	40	35	35	30	30	30	25
2′ 30″–2′ 59″	70	65	60	55	50	45	40	40	35	35	35
3′ 0″–3′ 29″	85	75	70	60	55	55	50	45	45	40	40
3′ 30″–3′ 59″	100	85	80	70	65	60	55	55	50	45	45
4′ 0″–4′ 29″	110	100	90	80	75	70	65	60	55	55	50
4′ 30″–4′ 59″	125	110	100	90	85	75	70	65	60	60	55
5′	130	115	105	95	90	80	75	70	65	65	60

Below 50 = Poor general physical fitness.
50–80 = Average general physical fitness.
Above 80 = Good general physical fitness.

OBSERVATIONS: EXERCISE FOR STUDENTS

....
....
....
....
....
....
....
....
....
....
....
....
....
....
....

Examination of Abdomen

PY 4.10*

Learning Objectives

After studying this practical the student should be able to:

1. Identify the anatomical parts of gastrointestinal tract.
2. Discuss the functions of gastrointestinal tract.
3. Know regarding the diseases of gastrointestinal tract.
4. Perform and clinically evaluate on examination of abdomen.

Brief Review of GIT

The gastrointestinal tract (GIT) is made up of a hollow muscular tube beginning from the oral cavity, proceed through the pharynx, esophagus, stomach and intestines to the rectum and anus. Various accessory organs such as salivary glands, liver, pancreas and gall bladder assist the gastrointestinal tract by secreting enzymes that helps breaking down food into its component nutrients. The food moves down and is propelled along the length of the GIT by peristaltic movements of the muscular walls.

The six primary processes of the digestive system include:

- Ingestion of food
- Secretion of digestive enzymes and fluids
- Movement and mixing of food and wastes through the body
- Digestion of food
- Absorption of nutrients
- Excretion of wastes.

Examination of Abdomen

It is a part of physical examination in medical practice and is done when patients present with signs and symptoms abdominal pathology.

The stages in which abdominal examination is to be conducted are as follows:

1. Positioning of the subject and their environment.
2. Inspection of the anterior and posterior abdomen.
3. Percussion of the subject's abdomen.
4. Palpation of the subject's abdomen and its organs.
5. Auscultation of abdomen

Positioning and Environment

A. Ask the subject to lie on the examination couch comfortably and the head resting on a pillow.
B. Ask the subject to bend knees so that the abdomen musculature is relaxed.
C. After draping the subject then should be exposed from the coastal margin above to pubic symphysis below.
D. Ensure adequate lighting and comfortable room temperature for examination.
E. Stand on the patient's right side.

*Competency achievement as per competency based Undergraduate Curriculum for the Indian Medical Graduate, 2018, 1; Medical Council of India.

189

Inspection

The subject's abdomen is examined for shape of abdomen normal contour and fullness (due to fat, flatus, feces), is it scaphoid (sunken) due to starvation as is malignacy, any growth and masses, lesions, scars and sinuses, any evidence of trauma, etc. Carefully observe for any signs of portal hypertension (caput medusae) and liver disease, oesophageal varices, venous distension and ascites.

Auscultation

Auscultation is performed prior to palpation of the abdomen as it is least likely to elicit pain. Listen to the bowel sounds for durations up to five minutes. Normal are intermittent, low pitch chucking. The grumbling bowel sounds or high-pitched noises are heard in bowel obstruction. Absence of sounds could be due to peritonitis.

Auscultate over renal arteries for bruits by listening in each upper quadrant, adjacent to and above the umbilicus.

Palpation

Palpate all nine areas of the subject's abdomen (Fig. 13.1). Perform, initially lightly and then deeply. The light palpation is done to explore for any palpable mass, rigidity, or pain. The deep palpation is done for and organomegaly, particularly enlargement of the liver and spleen. Hand is held flat and relaxed.

Liver: Palpate in the right upper quadrant around 10 cm below the rib margin in the mid-clavicular line. Gently push down (posterior) and towards the patient's head with your hand roughly placed parallel to the rectus muscle, as you feel the edge of the liver. Advance your hands a few cm upward till you reach the bottom margin of the ribs. Initial palpation is to be done lightly. Repeat the examination of the same region but push a bit more firmly so exploring the deeper aspects of the right upper quadrant, especially in subject's with a lot of subcutaneous fat.

Kidney: Place your right hand at the lateral and inferior border of the ribs, pushing down as one pushes up from behind with the left hand. Normally kidney is not palpable.

Spleen: Palpate near the belly button and move slowly towards the ribs. Exam is to be conducted superficially and then more deeply. Afterward start palpating around 10 cm below the rib margin and move upwards. Feel for enlargement of spleen in either direction. The normal spleen in not palpable.

Observe for any guarding (muscle contraction occurs as pressure is applied), rigidity (indicates peritoneal inflammation) and rebound pain on release.

Percussion

Percussion is performed by knocking the middle finger against the phalanx of the middle finger of the opposing hand resting over the surface of the abdomen in each of the nine qaudrants (Fig. 13.1). It may elicit a painful

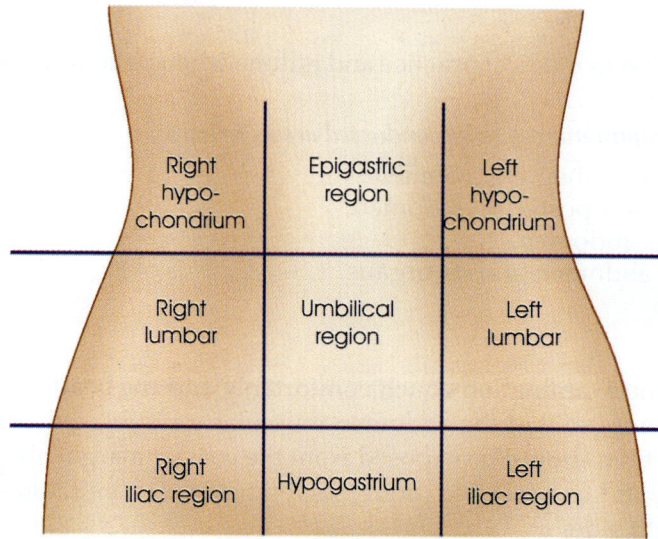

Fig. 13.1

response in the patient. Organomegaly may also be noted, including gross splenomegaly, hepatomegaly and urinary retention.

Percussing for organomegaly is carried out in a particular manner:

Spleen: Percuss for the spleen from the left iliac to the left hypochondrium, and the right iliac region to the right hypochondrium.

Liver: Percuss the liver from the right iliac region to right hypochondrium.

Other examination which can be carried out are examination of pelvic lymph nodes. Note that the abdominal examination is not complete without a digital rectal exam.

Observations

On inspection

On auscultation

On palpation

On percussion.

OSCE NON-SKILLED

Q1. Describe the types of intestinal motility movements within small and large bowel.

Ans. *These types of movements within the small and large bowel are of two types:*

Segmentation contractions: These are mixing contractions which churn the food (small intestine) to expose the chyme so that absorption is facilitated.

Propulsive contractions: It propels and pushes the food and stool forward. These are also known as peristaltic waves. These contractions are stimulated by stretch of the intestinal wall and occur as food, chyme or stool enters a portion of the small or large intestine. It also gets stimulated by the external input from the brain and spinal cord as well as various events occurring in other parts of the digestive tract.

VIVA VOCE QUESTIONS

Q1. What are the functions of GI system?

Ans. *The six primary processes of the digestive system include:*

- Ingestion of food
- Secretion of digestive enzymes and fluids
- Movement and mixing of food and wastes through the body
- Digestion of food
- Absorption of nutrients
- Excretion of wastes.

Q2. What are the functions of saliva?

Ans. *The functions of saliva are:*

- Saliva lubricates and moistens the food
- Saliva helps to control the body's water balance due to thirst sensation.
- Saliva reduces tooth decay and infection by removing food debris, dead cells, bacteria, and white blood cells.
- Saliva contains small amounts of the digestive enzyme amylase, which chemically breaks down carbohydrates into simpler compounds.
- Saliva aids in speech.

Q3. Enlist the secretions of GI tract and the amount secreted daily.

Ans. *The secretions of GI tract are*:

	Volume/day	Name of secretion
1. Esophagus	Small	–
2. Stomach	2000 ml	Gastric juice
3. Small intestine	1500 ml	Succus entericus
4. Large intestine	Small	Intestinal juice

ACCESSORY ORGAN SECRETIONS

	Volume/day	Name of secretion
1. Salivary glands	1500 ml	Saliva
2. Liver/gallbladder	500 ml	Bile
3. Pancreas	1500 ml	Pancreatic juice

Q4. Enlist the gastrointestinal system drugs classification.

Ans. *The major drug classifications are*:

Antiemetic

Acid-reducing agents

Laxatives

Antidiarrheals

Acid-reducing agents classifications; proton pump inhibitors and H_2 antagonists.

Q5. Enlist the names of GIT hormone.

Ans. *The main GIT hormones are*:
- Gastrin
- Somatostatin
- Secretin
- Cholecystokinin (CCK)
- Fibroblast growth factor 19 (FGF19)
- Incretins
- Ghrelin
- Neuropeptide Y (NPY)
- Peptide YY3-36 (PYY3-36).

The endocrine cells of the small intestine also secrete serotonin and substance P.

Q6. Discuss the secretions and functions of gastrin, somatostatin, secretin and cholecystokinin.

Ans. Gastrin is a mixture of several peptides containing 14 amino acids. Gastrin is secreted by cells in the stomach and duodenum. Gastrin stimulates the exocrine cells of the stomach to secrete gastric juice, hydrochloric acid and the proteolytic enzyme pepsin.

Somatostatin: It is the peptides; secreted by cells in the gastric glands of the stomach and it inhibits the release of gastrin and hydrochloric acid from stomach, the secretin and cholecystokinin from duodenum and glucagon from pancreas. Somatostatin is also secreted by the hypothalamus and the pancreas and inhibits insulin secretion also.

Secretin: It is a polypeptide of 27 amino acids. Secretin is secreted by cells in the duodenum when they are exposed to the acidic contents of the emptying stomach. Secretin stimulates the exocrine portion of the pancreas to secrete bicarbonate into the pancreatic fluid.

Cholecystokinin (CCK): It is an octapeptide containing 8 amino acids. It is secreted by cells in the duodenum and jejunum on being exposed to

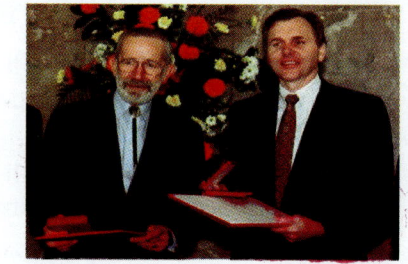

food. It acts on the gallbladder stimulating it to contract and force its contents of bile into the intestine, also stimulates the secretion and release of pancreatic digestive enzymes into the pancreatic fluid.

Q7. Enlist various disease associated with malabsorption.

Ans. The chronic diseases of malabsorption include the autoimmune coeliac disease, infective tropical sprue, and congenital or surgical short bowel syndrome. The rarer diseases affecting the small intestine include blind loop syndrome, Curling's ulcer, Milroy disease and Whipple's disease.

Q8. Discuss the gallbladder diseases.

Ans. The most common gallbladder disease includes gallstones. Gallstones are a common cause of inflammation of the gallbladder called cholecystitis. Inflammation of the biliary duct is called cholangitis, which may be associated with ascending cholangitis or autoimmune disease such as primary sclerosing cholangitis as a result of bacterial infection.

HISTORICAL UPDATE

Claudius Galen (circa 130–200) theorized that the stomach acted independently from other systems in the body, almost with a separate brain. Until the 17th century this fundamental was widely accepted.

Lazzaro Spallanzani, an Italian physician, in 1780 conducted experiments to prove the impact of gastric juice on the digestion process.

Philipp Bozzini in 1805 developed the Lichtleiter which was an instrument, which was used to examine the urinary tract, rectum and pharynx.

Adolf Kussmaul, a German physician, in 1868 developed the gastroscope, using a sword swallower to help develop the diagnostic process.

Rudolph Schindler popularly known as "father of gastroscopy," described many of the diseases involving the human digestive system in his illustrated textbook during World War I. Rudolph Schindler and Georg Wolf developed a semi-flexible gastroscope in 1932.

Hiromi Shinya a Japanese-born general surgeon, in 1970 delivered the first report of a colonoscopy to the New York Surgical Society.

Barry Marshall and Robin Warren in 2005 were awarded the Nobel Prize in Physiology or Medicine for their discovery of *Helicobacter pylori* and its role in peptic ulcer disease.

RECENT UPDATE

1. Barry Marshall and Robin Warren were awarded the Nobel prize in Physiology for their pioneering work discovery of the bacterium *Helicobacter pylori* and its role in gastritis and peptic ulcer disease in the year 2005. Peptic ulcer disease is no longer a chronic, frequently disabling condition, but a disease that can be cured by a short regimen of antibiotics and acid secretion inhibitors.

2. The gut microbiome is the characteristic distinction of symbiotic microorganisms in the human gastrointestinal system and their collective interacting genomes. Disease and disorders of the microbiome are associated with diverse human disease processes. Systems biology approaches are able to describe the gut microbiome at a detailed transcriptomic, proteomic and metabolic levels; especially at genetic and functional level. This specifies and marks the importance of the gut microbiome in the disease pathogenesis for numerous systemic diseases like obesity and cardiovascular disease, inflammatory bowel disease, etc. Exploring microbiome activity is necessary for potentially providing new targets for drug development.

OBSERVATIONS: EXERCISE FOR STUDENTS

....

....

....

....

....

....

....

14

Reproduction

PY 9.9*

SEMEN ANALYSIS

Learning Objectives

After learning the practical the students should be able to:

1. Count the numbers of sperm present in per milliliter (ml) of semen obtained from a single ejaculation.

2. They should be able to comment on the volume of semen present in one ejaculation, report the liquefaction time, measure of the percentage of sperm that have a normal shape (sperm morphology), measure of the percentage of sperm that can move forward normally (sperm motility) and evaluate pH.

3. Evaluate, summate and explain the results. They should be able to discuss the reason for altered sperm count and morphological variation.

Brief Review

Sperms are male gamete having capacity to fertilize an egg also known as an ovum or oocyte. They are formed in the seminiferous tubules of the testes. Sperm under a microscope appears to have a round head and a long tail. The head of a sperm has nucleus which has 23 chromosomes. The tail structure enables the sperm in motility and movement as it helps sperm propel forward from the vagina toward the uterus to reach the oocyte in the fallopian tubes and also aids sperm in binding and penetrating an ovum. As the sperm head penetrates the zona pellucida the 23 chromosomes of the sperm head join with the 23 chromosomes in the egg's nucleus to form an embryo with 46 chromosomes. The single cell embryo replicates further to produce 46 chromosome cells; eventually to form the foetus representing the end of the process of fertilization.

AIM OF THE EXPERIMENT/SEMEN EXAMINATIONS

Materials WBC pipette, microscope, improved Neubauer chamber, coverslips, slides and diluting fluid (5% sodium bicarbonate in 1% of phenol solution).

Procedure

1. The volunteer donor is instructed of abstinence from sexual activities for 48 hours period prior to giving his semen sample. He then should be asked to give a fresh sample of semen in Petri dish or small beaker.

2. Observe the sample for period of 20 to 30 minutes for liquefaction and measure its volume.

3. Sperm motility—take a clean glass slide and make a rim of small-sized circle of plasticine on the slide. Place a drop of semen on coverslip and invert it over the circle of plasticine. Observe the motility and specify percentage of motile sperms. The morphological features of sperms are to be studied.

4. Counting the sperm—clean and wipe the tip of WBC pipette, draw semen to 0.5 marks; and then the diluting fluid up to 11 marks. Gently mix the sample between the palms and charge as for WBC count the Neubauer chamber after five minutes. Count the sperms under high power in 4 WBC square.

*Competency achievement as per competency based Undergraduate Curriculum for the Indian Medical Graduate, 2018, 1; Medical Council of India.

Calculation

The sperm are counted in 64 squares as done for WBC.

Volume of 1 square = $1/160$ mm^3

Volume of 64 squares = $4/10$ mm^3

Dilution factor is 20.

Hence number of sperms in 1 mm^3 of undiluted semen = $N \times (10/4) \times 20$

Sperm count in 1 ml = $N \times 50 \times 1000$

Results—normal semen count is 60 to 120 millon/ml.

Observation

Note your results

Volume of semen ....

Liquefaction time ....

Sperm motility .... % of motile sperms

Sperm count ....

Precautions

1. Ensure clean and dry WBC pipette is used.
2. Ensure drawing semen up to 0.5 marks; and diluting fluid up to 11 marks.
3. Carefully count the sperms under high power in 4 WBC square.
4. Note the volume of semen, sperm morphology and sperm motility with accuracy.

Clinical Perspective

Male factor infertility occurs as a result of inability of man's sperm to fertilize an ovum leading to failure in conception. The various probable reasons include failure to produce a sufficient quantity of sperm; or produces sperm of a low quality (especially abnormally-shaped sperm). The sperm count helps in assessing male fertility, to verify whether the procedure of vasectomy was successful and also for screening of human donors during sperm donation.

OSPE (NON-SKILLED)

Q1. Enlist the normal results of a sperm count.

Ans. *The normal results of sperm count observed are:*

- **Sperm morphology:** Fifty percent and more of sperm are shaped normally.
- **Sperm motility:** More than fifty percent of sperm show normal motility.
- **Sperm volume:** More than 2 ml.
- **Liquefaction:** 20 to 30 minutes.
- **pH:** Between 7.2 and 7.8.
- **Sperm count:** 20 million to over 100 million per ml.
- **Appearance:** Whitish to gray opalescent.

Q2. Describe the normal shape of sperm.

Ans. The normal shaped sperm has an smooth, oval-shaped head (5–6 micrometers long and 2.5–3.5 micrometers wide), well-defined cap (acrosome) covering 40% to 70% of the sperm head, no visible abnormality of neck, mid-piece, or tail and does not have fluid droplets in the sperm head bigger than one half of the sperm head size.

Q3. Draw a well-labeled diagram of male reproductive system.

Ans.

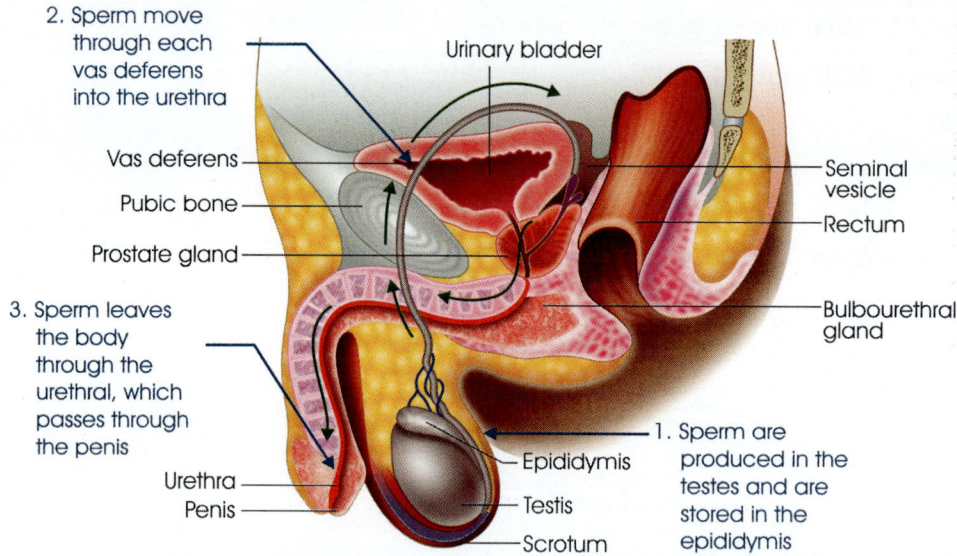

2. Sperm move through each vas deferens into the urethra

Urinary bladder

Vas deferens

Pubic bone

Prostate gland

3. Sperm leaves the body through the urethral, which passes through the penis

Urethra

Penis

Epididymis

Testis

Scrotum

Seminal vesicle

Rectum

Bulbourethral gland

1. Sperm are produced in the testes and are stored in the epididymis

VIVA VOCE QUESTIONS

Q1. Why chances of fertilization reduced in males with lower sperm count?

Ans. Males having low sperm count has lower concentration of sperm in the ejaculate as compared to normal healthy male semen. Moreover, the chance of one of the millions of sperm contained in the seminal fluid reaching the oocyte in the woman's fallopian tubes for fertilization gets greatly reduced in males with low sperm count.

Q2. What are the characteristic of low quality sperm?

Ans. The low quality sperm reduces the chance of fertilization as they are typically either immotile or abnormally shaped, or both. Immotile sperms are unable to travel up the vaginal tract and into the uterus, and thus unable to fertilize a mature oocyte. The abnormally-shaped sperm may be motile or immotile, or may be unable to bind to and penetrate ovum leading to failure in conception.

Q3. Explain the reasons for difficulty in process of ejaculating sperms.

Ans. In some males the sperm production may occur normally in the testicles, but there may be noted inability in the process of ejaculating sperm. This may be due to spinal cord injuries, injuries to the testicles, or in cases of cryptorchidism or testicular infections. In other cases such as obstructions in the epididymis and vas deferens (infections) the males may ejaculate, however, their seminal fluid does not contain sperm. In retrograde ejaculation male ejaculates into his bladder, and ejaculate is not expelled into female vagina.

Q4. Discuss the World Health Organization reference values for semen analysis testing.

Ans. *The World Health Organization reference values for semen analysis testing are:*

Characteristics	Reference value
Volume	> 2 ml
Sperm concentration	> 20 million/ml
Sperm number	> 40 million per ejaculate
Sperm motility	> 50% progressive or > 25% rapidly progressive
Morphology (strict criteria)	> 15% normal forms
White blood cells	< 1 million/ml
Mixed antiglobulin reaction test*	< 10% coated
Vitality	≥ 75% living
pH	≥ 7.2
Liquefaction time	< 60 minutes

*for antisperm antibodies

Q5. Discuss the terms azoospermia, normozoospermia and oligozoospermia.

Ans. Azoospermia: It is a condition in which semen contains no sperm.

Normozoospermia: In this condition the sperm count is more than 20 million sperm/ml of semen and no morphological or genetic defects in the sperm.

Oligozoospermia: In this condition the seminal fluid concentration of sperm is lower than 5–20 million sperm/ml of seminal fluid (indicating mild–moderate oligozoospermia) or concentration <5 million (indicating severe oligozoospermia).

RECENT UPDATES

Computer Assisted Semen Analysis (CASA) is being used for the assessment of sperm concentration and mobility characteristics, such as velocity and linear velocity with accurate results, and complete analysis within a few seconds. Raman spectroscopy performs characterization, identification and localization of sperm nuclear DNA damage more precisely nowadays.

Historical Updates

Edmund Beecher Wilson (19 October 1856—3 March 1939) and

Nettie Maria Stevens (July 7, 1861—May 4, 1912).

Edmund Beecher Wilson and Nettie Stevens discovered the chromosomal XY sex-determination system in 1905 (the fact that males have XY sex chromosomes and females have XX sex chromosomes).

OBSERVATIONS: EXERCISE FOR STUDENTS

Pregnancy Diagnostic Test

PY 9.10*

Learning Objectives

After learning the practicals students should be able to:

1. Discuss various pregnancy diagnostic tests, and understand that basis of tests is the detection of human chorionic gonadotropin (hCG) in urine or blood, the hCG produced in placenta in pregnancy.
2. Perform tests for detection of chorionic gonadotropin hCG by immunological tests that replaced the older tests on animal.
3. Educate the community regarding home-based pregnancy diagnostic tests.

Brief Overview

The confirmatory diagnosis of pregnancy is based on history and physical examination, laboratory evaluation, and ultrasonography. The diagnosis of **early pregnancy** is primarily based upon laboratory assessment of human chorionic gonadotropin (hCG) in urine or blood. The hCG is produced in placenta in pregnancy. With the development of the trophoblast cells from the early fertilized ovum, human chorionic gonadotropin is secreted by the syncytial trophoblast cells into the fluid of the mother. The secretion of this hormone can be measured in the blood as early as 8 to 10 days after ovulation, shortly after the blastocyst implants in the endometrium. The appearance of the hormone in urine forms the basis of the test for early pregnancy. Further the rate of secretion of hCG rises rapidly to reach a maximum at about 10 to 12 weeks of pregnancy and then decreases to a lower level by 16–20 weeks at which level it remains for remainder of pregnancy. The rapid immunological assay determining human chorionic gonadotropin (hCG) in the urine forms a very sensitive and appropriate for detection of early pregnancy. Results are read within a few minutes.

Immunological Test

Antibodies against hCG were prepared by injecting it into rabbit. Present day pregnancy test applies use of monoclonal antibodies selective for the beta area of the hCG molecule for detection of human chorionic gonadotropin in urine. The monoclonal anti-hCG antibody which after binding with the hCG (if present in the test sample) forms a fixed anti-hCG complex with an enzyme or other color producing molecule. The result is noted by the production of a visible marker.

The controls are routinely tested on the kits to confirm and verify the validity of patient results.

Urine Collection

Random urine specimen is appropriate for hCG testing, but the first morning urine is optimal because it generally contains the highest concentration of hCG.

Urine specimens should be collected in any clean, dry, plastic container. Specimens may be stored at room temperature for up to 8 hours prior to testing, or may be refrigerated (2 to 8°C) and run within 72 hours after collection.

Gravindex test also known as latex agglutination inhibition test: It is an agglutination inhibition test carried on a urine sample to detect pregnancy. Principle of the test is based on double antigen–antibody reaction. It identifies and detects the prevention of agglutination of hCG-coated latex particles by hCG present in the urine of pregnant female.

---

*Competency achievement as per competency based Undergraduate Curriculum for the Indian Medical Graduate, 2018, 1; Medical Council of India.

Materials: The kits available in market contain two reagents; Suspension of human chorionic gonadotropin (hCG)—coated latex particles, and solution of human chorionic gonadotropin (hCG) antibodies.

Procedure: Mix one drop of the urine with one drop of antibody solution for a minute on a black glass slide. Add one drop of the human chorionic gonadotropin (hCG) coated latex particles to the slide and observe for one minute.

- The antibodies will remain to agglutinate the human chorionic gonadotropin (hCG)-coated latex particles if the level of human chorionic gonadotropin (hCG) is too low. If agglutination occurs, the subject is not pregnant.
- The human chorionic gonadotropin (hCG) will bind to the antibodies, and thus no agglutination with the human chorionic gonadotropin (hCG)-coated latex particles occurs if the level of human chorionic gonadotropin (hCG) is high. If no agglutination occurs, the subject is pregnant.

ULTRASONOGRAPHY

It is a diagnostic technique and employs high-frequency sound waves to create an image of the internal organs. A screening ultrasound is done to check normal fetal growth and verify the due date in pregnancy. Two types of ultrasounds can be performed during pregnancy: Abdominal ultrasound and transvaginal ultrasound. The transvaginal ultrasound produces a sharper image and is often used in early pregnancy.

Results—Note the result and method carried out by you.

OSCE—NON-SKILLED QUESTION

Q1. What is screening test? Explain its implication in first and second trimesters of pregnancy.

Ans. Screening test is a procedure or a screening process which helps to determine the risk of the fetus of having certain birth defects.

First trimester screening includes

- Ultrasound test for fetal nuchal translucency screening with aid of an ultrasound examines the area at the back of the fetal neck for increased fluid or thickening.
- Maternal serum (blood) tests—the abnormal levels of pregnancy-associated plasma protein or human chorionic gonadotropin (hCG) are associated with an increased risk for chromosome abnormality.
- Pregnancy-associated plasma protein (PAPP-A) is a protein which is produced by the placenta in early pregnancy.
- Human chorionic gonadotropin (hCG) is a hormone produced by the placenta in early pregnancy.

Second trimester screening

It includes a maternal serum screen and ultrasound evaluation of the fetus for structure anomalies.

- **Maternal serum screen:** Estimation of levels of AFP (alpha-fetoprotein), hCG, estriol, and inhibin-A. This test helps to identify neural tube defects or chromosomal disorders such as Down syndrome in foetus and other chromosomal abnormalities.
- **Ultrasound:** A screening ultrasound is carried during the course of a pregnancy to check normal fetal growth and verify the due date.

VIVA VOCE QUESTIONS

Q1. What is amniocentesis?

Ans. Amniocentesis is a procedure in which a small sample of the amniotic fluid that surrounds the fetus is withdrawn to diagnose chromosomal disorders and open neural tube defects such as spina bifida. An amniocentesis is carried out in second trimester between the 15th and 20th weeks of pregnancy in females having increased risk for chromosome abnormalities (Females 35 years and above at delivery or having abnormal maternal serum screening test suggestive of chromosomal abnormality or neural tube defect.)

Q2. Discuss the test which detects pregnancy at the earliest after fertilization.

Ans. The rosette inhibition assay which detects early pregnancy factor (EPF) in blood within 48 hours of fertilization is the quickest and earliest test to confirm pregnancy after fertilization. The disadvantage of this test is that the EPF assay is expensive and time-consuming.

Q3. What is chorionic villus sampling (CVS)?

Ans. It is a prenatal test that involves taking a sample of placental tissue for diagnosing chromosomal abnormalities and some other genetic problems. Unlike amniocentesis, chorionic villus sampling does not provide information on neural tube defects. Those undergoing chorionic villus sampling need a follow-up blood test between 16 and 18 weeks of their pregnancy for screening neural tube defects.

Q4. Enlist the genetic disorders which can be diagnosed during screening.

Ans. The genetic disorders which can be diagnosed before birth are: Cystic fibrosis, haemophilia A, thalassemia, sickle cell anemia, Duchenne muscular dystrophy, polycystic kidney disease, Tay-Sachs disease, etc.

HISTORICAL UPDATES

These biological diagnostic tests were the earliest tests performed for the detection of pregnancy.

The tests performed for confirmation of pregnancy depend on the fact that placenta produces gonadotropins which are excreted in urine. The urine contains hormones and is injected commonly into immature female test animals the ovaries will undergo maturation. The first satisfactory test was done by Aschheim and Zondek in 1927-28. Most of the other biological tests are modification of the original.

Aschheim and Zondek test: Identifies the presence of hCG in urine. The urine is injected subcutaneously into an immature rat or mouse. In the case of pregnancy, the rat would show an estrous reaction with appearance of blood filled ovulatory follicle on fifth day confirming pregnancy.

Hogben test: Injection of urine containing hCG into the lymph space of adult female toads produces ovulation in around 18–20 hours.

Friedman rabbit test: Ovulation occurs in eighteen hours after injecting female rabbit intravenously with urine containing hCG.

Galli mainini frog test: Injection of urine containing hCG into the lymph space of male toad or frog produces shedding of sperms within three hours.

Judith Vaitukaitis (1940-till Date)

Judith L. Vaitukaitis: Was born in Hartford, Connecticut in the year 1940. She was a reproductive neuroendocrinologist and played a vital role in developing a biochemical assay in the early 1970s ultimately formulated home pregnancy test. She worked with Glenn Braunstein, to design accurate techniques for detection of elevated levels of hCG in the body which also was targeted towards diagnosing cancer. The researchers opined that a sensitive hCG assay will be able to detect pregnancy at an early stage. Vaitukaitis, Braunstein and Griff Ross published a landmark paper that described a new assay for detecting hCG.

Radioimmunoassay: A. R. Midgeley introduced a radioimmunoassay for hCG in 1966; but his technique could not adequately distinguish the alpha subunit of hCG from other commonly occurring hormones. Judith L. Vaitukaitis, Glenn Braunstein, and Griff Ross later in 1972 developed a sophisticated radioimmunoassay that could distinguish between the two substances.

Enzyme Linked Immunosorbent Assay (ELISA)

Monoclonal antibody test: A mixture of purified hCG linked to an enzyme is added to the test sample (blood or urine). If hCG is absent in the test sample, only hCG with linked enzyme binds. If more hCG is present in the test sample, the fewer enzymes linked hCG binds. The enzyme acts on substrate to produce blue colour. ELISA tests are very accurate tests, highly sensitive and specific as compared to radioimmunoassay (RIA) tests.

OBSERVATIONS: EXERCISE FOR STUDENTS

Examination of Central Nervous System

Learning Objectives

After learning the practical students should be able to:

1. Understand that recording of history is an important key part of the clinical examination in reference to central nervous system. The popular saying in clinical medical practice states that "History tells you what it is, and the examination tells you where it is", thus history and examination combo is very essential for treatment planning.
2. Describe the various tests for examinations of sensory system, motor system including deep and superficial reflexes and for cranial nerves.
3. Discuss the significance of the tests for assessing the type and extent of damage in the CNS.

Aim of Experiment

To extracted neurological history and perform detailed physical examination.

Procedure

The central nervous system examination proceeds with complete evaluation of higher functions, motor functions, sensory functions, cranial nerves and reflexes.

Apparatus: Stethoscope, gloves, tongue depressors, ophthalmoscope, a reflex hammer, and a tuning fork, a pin (Wartenberg) wheel, etc. Other test apparatus required for sensory and cranial nerve functions are pointed out in those sections.

Evaluation of Sensorial and Higher Functions

Mental status: Evaluate by testing memory, orientation, intelligence, and the other aspects of the patient's psychic state.

1. Observe whether the condition of the patient is alert or drowsy. In stupor the person although inaccessible does show some response to pain stimuli.
2. Memory can be judged during the course of discussion and by posing questions regarding his past health status, family history and personal history. Ensure whether patient's recent and remote memory functions are affected.
   In dementia (loss of memory) person is confused regarding time and place and shows impaired abilities but is awake and alert.
3. Orientation—ensure whether patient is well-oriented to time, place and person
4. Intelligence is to be tested by the ability to quickly and successfully apply previous knowledge to a new situation and to use reason in solving problems. This is subjective and can be evaluated by verbal interaction with patient. Additional information is gathered regarding patient's intelligence from his educational background and occupational history.
5. Evaluate his psychological frame of mind and find out if the patient is depressed or emotionally deprived.

Higher Functions Include Gait, Speech, and Mental Status

1. **Gait**—watch the patient carefully and observe his gait. It is attitude of a person in the upright position. A few abnormal types of gaits are described below.

   A. Hemiparetic gait (patient's of hemiplegia)

   B. Ataxic gait (the patient spreads his or her legs apart to widen the base of support to compensate for the imbalance while standing or walking). It is attributed to midline lesions of the cerebellum. When the lesion is unilateral, the patient may sway to the side of the lesion. In case of bilateral cerebellar involvement, the patient may fall to either side.

   C. Shuffling gait (the patient takes short steps but practically does not move forward or may make little progress). In addition some patients may exhibit tendency to accelerate (festinating gait) as he or she walks. Shuffling and festinating gaits are seen in Parkinson disease.

   D. Steppage gait—the patient takes high steps as if climbing a flight of stairs while walking on a level surface. The steppage gait is seen in chronic peripheral neuropathies and may also manifest due to the functional elongation of the legs due to bilateral drop foot.

   E. Spastic or scissor gait—patient's legs are held in adduction at the hip and the thighs rub against each other on walking. This is seen in patients of cerebral palsy.

2. **Speech**—observed for speech of the patient. The abnormalities of speech include dysphonia, dysarthria, and dysphasia or aphasia.

   A. Dysphonia—is the impairment or inability to phonate and the voice becomes hoarse. The causes of dysphonia are common cold (due to inflammation of the larynx), hypothyroidism (thickening of the vocal cords from amyloid deposits), unilateral recurrent laryngeal nerve paralysis and lesions of the vagus nerve.

   B. Dysarthria—is the inability to articulate spoken words. The paralysis of pharyngeal, palatal, lingual, or facial musculature may produce dysarthria. It is commonly seen in patients with cerebellar lesions.

   C. Dysphasia or aphasia—The ability to process language is impaired. It results in an inability to understand (sensory or Wernicke aphasia), transfer signals from the Wernicke to the Broca area (conduction aphasia), or properly execute speech (motor or Broca aphasia). The combination of Broca and Wernicke aphasias is referred to as global aphasia.

   D. Transcortical aphasias—the additional function that is impaired in sensory, motor, conduction or Broca's and Wernicke's combine aphasia is repetition. This feature is important in the diagnosis of transcortical aphasias.

   Record your observations:

   ....
   ....
   ....
   ....
   ....
   ....
   ....
   ....
   ....

OSPE

Q1. What are the functions of cerebellum in movements?

Ans. Coordination of voluntary movements, motor learning and planning and programming of movements.

Q2. Which part of the brain is involved in converting short term-memory to long-term memory?

Ans. Hippocampus is believed to be involved in conversion of short-term memory to long-term memory.

Q3. **Make a drawing to show the location of motor speech and sensory speech areas in the cerebral cortex.**

Ans.

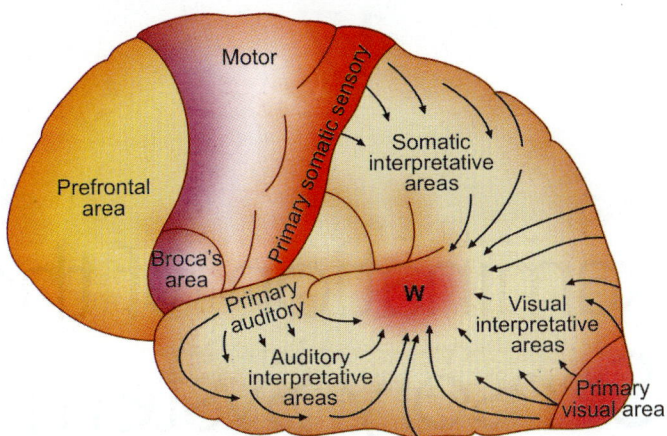

Q4. **Make a drawing showing the motor areas of the brain.**

Ans.

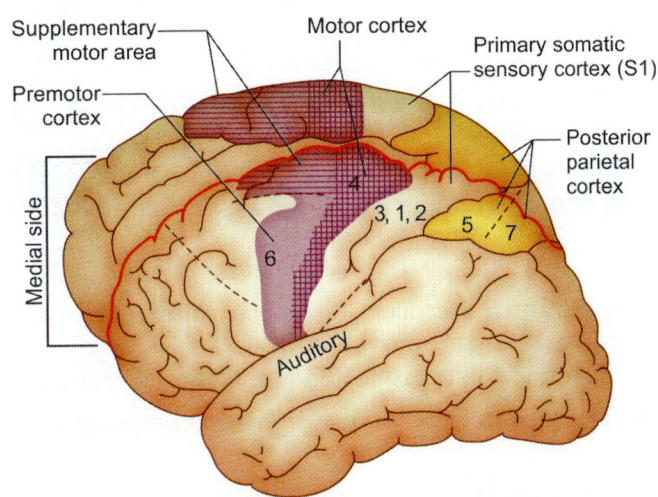

Q5. **How does categorical hemisphere differ from representational hemisphere?**

Ans. Categorical hemispheres specialized for language functions (called dominant hemisphere). The other hemisphere (non-dominant hemisphere), the representational hemisphere, is specialized in the area of spatiotemporal relation.

VIVA VOCE QUESTION

Q1. **Name the types of sleep.**

Ans. **Sleep is of two types:** REM (paradoxical sleep) and NREM (slow wave sleep).

OBSERVATIONS: EXERCISE FOR STUDENTS

....

....

....

....

17

Examination of the Sensory System

PY 10.3*

Learning Objectives

After learning the practical the student should be able to:

1. Accurately test and evaluate the sensory modalities by examination of the sensory system. Sensory system examination provides suitable clue of neurological deficit.
2. Explain the physiological basis of examination for detecting the sensory level of a lesion. It is an important assessment in patients having hemi-sectioning or sectioning of their spinal cord due to injury.

Aim of Experiment

To examine the various types of sensation: Exteroception (touch, temperature and pain), interoception (visceral sensation), proprioception (sense of position and movement).

(Teleception, distant sense, smell, sound, taste are tested along testing cranial nerves).

Apparatus: Cotton swabs, pins, tuning fork, two-point discriminator compass, coins, pencil, warm and cold water in test tubes.

Procedure

1. Record the health profile of volunteer person. Make the person comfortable to allay any anxiety.
2. Inform the volunteer regarding various tests which will be carried out during sensory examination.
3. Compare sensations on both sides of the body as well as adjacent dermatomes.

A. Touch

1. Take a swab of cotton wool and twist it into a small point.
2. Apply tip of tuned cotton swab over the volunteer individuals forehead and chest.
3. Confirm whether the individual identifies the touch.
4. Ask the individual to close his eyes and confirm for touch sensation on same places and also on both upper limbs and both lower limbs to compare and ask if sensation felt is equal on both sides. (Hypoaesthesia is diminished pain sensation.)

B. Pain (Fig. 17.1)

1. With eyes closed using a pin, lightly prick the volunteer individual on the forehead and chest, both upper limb and both lower limb by using sharp and blunt ends.
2. Ask the individual to close his eyes and repeat the test; confirm whether he perceives the sensation of both sharp and blunt ends and if the sensation is equally felt on opposite sides.
3. Note the areas of diminished pain sensation.

*Competency achievement as per competency based Undergraduate Curriculum for the Indian Medical Graduate, 2018, 1; Medical Council of India.

204

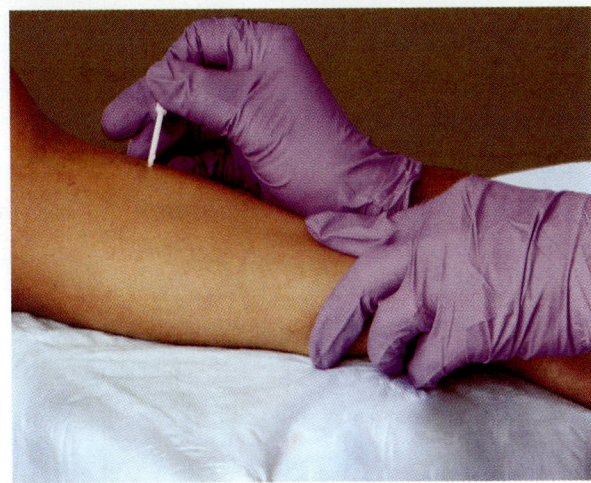

Fig. 17.1: Pain sense

Temperature

1. Apply hot and cold test tubes over forearm or along palm. Confirm whether the individual is able to confirm the temperature difference.
2. Ask the individual to close his eyes and evaluate patient again.

Deep Pain

1. Inform the procedure of the test to patient.
2. Firmly squeeze over the individuals muscles and tendons.
3. Ask the individual to confirm when pressure becomes painful.

Note: When examining a patient the doctor has to confirm if the force applied will be painful to normal people.

Deep pain can also be quantified using Algometer. (Analgesia is loss of pain sensation, hypoalgesia is partial loss of pain sensibility, hyperalgesia is a condition of exaggerated sensibility to pain).

Proprioception (Fig. 17.2)

The appreciation of passive movement. Hold the finger and fix the interphalangeal joint. Passively flex and extend the finger holding the joint, and leave it in some definite position. Ask the subject to keep the corresponding

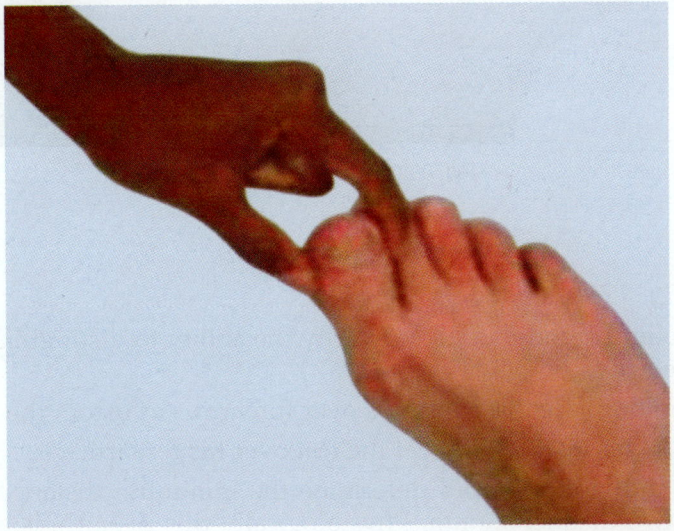

Fig. 17.2: Position sense

finger in similar position. Perform the test on all the upper and lower limbs, small and large joints (movements of less than 10° are appreciated at all the normal joints).

or

1. The test is carried over at the proximal interphalangeal joint of the big toe.
2. Grasp the proximal phalanx firmly in the finger and thumb by your left hand.
3. Grip the terminal phalanx on its lateral border by your thumb and forefinger of the right hand. Ensure second toe is not touched.
4. Move the terminal phalanx upward or downward.
5. The volunteer individual is made accustomed with the upward and downward movements.
6. Asked the volunteer individual to close his eyes. Repeat the test and confirm the positional movements on both sides of the body.

Vibration (Fig. 17.3)

1. Vibrate a tuning fork with a frequency of 128 cycles/sec (low frequency) by gently hitting on heel of your hand and then place the base of the tuning fork on forehead of volunteer individual.
2. Confirm perception and asked the volunteer individual to indicate the sensation.
3. Asked the individual to close his eyes and place the vibrating tuning fork over on bony prominences on the leg on each side.
4. Ask the individual to describe the sensation. The test is said to be positive if he perceives vibration and not touch or temperature.

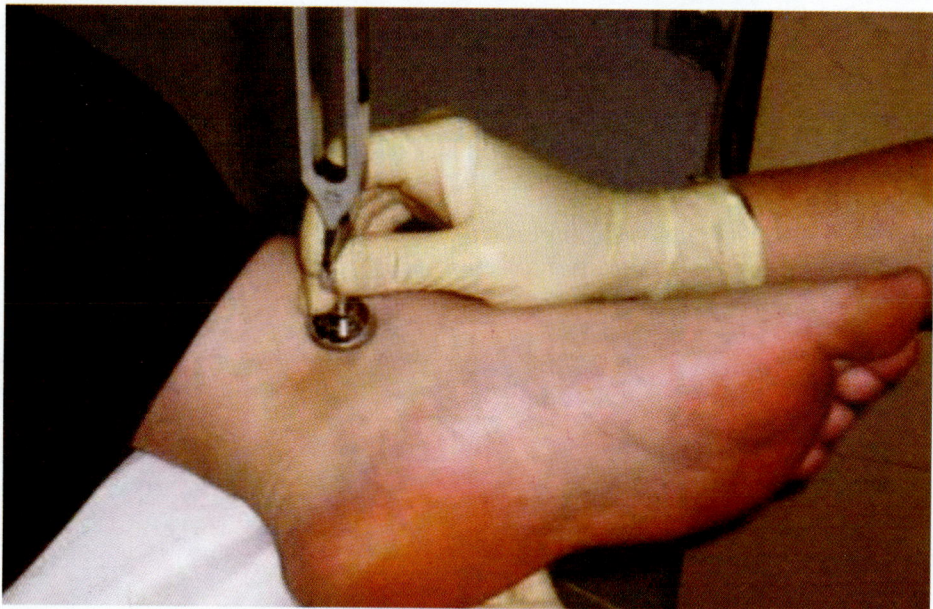

Fig. 17.3: Vibration sense

Cortical Sensation

Two-point Discrimination (Fig. 17.4)

1. Explain the test to the volunteer individual and verify the ability to distinguish the contact of two separate points applied simultaneously.
2. Use a compass separator and place the point tips over forearm. Accustom the individual with the test.
3. Ask the individual to close his eyes and repeat the test over his forearm.
4. Note that the volunteer individual should determine the minimum distance of separation at which two points are identified as two distinct stimuli. Physiologically this distance is around 3–5 mm in the finger pulps and 50–100 mm in the legs or back.

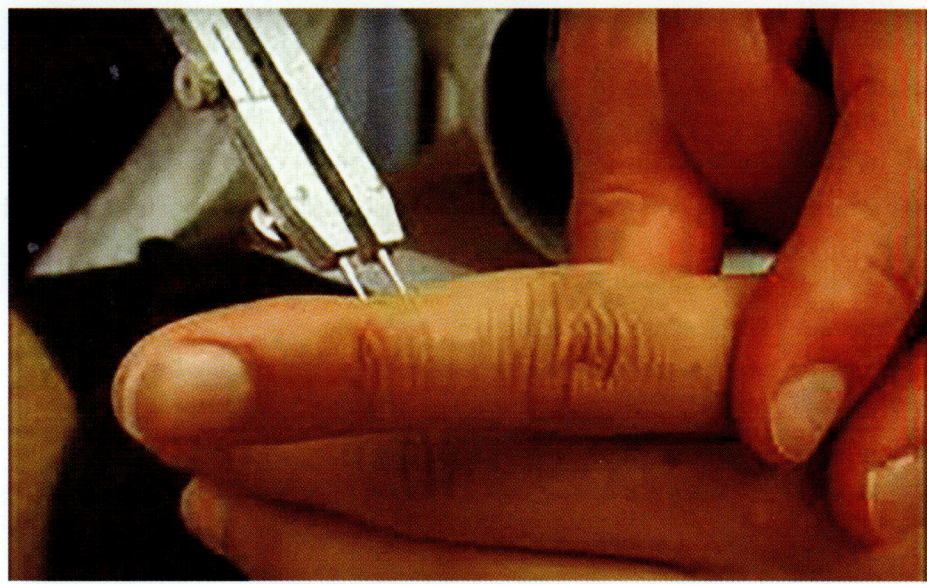

Fig. 17.4: Two-point disorimination

Stereognosis

1. Explain to the volunteer individual that the test is for checking the ability to identify objects by palpation.
2. Examine the individual by asking him to close his eyes and identify objects like coin and key. (The subject should identify the object by its shape, texture, size, etc. and should tell what it is).

Romberg's Sign

Ask the subject to stand with his feet close together and then to close his eyes. Swaying of the body from side to side will occur if the posterior column is affected. The position sense from the legs is lacking, hence the subject becomes unsteady on closing the eyes.

This is a test for the loss of position sense (*sensory ataxia*) in the legs. It is not at a test for cerebellar function. This is a test to differentiate sensory ataxia from cerebellar ataxia. In *cerebellar ataxia*, the subject is unsteady with his feet together even with eyes open.

Record your Observations

Name Age: Sex: Occupation:								
Sensation	Cervical		Thoracic		Lumbar		Sacral	
	Right	Left	Right	Left	Right	Left	Right	Left
Fine touch								
Crude touch								
Tactile localisation								
Two-point discrimination								
Joint and position								
Vibration								
Superficial pain								
Deep pain								
Temperature								
Cold								
Warm								
Stereognosis								
Romberg's sign								

OSPE

Q1. Name the sensations carried by anterior and ventral spinothalamic tracts. Are these sensations from the same side of the body?

Ans. The sensations are crude touch, pain and temperature from the contralateral side of body.

Q2. Name the sensations carried by dorsal columns. Are the sensations from same side of the body?

Ans. The sensations are fine touch, tactile localization, tactile discrimination, stereognosis, proprioception and vibration sense, from the same side of the body.

Q3. What is the purpose for testing sensory modalities?

Ans. **The purpose of testing sensory modalities is:** To identify the areas of abnormal sensation and define which modalities are involved within these limits.

Q4. Specify the equipment required for testing sensory modality.

Ans. *The equipment required for testing sensory modality is:*

A. Light touch	Tested with cotton wool
B. Temperature	Tested using warm/cool water filled into small glass tubes.
C. Pain	Tested with either a toothpick or a pin
D. Vibration	Tested with a vibrating tuning fork
E. Proprioception	Tested by changing joint positions.
F. Cortical localization Two-point discrimination Stereognosis	Tested with a divider or two toothpicks applied simultaneously Tested by giving an easily identifiable object like a key or coins of various denominations.

Q5. Discuss the types of sensation.

Ans. *The various types of sensation are:*
- Exteroception (touch, temperature and pain).
- Interoception (visceral sensation).
- Proprioception (joint position).
- Tele reception (smell, sound, taste).

QUESTIONS

Q1. What is a dermatome?

Q2. Name the receptors for pain.

Q3. What are the types of pain?

Q4. Name the sensations lost in posterior column lesions of the spinal cord.

Q5. What are cortical sensations?

Q6. What are Brodmann's area numbers for primary and secondary sensory area?

Q7. What is the frequency of the tuning fork used to test vibration sense?

Q8. What is astereognosis?

Q9. What are the sensations carried by dorsal columns?

Q10. What are the sensations carried by anterior and ventral spinothalmic tracts? Are these sensations from the same side of body or contralateral side?

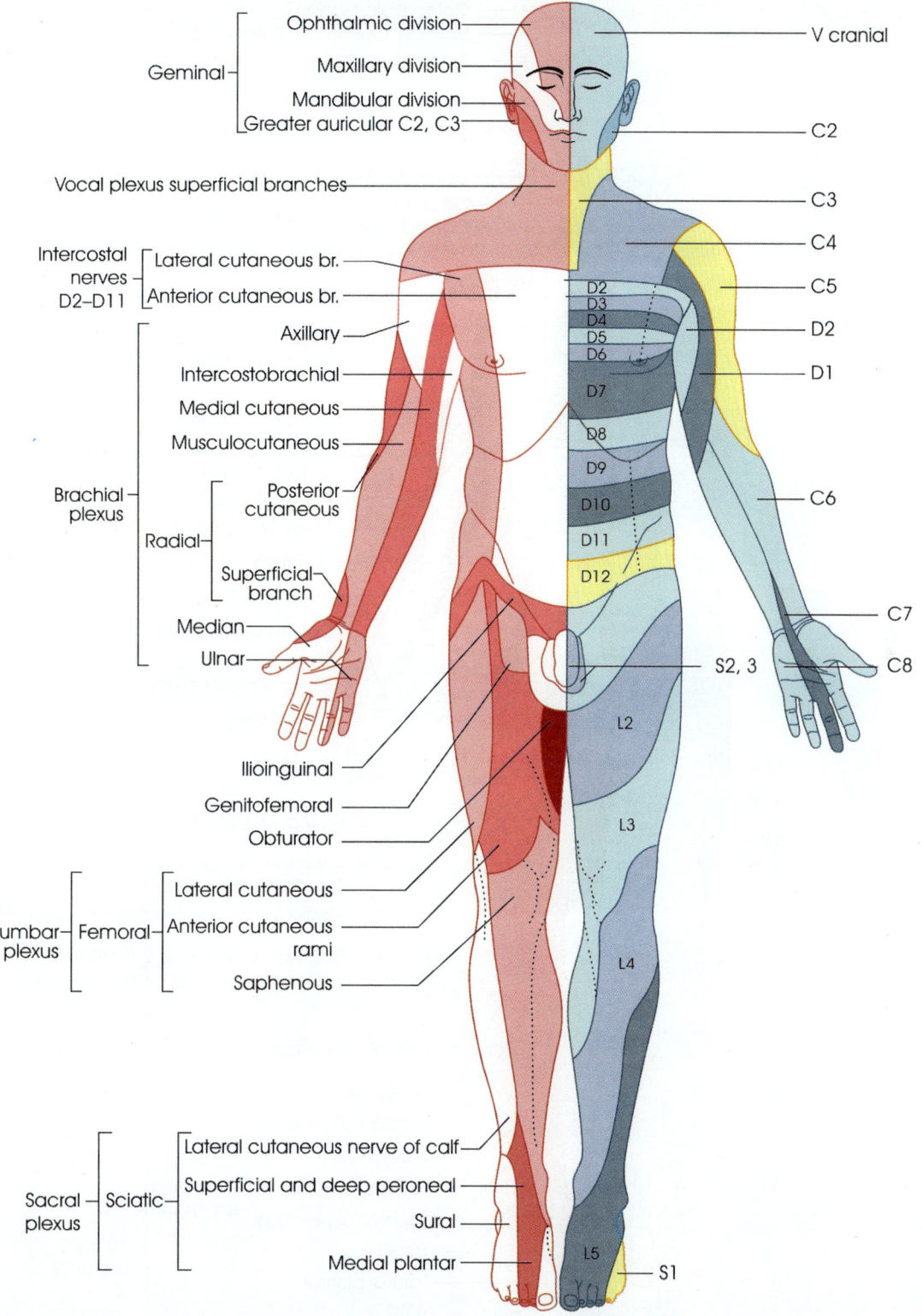

Ophthalmic division
Maxillary division
Geminal
Mandibular division
Greater auricular C2, C3

Vocal plexus superficial branches

Intercostal nerves D2–D11
Lateral cutaneous br.
Anterior cutaneous br.

Axillary
Intercostobrachial
Medial cutaneous
Musculocutaneous

Brachial plexus

Posterior cutaneous
Radial
Superficial branch

Median
Ulnar

Ilioinguinal
Genitofemoral
Obturator

Lumbar plexus
Femoral
Lateral cutaneous
Anterior cutaneous rami
Saphenous

Sacral plexus
Sciatic
Lateral cutaneous nerve of calf
Superficial and deep peroneal
Sural
Medial plantar

V cranial
C2
C3
C4
C5
D2
D1
C6
C7
C8
S2, 3
L2
L3
L4
L5
S1

D2
D3
D4
D5
D6
D7
D8
D9
D10
D11
D12

Fig. 17.5: Anterior view segmental innervations of the skin, dermatomes (left) and peripheral nerve supply (right)

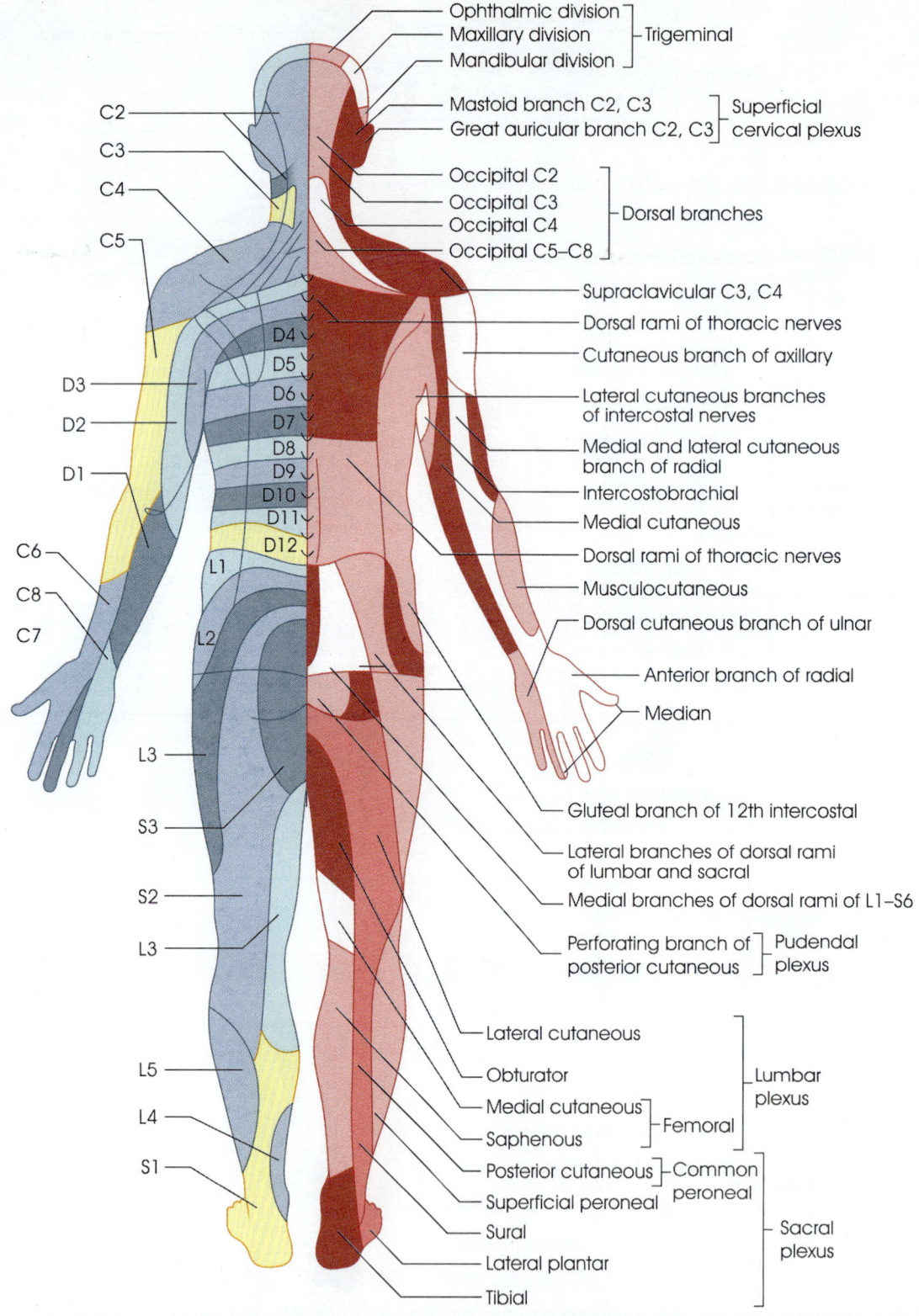

Fig. 17.6: Posterior view segmental in nervation of skin dermatomes (left) and peripheral nerve supply (right)

Examination of the Motor System

PY 10.4*

Learning Objective

After performing the tests students should be able to:

1. Describe the various tests conducted for examination of the motor system.
2. Perform a detailed examination of the motor system and evaluate muscle power.
3. Discuss the clinical signs observed in upper motor neuron lesions and lower motor neuron lesions.

Aim of the Examination

Test for:

I. Bulk of muscle
II. Tone of muscle
III. Strength of muscle
IV. Involuntary movements.

Procedure

I. Bulk of Muscle

Assess the bulk of muscle between both sides of the body in the volunteer individual. Measure the circumference of the limb at the same distance from a non-movable bony prominence on both the sides; using a measuring tape. The bulk of voluntary muscle varies with age, sex, state of nutrition, body buildup and muscular exercise. Observe your finding in upper limb (mid arm) (Fig. 18.1) and lower limb (thigh) muscles.

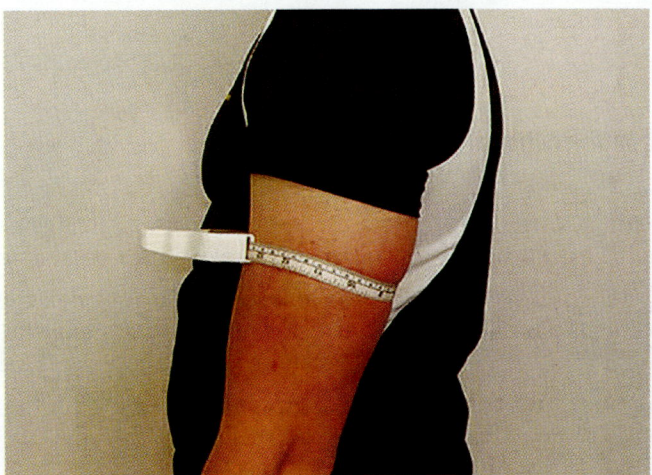

Fig. 18.1

*Competency achievement as per competency based Undergraduate Curriculum for the Indian Medical Graduate, 2018, 1; Medical Council of India.

The abnormal pathology includes atrophy and hypertrophy:

    a. Atrophy: The muscle wasting may be due to disuse, joint injuries or joint diseases or neurological disorders.

    b. Hypertrophy: The bulk of the muscle increases in muscular dystrophies. In pseudomuscular dystrophy the muscle bulk increases but these enlarged muscles are weak in spite of their increased size.

II. Tone of Muscle

Asked the individual to relax the muscle completely and then passively move the joints of the upper and lower extremities. The resistance offered by the muscle during passive movement represents the degree of muscle tone. Hypotonia is seen in lower motor neuron lesions, spinal shock, and some cerebellar lesions. Hypertonia may manifest as spasticity or rigidity.

Hypertonia: It is the increase in the muscle tone which may occur as:

    a. Spasticity—which occurs in upper motor neuron lesions. The muscle tone increases and is of clasp knife type, when tested by passively flexing a joint there is increased resistance at the beginning but as the movement is continued suddenly the resistance gives away.

    b. Rigidity:

        i. Cog-wheel rigidity—this is characteristic feature of extra-pyramidal lesion. The agonists and antagonists muscles contract alternately and regularly and there is alternate increase and decrease in resistance, hence the passive movement are jerky as of a cog wheel.

        ii. Lead pipe rigidity—this is characteristic feature of extra-pyramidal lesion both agonist and antagonist muscle contract and resistance is felt uniformly throughout the passive movement.

    c. Decorticate rigidity—in this condition the upper limb is flexed and the lower limb extended and is seen in cerebral cortical lesions.

    d. Decerebrate rigidity—in this condition there is extension of all limbs with internal rotation of the upper limb and plantar flexion of the feet.

Hypotonia: Decrease in muscle tone. There is decreased resistance to passive movement, there is increased range of movements in the limbs. This is seen in lower motor neuron lesion and cerebellar lesions.

III. Strength of the Muscle (Power)

The person tries to contract the muscle against resistance offered by the examiner and muscle strength is to be assessed using the scale below:

Score	Description
0	Absent voluntary contraction
1	Feeble contractions that are unable to move a joint
2	Movement with gravity eliminated
3	Movement against gravity
4	Movement against partial resistance
5	Full strength

IV. Tests for Strength of Muscle for Different Muscles

Upper limb

    1. Deltoids: Ask the individuals to raise both arms sidewards up as strongly as they can while you provide resistance to this movement. You will be comparing the strength of each arm.

    2. Biceps: Hold the individuals wrist from above and instructing him to flex the hand up to the shoulder. You have to provide resistance at the wrist. Observe the strength and repeat and compare to the opposite arm.

    3. Triceps: Ask the individual to extend the forearm against the resistance forced by you. Ensure that the patient begins their extension from a fully flexed position as this commencing movement is most sensitive to a loss in strength. The test is to be carried in both the arms.

    4. Forearm extensors (wrist extensors): Ask the individuals to extend their wrist while you resist the movement. The test is to be carried in both the arms. Wrist extensors are innervated by C6 and C7 nerve roots via the radial nerve. The radial nerve innervates all the extensor muscles in the upper and lower arm.

5. **Forearm flexors and the intrinsic hand muscles (thenar and hypothenar muscle):**
   a. Test the volunteer individuals grip by asking him to hold your fingers in the fist tightly and instruct him to continue holding tightly irrespective of your attempt to release them. You have to compare the hands for strength asymmetry. The finger flexion is innervated by the C8 nerve root via the median nerve.
   b. Test the intrinsic hand muscles also by having the volunteer individual abduct or fan out all of the fingers. Instruct him to resist examiner compression force. The finger abduction or "fanning" is innervated by the T1 nerve root via the ulnar nerve.

6. **Thumb opposition:** Test the strength of the thumb opposition by telling the volunteer individual to touch the tip of the thumb to the tip of his/her middle finger. You apply resistance to the thumb with your index finger. Repeat the test for other thumb. The thumb opposition is innervated by the C8 and T1 nerve roots via the median nerve.

Lower Extremities

1. **Hip flexion:** Ask the volunteer individual to lie down and raise each leg separately while you resist the movement. Repeat the test for other leg. This tests the strength of iliopsoas muscles. The hip flexors are innervated by the L2 and L3 nerve roots via the femoral nerve.

2. **Adductors of hip:** Place your hands on the inner thighs of the volunteer individual and ask the individual to bring both legs together. This tests the strength of the adductors of the medial thigh. The adduction of the hip is mediated by the L2, L3 and L4 nerve roots.

3. **Abductors of hip:** Place your hands on the outer thighs and asking the patient to move the legs apart. This tests the gluteus maximus and gluteus minimus for its strength. The abduction of the hip is mediated by the L4, L5 and S1 nerve roots.

4. **Hip extension:** Asked the volunteer individual to press down on your hand which is placed underneath the volunteer individual's thigh. Repeat the test in the other leg. This tests the gluteus maximus strength. The hip extensor is innervated by the L4 and L5 nerve roots via the gluteal nerve.

5. **Knee extensors:** Place one hand under the knee and the other on top of the lower leg of volunteer individual to provide resistance. Ask the volunteer individual to extend the lower leg at the knee. Repeat the test in other leg and compare to the other leg. This tests the quadriceps muscle strength. The quadriceps muscle is innervated by the L3 and L4 nerve roots via the femoral nerve.

6. **Knee flexors:** Hold the knee from the side and apply resistance under the ankle and instruct the volunteer individual to pull the lower leg towards the buttock as hard as possible. Repeat the test with the other leg. This tests the hamstrings strength. The hamstrings are innervated by the L5 and S1 nerve roots via the sciatic nerve.

7. **Dorsiflexion of the ankle:** Hold the top of the ankle and asked the volunteer individual to pull the foot up towards the face as hard as possible. Repeat the test with the other foot. This tests the muscles in the anterior compartment of the lower leg. The ankle dorsiflexor is innervated by the L4 and L5 nerve roots via the peroneal nerve.

8. **Ankle plantar flexion:** Hold the bottom of the foot and ask the ankle plantar flexion to press down as hard as possible. Repeat with the other foot and compare the results. This tests the gastrocnemius and soleus muscles strength in the posterior compartment of the lower leg. The ankle plantar flexor is innervated by the S1 and S2 nerve roots via the tibial nerve.

9. **Extensor halucis longus muscle:** Ask the volunteer individual to move the large toe against your resistance "up towards the face". The extensor halucis longus muscle is innervated by the L5 nerve root. This tests the extensor halucis longus muscle strength.

Involuntary Movements

The various involuntary movements which can be observed in patients are fibrillations, fasciculations, tics, myoclonus, dystonias, chorea, athetosis, hemiballismus, and seizures.

1. The fibrillations involuntary movements are not visible with naked eye except possibly those of the tongue.

2. Fasciculation involuntary movements may be seen under the skin as quivering of the muscle and are associated with neuromuscular disease and amyotrophic lateral sclerosis (ALS).

3. Tics—these are involuntary contractions of single muscle or groups of muscles leading to stereotyped movements. The Gilles de la Tourette syndrome manifests with multiple tics.

4. Myoclonus is a brief muscle jerk (<0.25 seconds) associated with various primarily generalized epilepsies. The dystonias are muscle contractions that are more prolonged than myoclonus and result in spasms.
5. Athetosis these are the spasms having a slow writhing character and occur along the long axis of the limbs or the body itself.
6. Chorea—these are quasi-purposeful movements affecting multiple joints with distal preponderance.
7. Hemiballismus—these are violent flinging movement of half of the body. It is associated with lesions of the subthalamic nucleus.
8. Seizures may result in repeated eye blinks or tonic or clonic motor activity.

Observations

I. Bulk of Muscle

Normal

Muscles tested ....
....
....
....

II. Tone of Muscle

Normal

Muscles tested ....
....
....
....

III. Strength of Muscle

Normal

Muscles tested ....
....
....
....

IV. Involuntary Movements

Any abnormal movements yes/No

Conclusion:

....
....
....
....

VIVA VOCE QUESTIONS

Q1. What is the characteristic type of hypertonicity of muscles seen in Parkinsonism?

Ans. The hypertonic muscles in Parkinsonism show lead-pipe type rigidity, it is because resistance to passive movement is sustained throughout the entire range of movement due to contraction of both agonist and antagonists.

Q2. Explain the clasp-knife effect present when the muscles are hypertonic (spastic) in upper motor neuron lesion.

Ans. Spasticity is characterized by a rapid building up of resistance to stretch and as the stretch is continued then there is sudden 'giving up' lessening the resistance produced because of stimulation of Golgi tendon organ receptors that produces inverse stretch reflex.

Q3. What are the features of upper motor neuron lesions?

Ans. Paralysis, spasticity of muscles, exaggerated deep reflexes, atrophy of muscles is minimal.

Q4. What do you understand by lower motor lesion?

Ans. When there is lesion of motor neuron or the nerve that supplies the muscle.

Q5. What are the features of lower motor neuron lesion?

Ans. Paralysis of flaccid type, absent reflexes and atrophy of muscles.

Clinical Perspective

The motor system evaluation is classified as body positioning, involuntary movements, and muscle tone and muscle strength. The muscle hypertrophy can be seen in response to muscular exercise training; physiologically in the dominant side of the body as opposed to the non-dominant side; in pathological conditions such as Duchenne Muscular Dystrophy where it is a pseudo hypertrophy also in other myotonic disorders. It is important for evaluating the muscle bulk in both sides of the body by a tape and then the bulk are to be compared. Motor examination will also help to differentiate between spasticity and rigidity. Spasticity is characterized by a rapid building up of resistance to stretch and as the stretch continues followed by sudden 'giving up' due to lessening of resistance (Clasp-knife effect). The rigidity is resistance to passive movement which is sustained throughout the entire range of movement (leadpipe rigidity).

OBSERVATIONS: EXERCISE FOR STUDENTS

....

....

....

....

....

....

....

....

....

....

....

....

....

Reflexes

PY 10.4*

Learning Objectives

After learning this practical the student should be able to:
1. Perform superficial and deep reflexes.
2. Clinically correlate the findings.

Aim of the Experiment

Perform superficial reflexes and deep reflexes.

Equipment Required

Petaller Hammer.

Procedure

Superficial reflex

1. Abdominal reflex—draw a line using blunt object away from the umbilicus along the diagonals of the 4 abdominal quadrants. The normal reflex draws the umbilicus toward the direction of the line that is drawn.
2. Cremasteric reflex is elicited in males by drawing a line using blunt object along the medial thigh and observe the movement of the scrotum. The normal reflex results in elevation of the ipsilateral testis.
3. Anal wink reflex is elicited by gently stroking the perianal skin with a pin. The response observed is puckering of the rectal orifice due to contraction of the corrugator-cutis-ani muscle.
4. Plantar response (Fig. 19.1) stroke the lateral aspect of the sole with a blunt rigid object or a key with a moderately strong stimulus. The normal response seen is plantar flexion of the great toe (this is considered as Babinski sign negative). Dorsiflexion of the great toe suggests an upper motor neuron lesion and is also referred to as a positive Babinski sign. The dorsiflexion of the big toe may also be associated with fanning out of the other toes. The presence of Babinski's sign is always abnormal in adults, but it is often present in infants, up to the age of about 1 year.

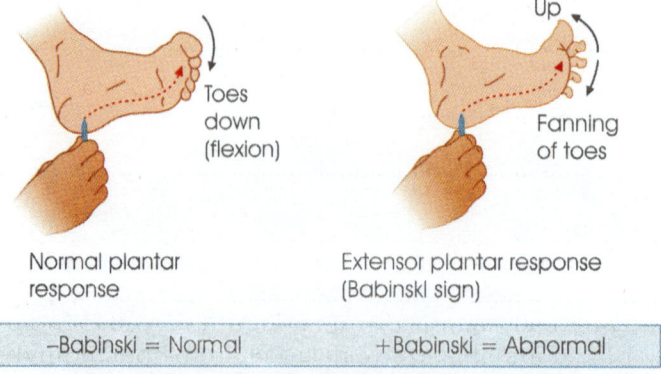

| −Babinski = Normal | +Babinski = Abnormal |

Fig. 19.1: Superficial reflex (protective reflex)

*Competency achievement as per competency based Undergraduate Curriculum for the Indian Medical Graduate, 2018, 1; Medical Council of India.

Deep Tendon Reflexes

Deep tendon reflexes are monosynaptic spinal segmental reflexes. If they are intact, integrity of cutaneous innervations, motor supply and cortical inputs to the corresponding spinal segment is confirmed. The upper motor neurons exert an overall inhibitory influence on these reflexes and when this influence is cut off the tendon reflexes are exaggerated. These reflexes include the biceps, brachioradialis, triceps, patellar, and ankle jerks. The deep tendon reflexes are often rated according to the following scale:

Reflex-grading system

Score	Reflexes
0	Absent
1	Hypoactive or present only with reinforcement
2	Readily elicited with a normal response
3	Brisk with or without evidence of spread to the neighboring roots
4	Associated with a few beats of unsustained clonus
5	Sustained clonus

Procedure

Deep tendon reflexes are elicited in all 4 extremities using a hammer. The reinforcement for better appreciating response is accomplished by asking the patient to clench their teeth, or if testing lower extremity reflexes, have the patient hook together their flexed fingers and pull apart. This is known as the Jendrassik maneuver.

Biceps reflex (Fig. 19.2): Place your thumb on the biceps tendon of the volunteer individual and strike your thumb with the reflex hammer. Observe for the arm movement. Repeat and compare your findings with the other arm.

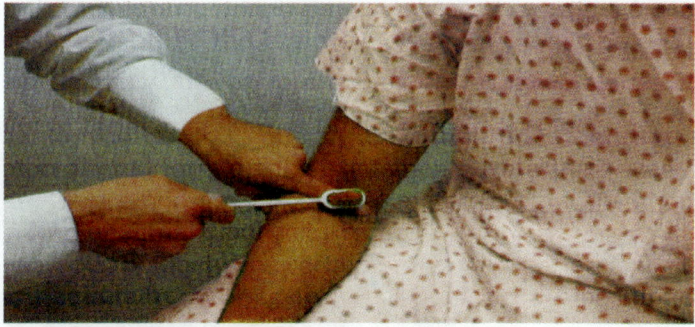

Fig. 19.2

Brachioradialis reflex (Fig. 19.3): Strike the brachioradialis tendon directly with the hammer as the volunteer individual's arm is resting. Strike the tendon roughly 2–3 inches above the wrist. Observe the reflex supination. Repeat and compare your findings to the other arm. The biceps and brachioradialis reflexes are mediated by the C5 and C6 nerve roots.

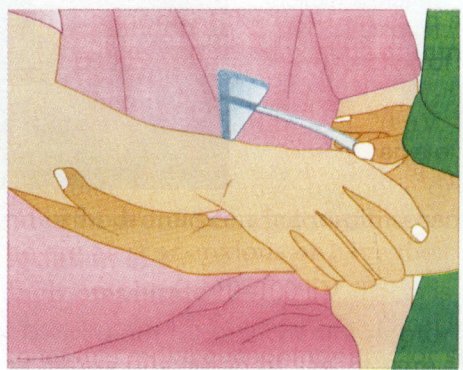

Fig. 19.3

Triceps jerk reflex (Fig. 19.4): Gently strike the short tendon of the triceps muscle close to its insertion near the tip of the elbow and elicit the reflex. The muscle will contracts in response and the forearm extends slightly. The triceps reflex is mediated by the C6 and C7 nerve roots, predominantly by C7.

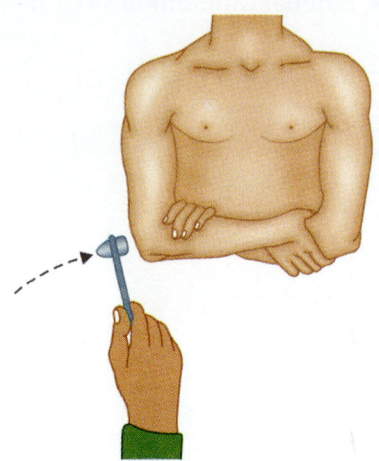
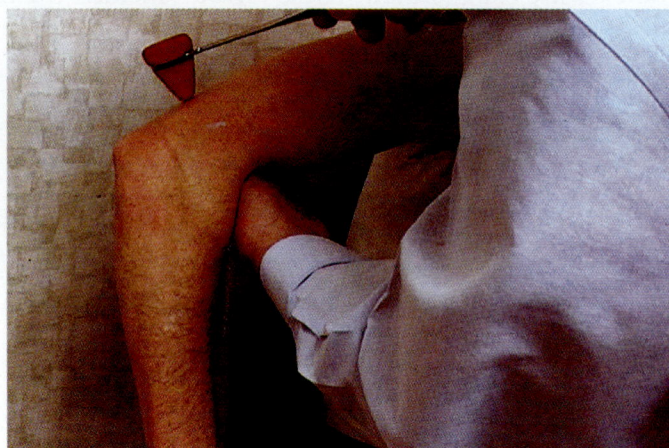

Fig. 19.4

Knee Jerk (Fig. 19.5): Ask the volunteer individual to keep the leg hanging freely off the edge of the bench. Test the knee jerk by striking the quadriceps tendon directly with the reflex hammer; the leg is normally extended once and comes to rest. Repeat the procedure and compare the result with that of the other leg. This reflex may be diminished or absent during sleep and in lower motor neuron lesion. The multiple oscillation of the leg (pendular reflex) is a sign of a cerebellar disease.

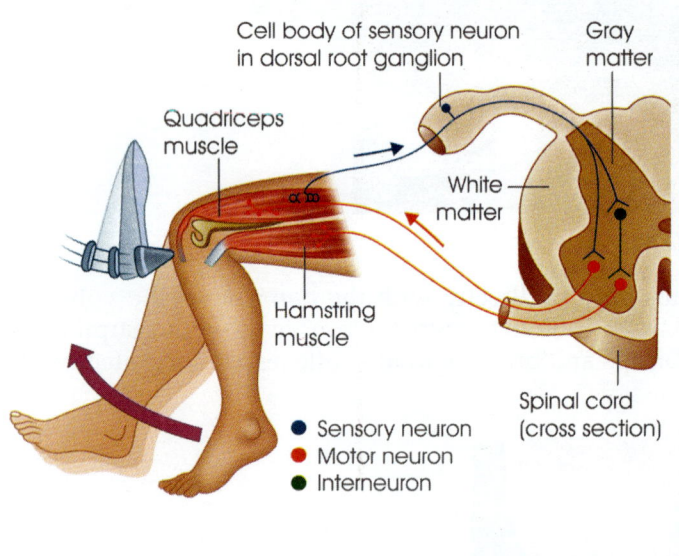
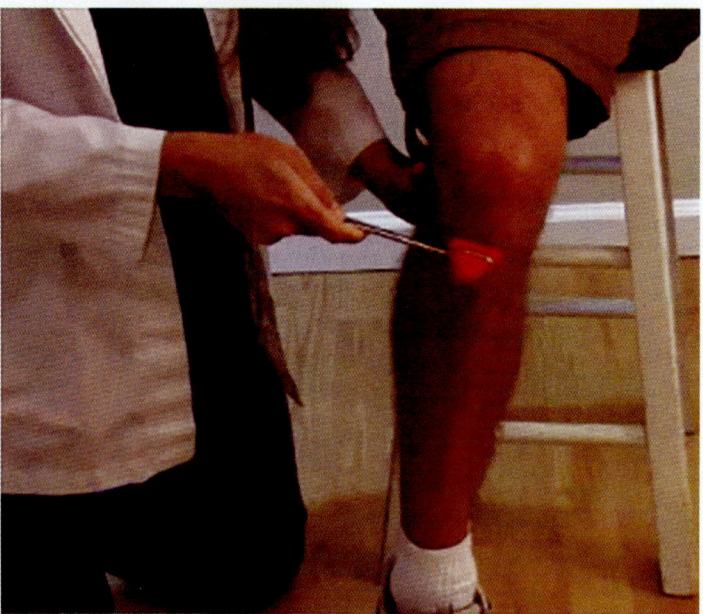

Fig. 19.5: Knee jerk reflex

Ankle Jerk (Fig. 19.6): The ankle reflex is elicited by hold on the relaxed foot with one hand and strike over the Achilles tendon with the hammer and note the plantar flexion. Repeat and compare your finding with other foot. The ankle jerk reflex is mediated by the S1 nerve root.

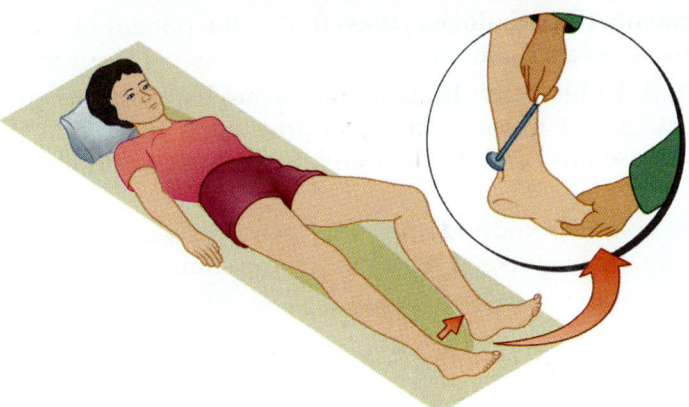

Fig. 19.6

Hoffman response: Hold the volunteer individual middle finger loosely and flick the finger nail downward. This causes the finger to rebound slightly into extension. If the thumb flexes and adducts in response, Hoffmann's sign is present. A positive Hoffman response is indicative of an upper motor neuron lesion affecting the upper extremity in question.

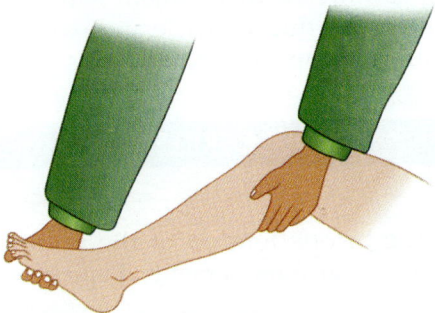

Fig. 19.7

Clonus (Fig. 19.7): If any of the reflexes appeared hyperactive, then hold the relaxed lower leg in your hand, and sharply dorsiflex the foot and hold it in dorsiflexed position. You will feel for oscillations between flexion and extension of the foot indicating clonus. Normally you are unable to feel any response.

Precautions while eliciting a reflex.
- Always compare one side to the other.
- Let hammer fall by gravity in most cases.
- Don't keep hammering a patient, if can't elicit a reflex.

If can't elicit a reflex, maneuvering can increase visibility by
- Clenching teeth.
- Jendrassik's maneuver:
- Patient clasps hands together tightly, or
- Gripping an object

Test for Cerebellar Function
Cerebellum is delivering unconscious regulation of muscle tone, equilibrium and coordination of voluntary movements. The signs suggesting cerebellar disease occur in several different aspects of the body.

Test
1. **Finger to nose and finger to finger test:**
   a. Ask the volunteer individual to fully extend arm, then touch nose.
   b. Ask the volunteer individual to touch his/her nose then extend the arm to bring his finger close as to touching your finger. If individual is unable to do so, he is having dysmetria.

2. **Rapid alternating movements (Dysdiadochokinesia):** Ask the patient to place one hand over the next and flip one hand back and forth as fast as he can.

3. **Rebound phenomenon:** Ask the individuals to pull your hand and then slip your hand out of their grasp. Normally the antagonist muscles contract and stops their arm from moving in the desired direction. In cerebellar disease this response is completely absent and limb continue moving in the desired direction.

4. **Heel to shin test:** Ask the volunteer individual to run their heel down the contralateral shin. The abnormal result occurs when they are unable to keep their foot on the shin.

Meningeal Signs

The signs of meningeal irritation indicate inflammation of the Dura.

These signs are tested as follows:

1. Nuchal rigidity (neck stiffness): Place your hand under the volunteer individual head and gently try to flex the neck. If you observe undue resistance, it is because of diffuse irritation of the cervical nerve roots from meningeal inflammation.

2. Brudzinski sign: There is flexion of both knees during the maneuver to test nuchal rigidity and this specifically indicates diffuse meningeal irritation in the spinal nerve roots.

3. Kernig sign: Ask the individual to flex the hip and knee on one of the sides while he is supine; further ask him to extend the knee while the hip is still flexed. In patient with meningeal inflammation there is spasm of hamstring resulting in pain in the posterior thigh muscle and patient finds it difficult to extend the knee. In case of severe meningeal inflammation the opposite knee flexes during the test.

OSCE SKILLED

Q1. Demonstrate bicep jerk.

Ans. **Biceps reflex:** Place thumb on the biceps tendon of the volunteer individual and strike on thumb with the reflex hammer. Observe for the arm movements. Repeat and compare your findings with the other arm.

Q2. Demonstrate triceps jerk.

Ans. **Triceps jerk reflex:** Gently strike the short tendon of the triceps muscle close to its insertion near the tip of the elbow and elicit the reflex. The muscle contracts in response and the forearm is extended slightly.

Q3. Demonstrate knee jerk.

Ans. **Knee jerk:** Ask the volunteer individual to keep the leg hanging freely off the edge of the bench. He strikes the quadriceps tendon directly with the reflex hammer. The leg extends once and comes to rest. Repeat the procedure and compare the result with that of the other leg.

Q4. Demonstrate ankle jerk.

Ans. **Ankle jerk:** Hold the relaxed foot with one hand and strike over the Achilles tendon with the hammer and notes the plantar flexion. Repeat and compare your finding with other foot.

VIVA VOCE QUESTIONS

Q1. What are the key components of motor system?

Ans. *The motor system is divided into:*

The peripheral apparatus consisting of the anterior horn cell and its peripheral axon, neuromuscular junction and muscle.

The more complex central apparatus consisting of the descending pyramidal tracts involved in control and the systems involved in initiating and regulating movement (the basal ganglia and cerebellum).

Q2. Which are the key components of motor examination?

Ans. The key components in motor examination include assessment of strength, muscle tone, muscle bulk, coordination, abnormal movements and various reflexes.

Q3. How is the grading of muscle strength done?

Ans.

Grade	Muscle strength
5+	Normal
4+	Slightly less than full power against strong resistance
4	Able to overcome moderate resistance
4–	Able to overcome mild resistance
3	Able to accomplish full resistance of muscle against gravity
2	Able to accomplish full resistance of muscle with gravity eliminated
1	Only trace muscle contraction, may only be palpable
0	Flaccid

Q4. How are reflexes graded?

Ans. *The reflexes are graded as follows*:

0 = Reflex is absent; 1+ = Reflex is diminished; 2+ = Reflex is normal; 3+ = Reflex is hyperactive; 4+ = Reflex is hyperactive with clonus.

Q5. Give the root value at spinal cord for various reflexes.

Ans. *The reflexes and their spinal cord level control are as belows*:

Upper extremity	Level	Lower extremity	Level
Pectoral	C4-5	Patellar	L2-4
Biceps	C5-6	Achilles	S1-S2
Triceps	C6-7	Hamstrings	L4-5 S1-2
Brachioradialis	C5-6	Cremasteric	L1-2
Upper abdomen	T6-9	Bulbocavernosis	S3-4
Lower abdomen	T10-12	Anal wink	S3-5

Q6. Enlist various tests employed to test cerebellar function.

Ans. *The various cerebellar function tests are*:

Finger nose test, heel-to-shin test, rapid alternating movement test (e.g. touch each fingertips with thumb; supinate/pronate hand; tap floor with foot, etc.) Romberg test—[the patient is asked to stand with feet together—the patient with vestibular deficit will report vertigo (close eyes if proprioceptive deficit, patient will sway ⇒ +ve Romberg's)] and tandem gait (heel-toe walking) test.

Q7. What precautions should be taken while eliciting a reflex?

Ans. *The precautions should be taken while eliciting a reflex are*:

- Always compare one side to the other.
- Let hammer fall by gravity in most cases.
- Don't keep hammering subject, if can't elicit a reflex.

Q8. If can't elicit a reflex, which maneuvering can increase its visibility?

Ans. *If you can't elicit a reflex, you can increase its visibility by*:

- Clenching teeth.
- Jendrassik's maneuver
- Patient clasps hands together tightly.
- Gripping an object.

Q9. How will you elicit best supinator, biceps, triceps and knee jerk?

Ans. *The following precautions can be taken to elicit best reflex response:*

Supinator/brachioradialis (C5-6): Patient's elbow should be at 90° and kept relaxed, hand exactly pronated [thumb exactly in the arc of flexion] and resting and ensure that hammer falls on distal end of radius.

Biceps (C5-6): Patient's elbow should be at 90° and kept relaxed, physicians should place finger over biceps tendon and ensure that hammer falls on physicians finger.

Triceps (C6-7): In seated position—Patient's arm crossed over, onto chest, hammer to be held vertically, with mallet at bottom, swing into triceps tendon.

Supine: Patient's arm crossed over, onto chest, hammer to be held with physicians hand, and mallet at elbow, swing into triceps tendon.

Knees (L3-4) supine: Physicians should lift both knees with one arm, flexing legs slightly and ensure hammer falls on patellar tendon.

Seated: Patient's leg should be hanging, reflex to hold hammer with mallet at bottom, and let it swing into patellar tendon.

Q10. What is the Lasègue or straight-leg raising (SLR) sign?

Ans. Lasègue or straight-leg raising (SLR) sign is elicited by passively flexing the hip as the knee is kept straight while the patient is in the supine position. The limitation of flexion due to hamstring spasm and, or pain signifies local irritation of the lower lumbar nerve roots. The reverse SLR is elicited by passively hyper-extending the hip as the knee is kept straight while the patient is in the prone position. Limitation of extension due to spasm and or pain in the anterior thigh muscles indicates local irritation of the upper lumbar nerve roots.

Q11. What are the signs of upper motor neuron lesion?

Ans. The signs of upper motor neuron lesion are muscular weakness or paralysis with a characteristic distribution, increase in tone (spastic type), exaggerated tendon reflexes, extensor plantar response, and loss of abdominal reflexes, no or little muscle wasting and normal electrical excitability of muscle.

Q12. What are the signs of lower motor neuron lesion?

Ans. The signs of lower motor neuron lesion are muscle paralysis, muscle wasting, hypotonia, loss of reflexes, fasciculation, contractures of muscle and trophic changes in skin and nails.

Q13. What are primitive reflex?

Ans. The primitive reflex includes the glabellar tap, rooting, snout, sucking, and palmomental reflexes. These signs are generally absent in adults. When present in the adult, they signify diffuse cerebral damage, particularly of the frontal lobes.

Q14. What are superficial reflex?

Ans. The superficial reflex is segmental reflex responses indicating the integrity of cutaneous innervations and the corresponding motor outflow.

Examples: The corneal, conjunctiva, abdominal, cremasteric, anal wink, and plantar (Babinski) reflexes.

Q15. What are the clinical findings in upper and lower motor neuron lesion?

Ans. The upper motor neuron lesions are characterized by weakness or paralysis, spasticity, hyperreflexia, primitive reflexes and the Babinski sign positive. Lower motor neuron lesions are characterized by weakness or paralysis, hypotonia, hyporeflexia, atrophy and fasciculations.

HISTORICAL ASPECTS

The history of clinical medicine depicts the slow and gradual evolution of biomedical sciences. Despite the mega advances in the biomedical sciences during the last century the complexities of disease processes with changing environment earmarks that the clinical medicine still is a mix of applied science and the art of healing. The Greek and Roman believed that diseases are believed to reflect an imbalance of the humors. This thought prevailed for two centuries. In the Renaissance period the humoural basis of disease was discarded and the fields of anatomy, surgery and chemistry began to influence the development of medical practice. In the seventeenth century there were rapid and huge advances in the understanding of human physiology and so also the importance of clinical practice at the bedside was recommended over then. During the eighteenth and nineteenth centuries the scientific basis proven with statistical approaches to its applications developed. During the twentieth and early years of the twenty-first centuries there were overall advances in all aspect of scientific medicine especially diagnosis and description of diseases based over at the molecular level.

RECENT ADVANCES

A clinical decision support system (CDSS) is designed health technology system to assist medical doctors and other health professionals with clinical decision making tasks. Clinical decision support systems link health observations with health knowledge to influence health choices by clinicians for improved health care. Large number of medical institutions and software companies are trying to produce viable CDSSs to support all areas of clinical tasks. The two sectors of the healthcare where CDSSs has a large impact are the pharmacy and billing sectors. CDSS is commonly used in pharmacy and prescription ordering systems that conducts batch-based checking of orders for negative drug interactions and report warnings to the prescribing professionals. As many hospitals rely on medical reimbursements; several systems are designed to help examine both a proposed treatment plan and the current rules of health care to suggest a plan attempting to resolve the care of the patient and financial needs of the institution. CDSSs aimed at diagnostic tasks have also found success in the markets but have been limited in deployment and scope. CDSS must demonstrably improve clinical workflow or outcome for its successful intervention.

OBSERVATIONS: EXERCISE FOR STUDENTS

Cranial Nerves

PY 10.20*, PY 10.16*, PY 10.17*

BRIEF REVIEW OF FUNCTIONS

There are twelve cranial nerves and their functions are as follows:

1. I: Smell
2. II: Visual acuity, visual fields, colour vision and ocular fundi
3. II, III: Pupillary reactions
4. III, IV, VI: Extra-ocular movements, including opening of the eyes
5. V: Facial sensation, movements of the jaw, and corneal reflexes
6. VII: Facial movements and gustation
7. VIII: Hearing and balance
8. IX, X: Swallowing, elevation of the palate, gag reflex and gustation
9. V, VII, X, XII: Voice and speech
10. XI: Shrugging the shoulders and turning the head
11. XII: Movement and protrusion of tongue.

TESTING FOR FUNCTIONAL STATUS OF CRANIAL NERVE

Cranial Nerve I: Olfactory Nerve

1. Ask the subject to breathe in through the nose and observe for patency of the nasal passages bilaterally.
2. Ask the subject to close their eyes. Occlude one of his nostrils and expose the patient's nostril to garlic paste or a small bar of soap or any fragrant or pungent smelling substance such as lemon, clove or asafetida can be used.
3. Ask the patient to smell the object and identify the smell.
4. Switch nostrils and repeat the test.

Record Your Results

Right nostril

....
....
....
....

Left nostril

....
....
....
....

---

*Competency achievement as per competency based Undergraduate Curriculum for the Indian Medical Graduate, 2018, 1; Medical Council of India.

VIVA VOCE QUESTIONS

Q1. What is meant by anosmia?

Ans. Loss of sense of smell is called anosmia.

Q2. Name some conditions in which anosmia may be present.

Ans. Subfrontal meningiomas can cause unilateral or bilateral anosmia. Head injury may cause permanent anosmia if the olfactory nerve fibres passing through the cribriform plate are sheared as a result of injury. Anosmia is commonly neurodegenerative occurring in Lewy body disease so may be present in Parkinsonism and often the test is performed in Kallman's syndrome.

Q3. What is meant by parosmia?

Ans. Preversion of smell is called parosmia.

Q4. Name some conditions of parosmia.

Ans. It can be psychological in origin, may occur following partial recovery of the olfactory nerve after trauma, certain drugs, and sinus infections can cause it.

CRANIAL NERVE II—OPTIC NERVE

A. Visual Acuity

1. Test visual acuity by using Snellen chart.
2. Ask the volunteer individual to sit comfortably on examination stool at 6 metre (i.e. 20 feet) distance.
3. Ask subject to cover one of his eyes completely with hand and read the lowest line on the chart that is possible. Repeat the test covering the opposite eye too. Note the visual acuity for each eye.

Note: The results are expressed as a fraction. The numerator of the fraction is 20 or 6 the distance at which the subject reads the chart. The denominator is the lowest line that subject reads and its number represents the greatest distance from which the healthy individual can read this line.

(Less than 6/60 is severe loss of acuity, if so then ask to count fingers at 1 metre distance, still unable to do that patient asked to perceive hand movements, if unable then ask for perception of light or no perception of light).

Near vision is tested by asking the subject to read from Jaeger's chart at ordinary reading distance noting the smallest print the subject can read.

Record your result.

....
....
....
....

B. The Colour Vision is Tested Using Ishihara Plates

The different plates have figures written in colour in the background of colours. Some figures normal individuals can read not colour bind, on other charts, figures blind individuals but not normal can read.

Record your result

....
....
....
....

C. Field of Vision

The visual fields are tested by confrontation method.

1. Ask the volunteer individual to sit on stool at one foot distance directly facing you.
2. Ask the volunteer individual to cover the right eye with right hand and look into your eyes till test is over.

3. Explain the test to the volunteer individual and ask to observe your index finger as it enters from out of sight into his peripheral vision.
4. Cover your left eye with your left hand (the opposite to eye of the subject) and beginning with your hand and arm fully extended, slowly bring the outstretched fingers centrally, and notice when your fingers enter volunteer individual's field of vision.
5. Ask the volunteer individual to inform at the same time when sees your finger.
6. Repeat this maneuver once for every 45 degrees out of the 360 degrees of peripheral vision.
7. Repeat the same maneuver with the other eye.

Record your results

Field of vision left eye   *Normal/restricted*
....
....
....

Field of vision right eye   *Normal/restricted*
....
....
....

D. Fundus Examination

1. Observe the retinal vessels, optic disc, physiological cup and fovea using an ophthalmoscope.
2. You should observe for blurring of the optic disc margin, pulsations of the optic vessels and also for change in the optic disc's colour from its normal yellowish orange.

Note: The loss of pulsations of the retinal vessels followed by blurring of the optic disc margin and possibly retinal hemorrhages is seen in patient with increased intracranial pressure.

Record your result.
....
....
....
....

VIVA VOCE QUESTIONS

Q1. How is colour vision tested as a bedside test?

Ans. Ishihara plates provide a sensitive bedside test for colour vision.

Q2. What do you understand by protanopia and protanomally.

Ans. Protanopia is blindness to red colour and protanomally is weakness to red colour perception.

Q3. What is deuteranopia or deuteranomally?

Ans. Blindness to green colour is deuteranopia and weakness to perception of green light is called deuteranomally.

Q4. How to distinguish whether the colour blind individual is red colour blind or green colour blind since both confuse between these colours?

Ans. Ishihara plates have been so made to enable the distinction.

Q5. Why is it important to check for colour blindness?

Ans. Checks are required for drivers so that signals can be read.

Q6. Can unilateral loss of colour vision be present?

Ans. Acquired unilateral loss of colour vision is a chracteristic feature of optic neuropathy and can occur even when visual acuity is well preserved.

Q7. What are the tests used for testing field of vision?

Ans. Simple confrontation field testing is often used comparing the subject's field with examiners own assuming their own is normal. In the ophthalmic clinic a perimeter (often automated type) is used.

Q8. What do you mean by hemianopia? What type of lesion produces homonymous hemianopia.

Ans. Loss of half field of vision is hemianopia. If the loss for both eyes is of the same half field of vision it is homonymous hemianopia, it occurs with lesion of optic tract, optic radiations and cortical area.

Q9. What do you understand by heteronymous hemianopia and what is the site of lesion that produces it?

Ans. Different but half field of vision for both eyes is blind.

Q10. Define visual acuity.

Ans. The degree to which the details and contours of objects are perceived and identified. It is the shortest distance by which two lines can be separated and still perceived as two lines.

Q11. What is the defect in myopic eye and how is it corrected?

Ans. Eye ball is too long for refractory power of the eye. Corrected by concave lens.

Q12. What is the defect in age-related macular degeneration?

Ans. It is a degeneration disease in which sharp central vision is gradually destroyed.

CRANIAL NERVES II AND III (OPTIC AND OCULOMOTOR)

Test:

1. Ask the volunteer individual to focus on an object in the distance. Observe for the diameter of the pupils and note the symmetry between the pupils.
2. Focus pen torch or ophthalmoscope light into one eye at a time and check for direct and consensual light responses in each pupil. Note for the rate of the reflexes.
3. If direct and consensual light responses are sluggish or absent, then test for pupillary constriction via accommodation.
4. Ask the volunteer individual to focus on the light pen while the examiner moves it closer and closer to their nose. The eyes accommodates to the near object the pupils constrict.

Afferent pupillary defect

In a patient with severe lesion of the anterior visual system in one eye (an ophthalmological disorder or optic nerve disorder such as severe optic neuritis or an ischaemic optic neuropathy) will have afferent pupillary defect, failure of constriction of either pupil to light shown into the affected eye. If visual system on other side is unaffected light shown into the normal eye will lead to a normal direct pupillary response and there will also be a consensual papillary response in the visually impaired eye, assumimg the efferent pathway is intact.

Efferent papillary defect (part of 3rd nerve lesion)

A lesion of the pupilloconstrictor nerve fiber in oculomotor nerve will lead to dilation of the ipsilateral pupil (due to unrestricted effect of sympathetic supply). There will be failure of constriction of the pupil to light although the consensual response in the other eye will be preserved. Light shown into contralateral eye will elicit a normal direct response but no consensual response.

Record your results

....
....
....
....
....
....

Q13. Define near response in the eye.

Ans. The nearest point to the eye at which an object can be brought to clear focus by accommodation is called near point of vision.

Q14. What is the pathway for light reflex, consensual light reflex and accommodation reflex?

Ans. The optic nerve fibers for pupillary reflex leave the optic tract near the lateral geniculate bodies on each side, enter the midbrain via superior colliculus and terminate in the pretectal nucleus from where the fibres project to the ipsilateral and contralateral Edinger-Westphal nuclei that contain preganglionic parasympathetic neurons of the oculomotor nerve that terminate in the ciliary ganglion from which postganglionic nerves project to the ciliary muscles. The pathway is dorsal to the pathway for near response and hence light response is sometimes lost but response to accommodation remains.

Q15. What is Argyll Robertson pupil?

Ans. These are small irregular unequal pupil which do not react to light but react with accommodation. They were seen in advanced syphilis. Without the irregularity but with the other features diabetic small vessel disease is now the most important cause.

Q16. What is presbyopia? How is it corrected?

Ans. In old age the lens gradually becomes hard due to loss of elasticity resulting in loss of accommodation for near work. By the age of 40–50 years a normal individual requires reading glasses with biconvex lens.

CRANIAL NERVES III, IV AND VI (OCULOMOTOR, TROCHLEA AND ABDUCENT NERVE)

Terminology of eye movements

Horizontal movements of the eye outwards (laterally) abduction and inward movement (medially) is adduction. Vertical movements upwards is elevation and downward is depression. Diagonal movements at any intermediate angle are also done and rotary movements are those in which the eye twists on the anterior-posterior axis. Intorsion is rotation such as upper part of the eye moves medially and the lower part of the eye moves laterally. Extorsion is opposite. Convergence refers to adduction of both the eyes to fix on a near object. A squint is when eyes point in different direction and described as convergent or divergent strabismus depending on whether the eyes point towards or away from each other. Saccades are abrupt rapid small movements of both the eyes such as those needed to shift fixation from one object to the another, Nystagmus denotes rhythmic oscillations of one or both eyes. In pendular nystagmus the movement is slow in both directions. In jerk nystagmus there is slow phase in one direction and a fast phase in the opposite direction. By convention the direction of nystagmus is the direction of fast phase but the defect is in the slow phase.

Lateral rotation of the head causes reflex movements of the eyes in the opposite direction (abduction of one eye abduction of the other).

Actions of eye muscles

Table 20.1: Actions of the eye muscles

Nerve	Muscle	Action With eye abducted	With eye adducted
Abducens—VI	Lateral rectus	Abduction	Abduction
Oculomotor—III	Inferior rectus	Depression	Depression; extorsion
Oculomotor—III	Inferior oblique	Extorsion; elevation	Elevation
Oculomotor—III	Medial rectus	Adduction	Adduction
Oculomotor—III	Superior rectus	Elevation	Elevation intorsion
Trochlear—IV	Superior oblique	Intorsion; depression	Depression

The eye is offset laterally in relation to the apex of the orbit which accounts why the superior and inferior rectus muscles have only purely vertical action when the eye is abducted. Adduction of the eye turns the superior and inferior oblique muscles into a pure depressor and elevator, respectively.

Examination of eye Movements

The eye is offset laterally in relation to the apex of the orbit, hence the superior and inferior rectus muscles have only purely vertical actions when the eye is abducted; adduction of the eye turns superior and inferior oblique muscles into pure depressor and elevator respectively (Fig. 20.1).

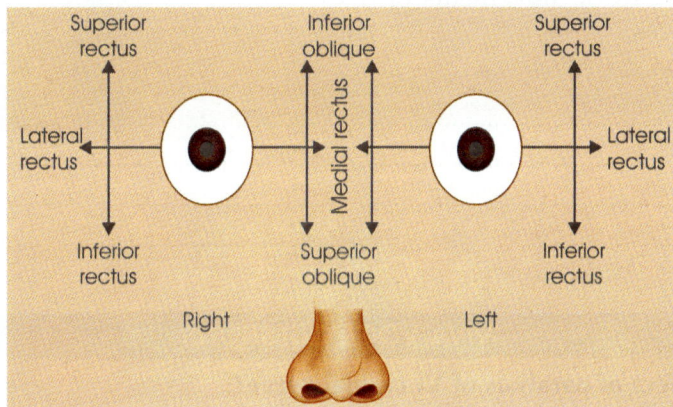

Fig. 20.1

The details of eye movements are examined when symptoms are present or abnormal signs are likely to be present. Ask the subject to keep head still assist yourself by putting your left hand on the head to steady it. And then to look at your right index finger held directly in front of the eyes at about half a metre away. Look for any visible abnormality of the alignment of the eyes and for any nystagmus. Move your finger to the right and left and up and down. Eye movements which are broken up into series of short saccades indicate a brainstem or cerebellar lesion affecting eye movement control. If there is diplopia it would be experienced at some point or all along. When looking for nystagmus not to get to far away in any direction. Look for nystagmus at about 30 degrees away from the primary position of gaze. (Nystagmus can normally appear if the patient struggles to deviate his eyes beyond what is possible.)

A third nerve lesion produces complete ptosis on the affected side and with paralysed eyelid raised paresis of adduction is seen when attempting to gaze on the other side. The other features of third nerve lesion are paresis of elevation of the eye and intorsion of the eye on attemting to look down due to action of superior oblique on the eye that cannot be adducted.

Procedure for examination

A. Inspect for presence of ptosis, squint, nystagmus, retraction of upper eyelid, size of pupil (whether equal on both sides) shape.

B. Tests

1. Instruct the volunteer individual to follow the penlight with their eyes without moving their head.
2. Move the penlight slowly at eye level, first to the left and then to the right.
3. Repeat this horizontal sweep with the penlight at the level of the patient's forehead and along chin.
4. Note for the extraocular muscle palsies and horizontal or vertical nystagmus. The students should note that the limitation of movement of both eyes in one direction is called gaze palsy or a conjugate lesion. It is indicative of a central lesion. The disconjugate lesions (where the eyes are not restricted in the same direction or if only one eye is restricted) are due to more peripheral disruptions in cranial nerve nuclei, cranial nerves or neuromuscular junctions exception to this is isolated impairment of adduction of one eye due to an ipsilateral median longitudinal fasciculus lesion.

C. Examine the pupils for

1. Size
2. Shape
3. Mobility
4. Reaction to light
5. Reaction to accommodation.

D. Diplopia

The image of the object if it does not fall on the corresponding points in the retina of the two eyes diplopia is produced. Diplopia is produced even with slight misalignment of the eyes.

If there is complaint of double vision the diplopia can be monocular or true diplopia that is binocular that can be due to paresis of movements of one or both eyes. Diplopia can even develope with small misalignment of the eyes.

Record your results

....

....

....

....

VIVA VOCE QUESTIONS

Q1. What would be the effect of paralysis of VI cranial nerve?

Ans. Inability to move the eye laterally (abduction). Horizontal diplopia.

Q2. What would be the effect of paralysis of III cranial nerve?

Ans. Third nerve lesion may result in ptosis (levator palpebrae superioris is innervated by third cranial nerve), elevation and adduction of the eye may be effected and may produce pupillary dilatation.

Q3. What would be the effect of paralysis of fourth cranial nerve?

Ans. Extorsion of the eye due to unopposed action of inferior oblique leads to diplopic.

CRANIAL NERVE V (TRIGEMINAL)

It is a mixed motor and sensory nerve. The cutaneous distribution of the three divisions of trigeminal nerve are by ophthalmic, maxillary and mandibular. These nerves also mediate general sensations inside the mouth and nose and proprioception. Afferents mediating touch sensation pass to the principal sensory nucleus of the trigeminal nerve in the pons. Pain and temperature afferents enter spinal tract and pass into medulla and into spinal nucleus of the trigeminal nerve. Thus lesions in the medulla can give rise to dissociated sensory loss in the trigeminal area (loss of pin prick sensation with preserved light touch). Motor component of the trigeminal nerve from the motor nucleus in the pons run in the motor root of the trigeminal nerve and enter mandibular nerve. They supply the muscles of mastication; masseter, temporalis and the lateral pterygoids.

Test

1A. Instruct the volunteer individual to clench teeth (or bite down hard) and palpate the masseter muscles, these should stand out with equal prominence on each side. If there is paralysis on one side the muscles on affected side will fail to become prominent.

1B. Note for any masseter wasting.

2. Ask the volunteer individual to open mouth against resistance as you apply resistance at the base of the volunteer individual's chin. When the subject opens mouth lateral pterygoid muscles on each side draw the mandible forward. (In severe lesion of the trigeminal nerve will lead to a deviation of the jaw towards the side of the lesion due to weakness of the pterygoid muscles on the affected side.) The pterygoid muscles may be tested further by asking the subject to push the jaw sideways against your hand.

3. Test the gross sensation of the trigeminal nerve (Fig. 20.2), explain the test with needle to the volunteer individual to alleviate fear of being hurt. Asked the volunteer individual to close the eyes and inform whether the touch of a needle is sharp or dull when the volunteer individual feels an object touching the face.

4. Test touch sensation of the volunteer individual with collon wool (or using von Frey's asthesiometer) above each temple and along the nose and chin bilaterally. Ask the volunteer individual to also compare and report the strength of the sensation of both sides.

5. If the volunteer individual is unable to distinguish pinprick and light touch, then check temperature and vibration sensation using the vibration fork.

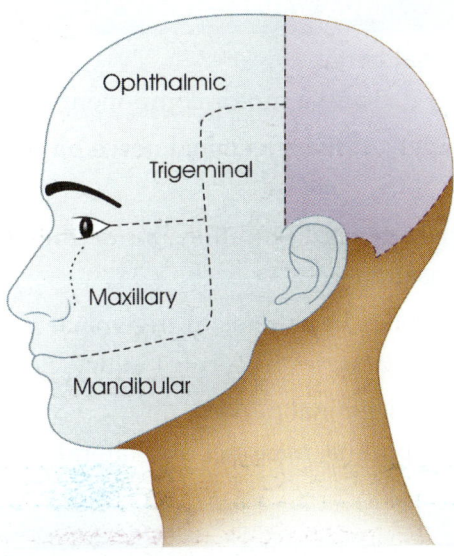

Fig. 20.2: Sensory areas of three divisions of trigeminal nerve

6. *Corneal reflex:* Ask the subject to look at a distant object. Then touch the limbus (sclerocorneal junction) with a sterile cotton (Fig. 20.3) wool brought from the side of the subject. Test both the eyes.

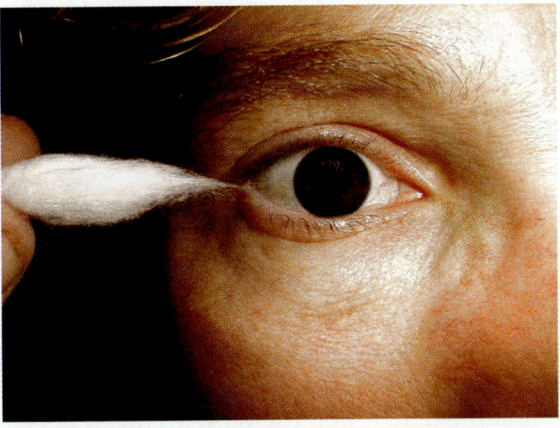

Fig. 20.3

The corneal reflex

A sensory stimulus applied to the cornea causes blink which cannot be suppressed. In coma a drop of saline is used. The test is uncomfortable and not a part of routine neurological examination.

If there is ipsilateral facial paralysis (e.g. Bell's paralysis), the reflex will be absent on the affected side, but readily seen on the other side.

Response: Closure of both eyes

Afferent: 5th cranial nerve.

Efferent: 7th cranial nerve.

Jaw jerk: Ask the subject to let his jaw sag and open slightly. Place the left thumb over the chin and tap with the knee hammer.

Response: Closure of mouth.

Afferent and efferent: 5th cranial nerve.

Record your results.

....

....

....

VIVA VOCE QUESTIONS

Q1. Name the components of trigeminal nerve.

Ans. Sensory three divisions as in Fig. 20.3 and a motor component.

Q2. What are the areas of sensory supply of the trigeminal nerve on the face?

Ans. Refer to Fig. 20.3.

Q3. Does trigeminal nerve also mediate general sensations inside the mouth and nose and proprioception.

Ans. Yes it is responsible for these sensations.

Q4. Is it important to test for corneal reflex in patients of trigeminal nerve lesions?

Ans. Patients with anaesthetic cornea are at a risk of corneal injury, hence it should be tested.

Q5. What are the muscles supplied by trigeminal nerve?

Ans. Trigeminal nerve supplies the temporalis, masseter and lateral pterygoid muscles.

OSCE

1. Tested sensations of touch pain on one side of the face. (Yes/No)
2. Tested sensations on the opposite side of the face. (Yes/No)
3. Look for the wasting of temporalis and masseter muscles. (Yes/No)
4. Feel for the contraction of masseter muscle when asked to clench jaws. (Yes/No)
5. Ask the subject to open the jaw. (Yes/No)

CRANIAL NERVE VII (FACIAL)

It supplies all muscles of face and scalp except the levator palpebrae superioris. Hence it is responsible for facial expression. If there is paralysis the person gives history that is unable to whistle. Food is apt to collect between the teeth and gums and saliva or any fluid escapes from the affected angle of the mouth.

A. Inspect and look for:

1. Inspect the face for any facial asymmetry particularly sagging, drooping of the facial creases. Depth of nasolabial folds on each side. Furrows of forehead, width of palpebral fissure, symmetry of angles of mouth.

B. Test

1. Ask the volunteer individual to raise their eyebrows, clinch teeth, frown and puff out both cheeks (If one or both sides of the facial muscle are weak in patient they will have difficulty holding the air in). Note for any asymmetry and difficulty encountered while performing these maneuvers. Observe for any weakness. The most notable deficit in patients with facial nerve damage is weakness of muscles of facial expression.
2. Ask the volunteer individual to close eyes strongly and resist examiners attempt to pull them open. In normal physiological state the patient's eyes cannot be opened by the examiner. The common cause of facial weakness is Bell's palsy. It is an idiopathic condition resulting from viral infection-induced inflammatory swelling of the facial nerve in its canal.
3. Ask the subject to whistle, note if able to do it or whether the air tends to escapes from weak side.
4. Ask the subject to show teeth. Note position of angles of mouth.
5. Ask to inflate mouth with air and tap lightly on either cheek. He is able to retain the air in the mouth (Fig. 20.4).

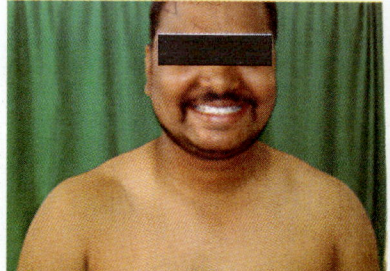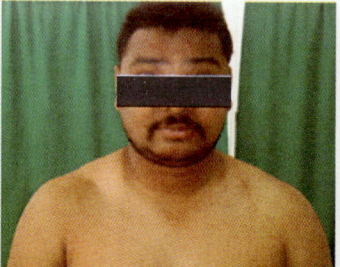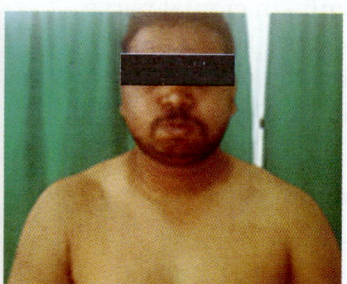

Fig. 20.4: Subject asked to clinch teeth, raise eyebrows and puff out both cheeks

6. Taste sensation: Cranial nerve VII is also responsible for carrying taste sensations from the anterior 2/3 of the tongue. Test for taste sensation in anterior part of tongue by placing a drop of sugar solution on a papter on the protruded tongue. (While testing for taste sensation avoid stimulationg V cranial nerve fibres).

7. Hyperacusis which produces increased auditory volume in an affected ear is observed with pathology involving the seventh cranial nerve. The seventh cranial nerve innervates the stapedius muscle in the middle ear which damps ossicle movements and decreases its volume.

A lower motor lesion affecting the whole of the facial nerve nucleus or the whole of the facial nerve will cause weakness of all muscles on the affected side of the face. An unilateral upper motor neuron lesion will cause weakness of the lower half of face with sparing of upper half of the face because of bilateral representation of the upper half of the face in the motor cortex.

Record your results.

....
....
....
....
....
....
....

VIVA VOCE QUESTIONS

Q1. Mention the functions of facial nerve.

Ans. Innervates facial muscles, carries taste fibres from anterior 2/3rd of tongue and supplies stapedius muscle.

Q2. Why in some cases of facial nerve paralysis the muscles of the lower part of face are paralysed and not of the muscles of the upper part of the face?

Ans. In cortical lesion involving facial area there is bilateral representation.

Q3. What is the role of facial nerve in taste and sound perception?

Ans. Taste perception in anterior 2/3 tongue is by facial nerve. Facial nerve supplies stapedius muscle which damps loud sounds.

Q4. What are the parasympathetic functions of the facial nerve?

Ans. Innervation of lacrimal and salivary glands.

Q5. What is Bell's palsy?

Ans. Paralysis of facial nerve on the affected side.

OSCE

1. **Look for facial symmetry and for nasolabial folds. (Yes/No)**

2. **Ask the subject to clinch the teeth. (Yes/No)**

3. **Ask to raise eyebrows. (Yes/No)**

4. **Ask to puff out both cheek. (Yes/No)**

5. **Test taste sensation in the anterior part of tongue. (Yes/No)**

CRANIAL NERVE VIII (AUDITORY)

A. Test for cochlear function (auditory function)

1. The hearing can be assessed by instructing the individual to close the eyes and respond with yes or no as the sound is heard in the respective ear.

2. Rub your index finger and thumb together close to the subjects ear or whisper numbers close to the ear with contralateral ear occluded (alternatively test by watch test standing behind the subject starting from outside the range of hearing bring a watch gradually nearer, subject is asked to say yes on hearing, comparison is made with the other side). Confirm if the sound was the same in either ears or louder in a particular ear. If lateralization or hearing abnormalities are noted, then perform the Rinne and Weber tests using the 256 or 512 Hz tuning fork (not lower frequency tuning fork 128 used for vibration sense).

3. Rinne test (Fig. 20.5). It compares air conduction to bone conduction. Gently hit the tuning fork firmly on palm and place the butt on the mastoid eminence firmly. Ask him to raise his finger immediately after he stops hearing the vibration. When the individual says "now", remove the butt from the mastoid process and place the U of the tuning fork near the ear without touching it. The individual informs by saying 'now' when he is able to hear anything. In normal persons the air conduction is better than bone conduction. If the bone conduction is the same or better than the air conduction, there is a conductive deafness on that side. If there is a sensi-neuronal hearing loss, then the vibration is heard longer in the air than on bone.

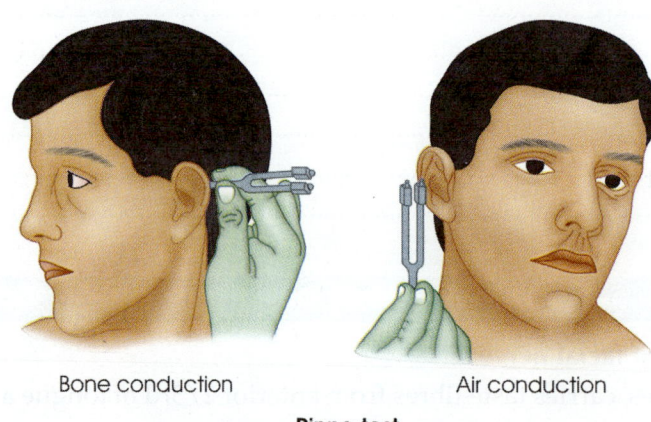

Bone conduction   Air conduction

Rinne test

Fig. 20.5: Demonstration of Rinne test in the subject

4. Weber test (Fig. 20.6): Gently hit the tuning fork strongly on your palm and then place the butt of the tuning fork at the centre of individual's forehead and ask the individual if hears the sound. In healthy individual the sound is equally in both ears. In conductive deafness sound is better heard in affected ear because masking effect of environmental noise is absent on disease side. In sensorineural deafness sound is better heard in normal ear.

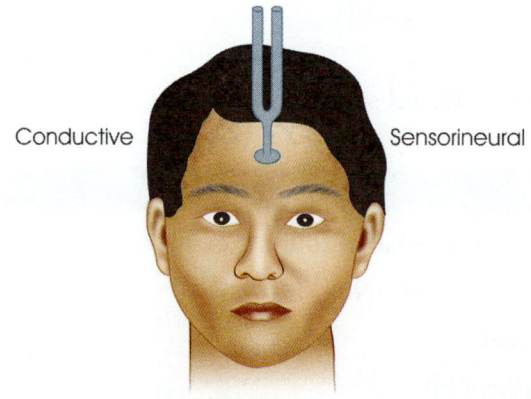

Conductive   Sensorineural

Weber's test

Fig. 20.6: Demonstration of Weber's test in the subject

B. Vestibular Function:

Ask for history of vertigo or nystagmus

Vestibular function tests are performed if the subject has vertigo.

Note your results

....

....

....

....

....

....

Q1. What is the test used to detect if the deafness is due to lesion in the middle ear or due to inner ear lesion.

Ans. Rinne test.

Q2. What should be the frequency of tuning fork to be used for Rinne's test?

Ans. 256 or 512 Hz

CRANIAL NERVES IX AND X (GLOSSOPHARYNGEAL AND VAGUS)

There are anatomical and functional relationships between the glossopharyngeal nerve, vagus nerve and cranial component of the accessory nerve. The nucleus ambiguous in the medulla contains the motor neurons which innervate striated muscle of the palate, pharynx, larynx and upper oesophagus, fibers running partly in the glossopharyngeal nerve mainly in the vagus nerve and partly in the cranial portion of the accessory nerve. Situated more dorsally in the medulla the dorsal motor nucleus of the vagus and the inferior salivary nucleus (whose fibers join the glossopharygeal nerve) contain parasympathetic neurons which control glands and smooth muscle. Special visceral afferents (taste fibres from the intermediate nerve and the glossopharyngeal nerve) enter the solitary tract to end in the nucleus of the solitary tract in the medulla. General somatic sensory afferents in the glossopharyngeal and vagus nerve join trigeminal sensory nuclei.

The glossopharyngeal nerve mediates somatic sensations of the palate and pharynx and gustatory sensations from the posterior third of the tongue, it contains autonomic secretomotor fibers for the parotid gland and supplies the stylopharyngeus muscle which cannot be tested clinically.

Testing of Nerves

These nerves are responsible for phonation, swallowing, guttural and palatal articulation. Glossopharyngeal nerve also supplies posterior one-third of the tongue and is responsible for general sensations and taste impulses from the posterior third of the tongue.

Glossopharyngeal nerve is not tested in routine neurological examinations. In stuporous or comatosed patients testing of gag reflex may be useful, the afferent component is by glossopharyngeal nerve.

Testing Vagus Nerve

Vagal motor efferents supply pharyngeal muscles. The superior laryngeal nerve supplies the sensation from the larynx, recurrent laryngeal nerve supplies the laryngeal muscles but not the cricopharyngeus visceral efferents and afferents of the vagus nerve cannot be tested.

A. Ask: For any history of regurgitation of fluids through nose when subject tries to swallow.

B. Test:

1. Ask the volunteer individual to open his mouth and say 'AH'. Observe for the palatal movements. Vagal motor efferents supply pharyngeal muscles.
2. Observe and assess the gag reflex by gently stroking the soft palate on each side.
3. Assess swallowing by giving him water to drink.
4. Observe if there is any nasal quality in speech.

Normal response: The palate elevates symmetrically when sustaining an 'AH' and in response to stimulation on either side. Some patients do not have a gag response but this is observed bilaterally. In unilateral palatal weakness the palate fails to elevate on the weak side and gag reflex is absent on that side (Fig. 20.7).

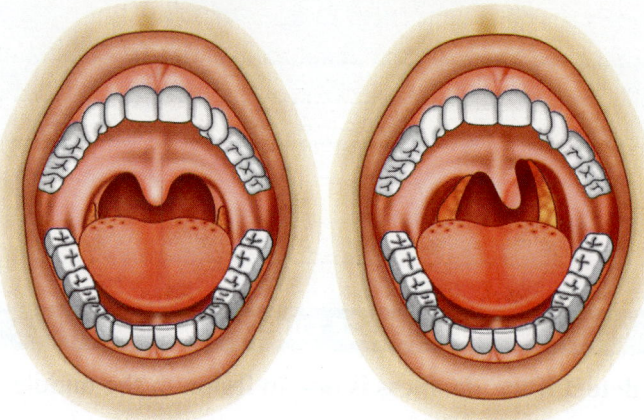

Fig. 20.7

Note your results

....

....

....

....

CRANIAL NERVE XI (ACCESSORY NERVE)

1. Ask the volunteer individual to shrug their shoulders as strong as they possible as you resist this motion by pressing down on his shoulders with your hands (Fig. 20.8).

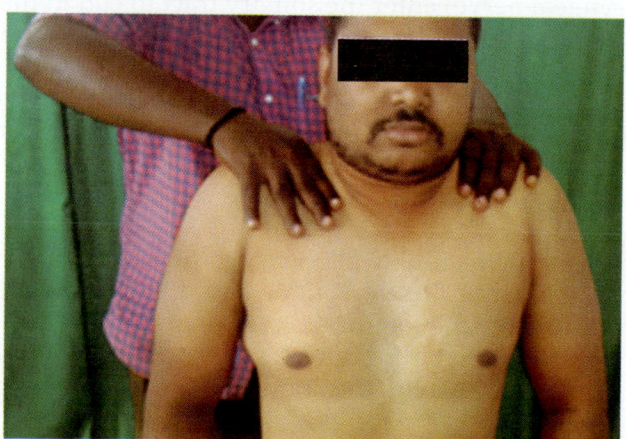

Fig. 20.8; Photograph demonstration of examination of spinal accessory nerve

2. Ask the section to turn their head to the opposite side against resistance, watch and palpate the sternocleidomastoid muscle.

3. Test other side and ask the patient to turn their head to the opposite side against resistance, both watch and palpate the sternocleidomastoid muscle.

4. Asked the patient to flex the head forward against resistance. Ensure you place your hand behind individual's head to support his head if there is any weakness.

5. The subject should normally overcome the resistance applied by the examiner.

Note your results

....

....

....

....

CRANIAL NERVE XII (HYPOGLOSSAL NERVE)

The hypoglossal nerve is motor to the tongue. Observe the tongue for any atrophy or enlargement. Ask the individual to protrude the tongue and move the tongue from side to side. Normally the volunteer individual will be able to protrude it straight (Fig. 20.9A). If case of hypoglossal nerve damage, tongue will deviate towards the affected side. In unilateral paralysis, the tongue will be deviated towards the paralysed side on protrusion (Fig. 20.9B). The muscles of the healthy side push the tongue to the paralysed side (Fig. 20.9B).

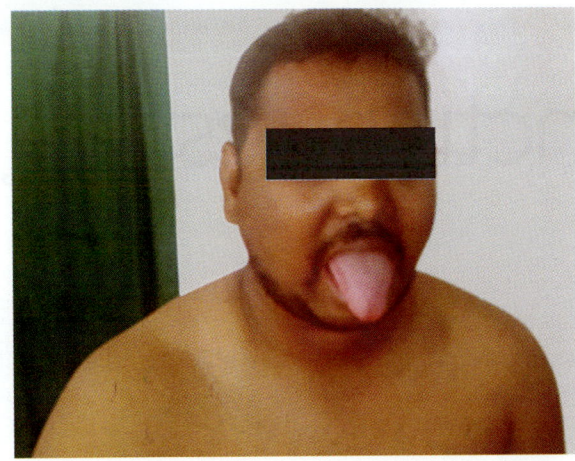
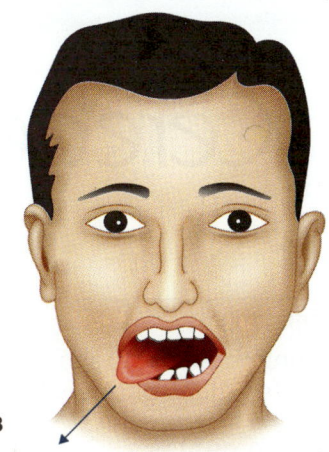

Fig. 20.9A and B

In bilateral paralysis, the person will not be able to protrude the tongue *fn*.

In LMN type of paralysis, wasting, fasciculation and flaccidity of the tongue are present. In UMN type of paralysis, the tongue may be small and spastic.

Note your results

....
....
....
....

Q1. What are the effects of paralysis of the VII cranial nerve?

Ans. Loss of expression and asymmetry of face, furrows over forehead and nasolabial folds disappear and smoothen out. Ala nasi does not function properly during respiration. The angle of the mouth is drawn upwards and deviated to the opposite side. Eyes are wide open, eye brows drop down.

Paralysis of the buccinators causes food to accumulate between cheek and teeth and it dribbles along with saliva from the angle of mouth.

Paralysis of stapedius, the subject complains of loudness of sound called hyperacusis.

Paralysis of sensory fibers lead to loss of taste sensations from anterior two-thirds of tongue. The effect is better appreciated in bilateral paralysis.

The paralysis of secretomotor fibres produces decrease in tear formation, also dryness of conjunctiva (xerosis) or xerophthalmia, decrease in salivary secretion resulting in difficulty in swallowing.

OSPE

1. Look for the facial symmetry, nasolabial folds, and furrows over the head. (Yes/no)

2. Look for angle of the mouth both sides. (Yes/no)

3. Look for width of palpaberal fissure compare with other side. (Yes/no)

4. Ask the subject to show upper teeth. (Yes/no)

5. Ask the subject to close the eye tightly as he can try to open passively. (Yes/No)

21

Cerebellar Function Tests

PY 10.7*

Aim of the Experiment

To test the functions of cerebellum.

Procedure

The functions of the cerebellum are tested under the following headings:

- Tone
- Coordination of movements
- Reflexes
- Speech
- Gait
- Involuntary movements.

1. TONE

Muscle tone is the state of partial contraction found in healthy muscles at rest. It is the degree of tension present in a muscle at rest. It is assessed by passive movements.

Method of eliciting tone:

Instruct the subject to keep his limbs relaxed. Move the limbs passively at the joints and assess the resistance offered by the muscles.

2. COORDINATION

The coordination of movements means smooth recruitment, interaction and cooperation of a group of muscles to carry out a precise and definite motor act.

Tests of Coordination in the Upper Limbs

a. The Finger-nose Test *(Fig. 21.1)*

Ask the subject to keep his right upper limb outstretched and then to touch the tip of his nose with his forefinger. Ask him to do this few times and check if he is able to perform it smoothly.
   Repeat this in the opposite limb.
   In cerebellar lesions, there will be overshooting of the finger (past pointing). This is known as dysmetria.

b. The Finger-finger Nose Test *(Fig. 21.1)*

The subject is instructed to touch the examiner's finger first and then touch his nose. Ask him to do this few times. Repeat this in the other limb.

---

*Competency achievement as per competency based Undergraduate Curriculum for the Indian Medical Graduate, 2018, 1; Medical Council of India.

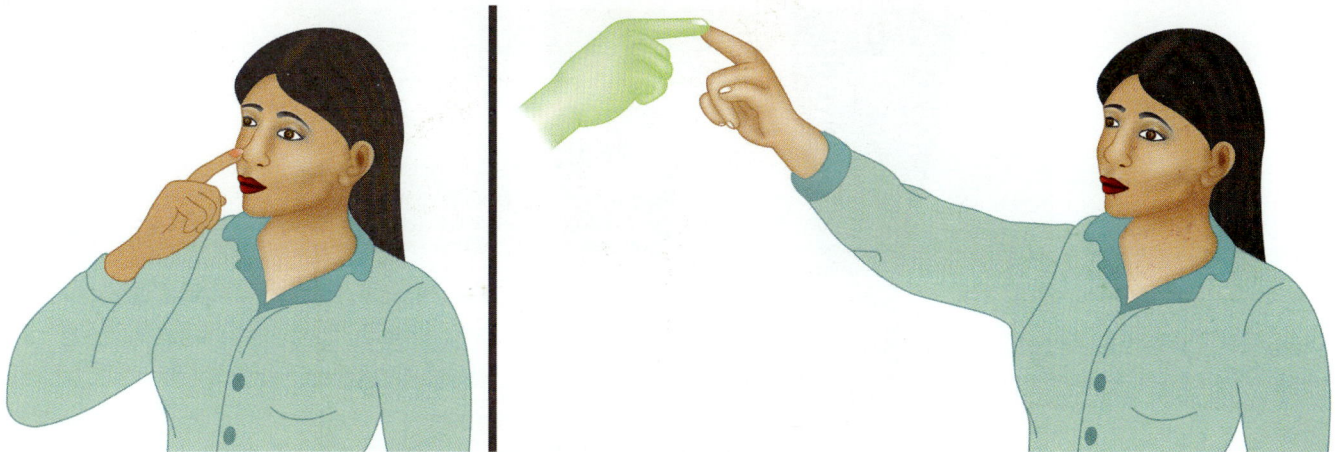

Fig. 21.1: Finger nose test and finger-finger nose test

c. Drawing a Circle in the Air

In cerebellar lesions, there will be overshooting of the finger (past pointing). This is known as dysmetria.

d. Diadochokinesia (Fig. 21.2)

Ask the subject to carry out rapid alternating movements of supination and pronation of one forearm and hand over the palm of the other hand. Difficulty in performing such rapid alternate movements is called dysdiadochokinesia.

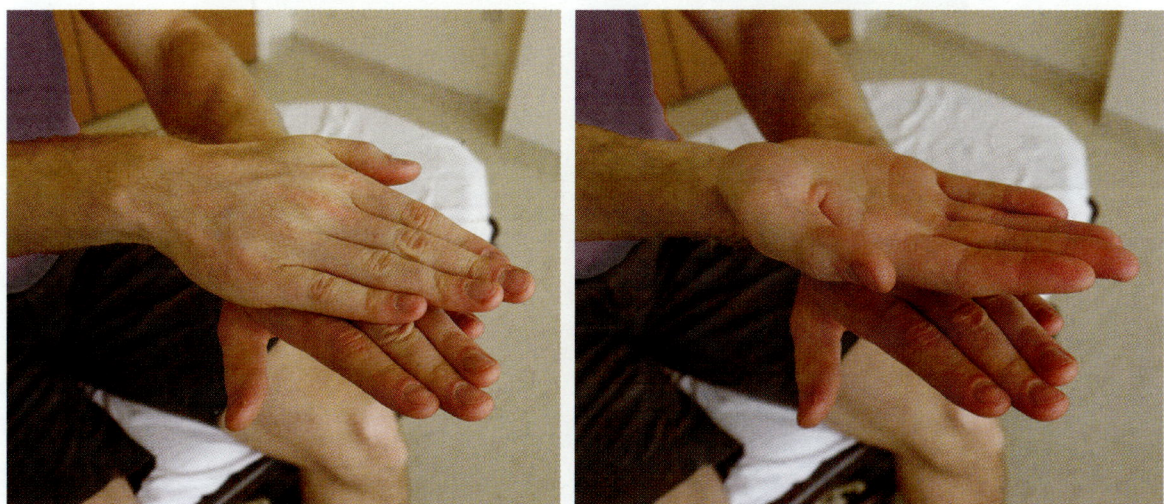

Fig. 21.2: Testing for diadochokinesia

Rebound Phenomenon

Ask the subject to flex his forearm against resistance offered by the examiner. Withdraw the resistance suddenly and check for rebound phenomenon. Repeat the test on the other side. Normally he should be able to put a brake on the movement. In cerebellar lesions, there is inability to terminate the movement all of a sudden due to which he may even hit his own face.

Tests of Coordination in the Lower Limbs

a. Tandem Walking (Fig. 21.3)

Ask the subject to walk in a straight toe to heel. In cerebellar lesions, he will deviate to one side or the other depending on the side of lesion.

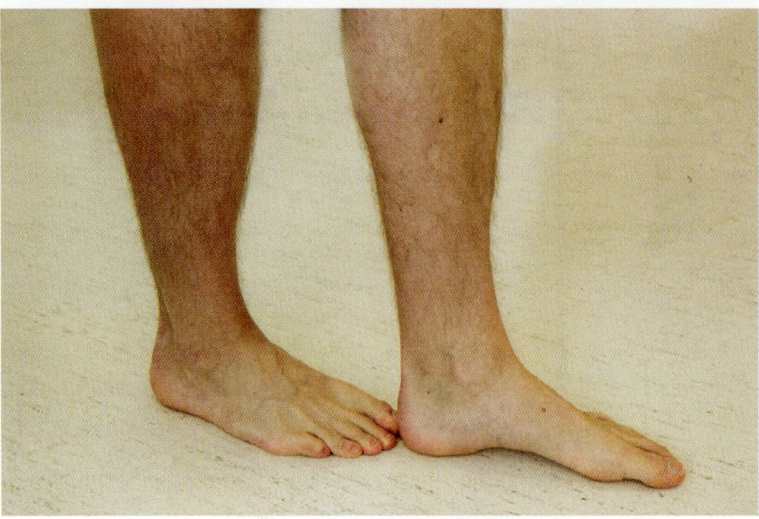

Fig. 21.3: Tandem walking

b. Heel Knee Test *(Fig. 21.4)*

In supine position, ask the subject to place the heel of one leg on the opposite knee and then to slide it down along the shin of the tibia towards the ankle. Ask him to repeat the procedure few times in quick succession. Repeat the test for the other leg also. In cerebellar lesions, the subject will have difficulty in performing the test smoothly.

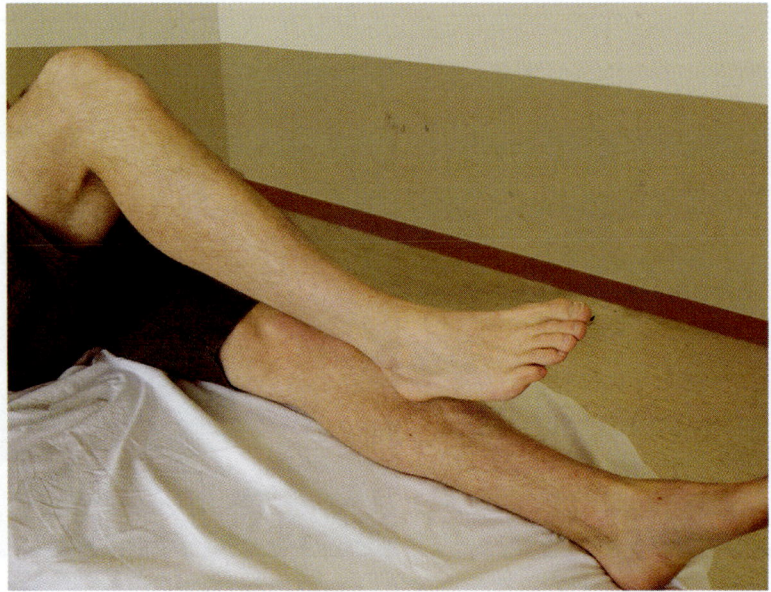

Fig. 21.4: Performing the heel shin test

c. Drawing a Circle in the Air

Ask the subject to draw a circle in the air with his great toe. Test the other leg also.

3. DEEP REFLEX—KNEE JERK

Perform knee jerk on both sides in the sitting position with legs hanging down freely. In cerebellar lesion, pendular knee jerk response is observed.

4. SPEECH

Ask the subject to pronounce "RAJAGOPALACHARI"/"RHINOCEROUS". In cerebellar lesion, there will be dysarthria. (Scanning speech/staccato speech).

5. GAIT

Ask the subject to walk barefoot for at least 9 metres and then turn around and walk back to the starting point. Observe the gait. In cerebellar lesion, the gait is broad based with feet apart, staggering or reeling towards the side of the lesion. This is called, 'ataxic or reeling or drunken gait'.

6. INVOLUNTARY MOVEMENTS

Tremor: Tremor may be defined as involuntary, regular, rhythmic, purposeless movements due to alternate contraction and relaxation of the agonist and antagonist muscles.

In cerebellar lesion, coarse tremor occurs when the subject intends to do something or attempts to pick up an object. This is called intention tremor.

7. LOOK FOR NYSTAGMUS

Nystagmus is involuntary, jerky, to and fro, often rhythmical oscillations of the eyeball. In lesion, nystagmus is seen towards the side of the lesion.

Observations and Result

Tone

Coordination of movements

Speech

Gait

Involuntary movements

....

....

....

....

OSPE

Q1. What type of tremor is seen in cerebellar lesions? When does the tremor appear?

Ans. In cerebellar lesions intention tremor appears. The tremor is there when patient attempts to perform some work.

Q2. What is the role of cerebellum in movements?

Ans. Cerebellum coordinates voluntary movements.

Q3. What is the type of gait the patients with cerebellar lesions would have?

Ans. Wide-based, unsteady, drunken gait

VIVA VOCE QUESTIONS

Q1. What are the functions of cerebellum?

Ans. Maintains body posture, coordinates movements, has a role in motor learning and planning and programming of movements.

Q2. What is dysdiadochokinesia?

Ans. Inability to perform rapid alternating movements.

Q3. Name the gait seen in cerebellar lesion.

Ans. A wide-based drunken gait.

Q4. How does tremor in cerebellar lesions differ from that of Basal Ganglia lesions?

Ans. Tremor in cerebellar lesion is intention tremor as appears during movement while in basal ganglia lesion it is rest tremor that disappears during movement.

Perimetry

PY 10.18*

Learning Objectives

After learning the practical the student should be able to:

1. Explain the indications for doing perimetry.
2. Examine and chart the field of vision in the subject
3. Able to interpret and discuss the finding of perimetry charting.

Brief Review

Field of vision is the field which the eye sees all around a fixation point though the eye is fixed on a point. The sum of the objects that form images upon the retina while the eye is gazing in one particular direction is called the field of vision. Although the field of vision differs with each different act of fixation the peripheral limits are the same and are largely determined by the orbit, nose and cheek. Figure 22.1A shows the visual pathway from retina to the visual cortex.

Note that temporal field of each eye is seen by nasal part of retina of each eye and temporal part of retina views the nasal field of the eye (Fig. 22.1B).

The visual field is not circular as it is restricted by bones. In each eye the temporal field is more than nasal field as nasal field is obstructed by nasal bones and upper field is less than the lower field as upper field is restricted by orbital bone.

Monocular visual fields are slightly irregular and they extend from fixation point, approximately 60 degrees nasally and above to 70 degrees below and 90 degrees temporally.

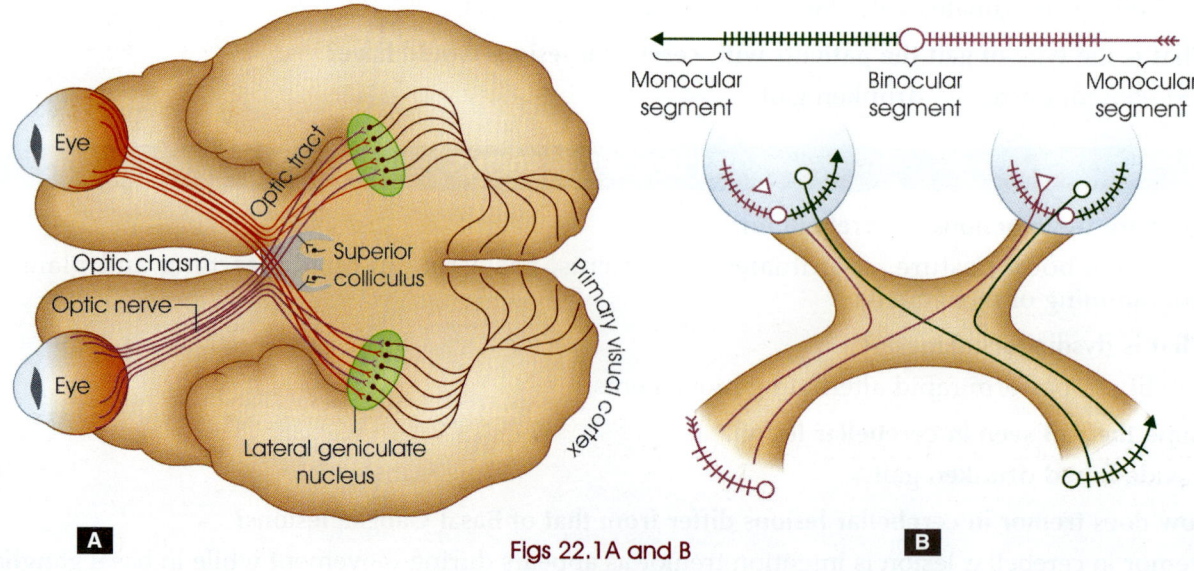

Figs 22.1A and B

*Competency achievement as per competency based Undergraduate Curriculum for the Indian Medical Graduate, 2018, 1; Medical Council of India.

In front there is a cone-shaped area in which the two fields overlap and enjoy binocular vision (Fig. 22.1B). The visual fields of both eyes for blue, red and green are progressively smaller (Fig. 22.4).

Lesion of the optic nerve causes blindness of that eye (Figs 22.2 A and B–a), lesion of the left optic tract (Fig. 22.2A) which is carrying fibers from the lateral half of the left retina, and medial half of right retina, results in blindness in the right field of both eyes (Fig. 22.2 B–c), resulting in right hemianopia (hemianopia, because half field of vision of eye is blind); and left field of vision would be lost if there is lesion of the right optic tract.

Hemianopia means half field of vision is blind; if the **same field of vision** for both eyes is blindness is it is called homonymous hemianopia, as in optic tract lesions; if there is lesion in optic chiasma as with pituitary tumor, the medial fibers from both the retina are affected and the hemianopia is heteronymous and bitemporal (Figs 22.2A and B–d). Heteronymous as field affected in each eye is not common for both eyes and bitemporal as temporal fields are affected in both the eyes.

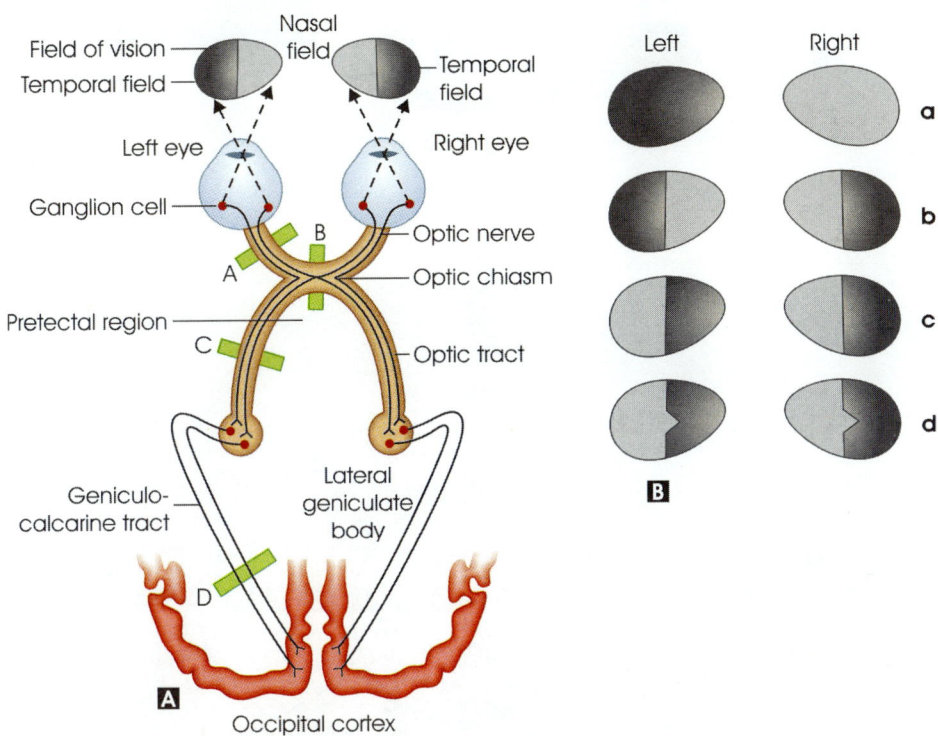

Figs 22.2A and B

Visual field testing is carried out clinically by asking the subject to keep his eye fixed while presenting objects at various places within the field of vision. The simple manual equipment used is tangent screen test but for more accurate result a perimeter is used. The test is performed manually or by an automated machine. The machine-based automated tests aid in diagnosis and a detailed print out of the patient's visual field is obtained.

Aim of Experiment

Charting the uni-ocular visual field by Lister's perimeter.

Note: Field of vision is the visibility of all the objects that form images on the retina as eyes look forward and is fixed at a particular point.

Instrument and Materials

Perimeter (Fig. 22.3) consists of metal arc which is graduated in degrees. The metal arc is projected towards subject side. The holder sliding in the arc carries forward a test object, which glides along the length of the arc. The arc is pivoted at the centre. Arc can be rotated through various angles. The test object of different colors and sizes are used for testing the field of vision.

Perimetry chart: The concentric circles around the centre (point corresponds with visual axis) represents points of equal visual acuity called isopters. Therefore, all points on one particular concentric line subtend the same

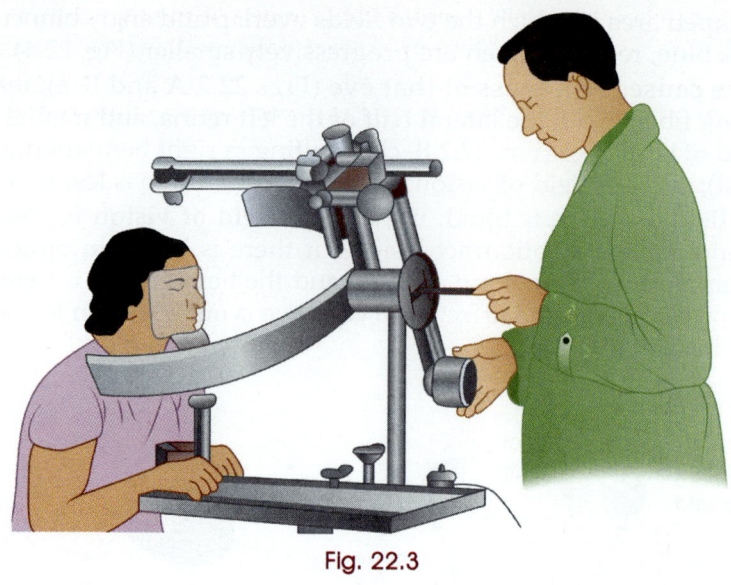

Fig. 22.3

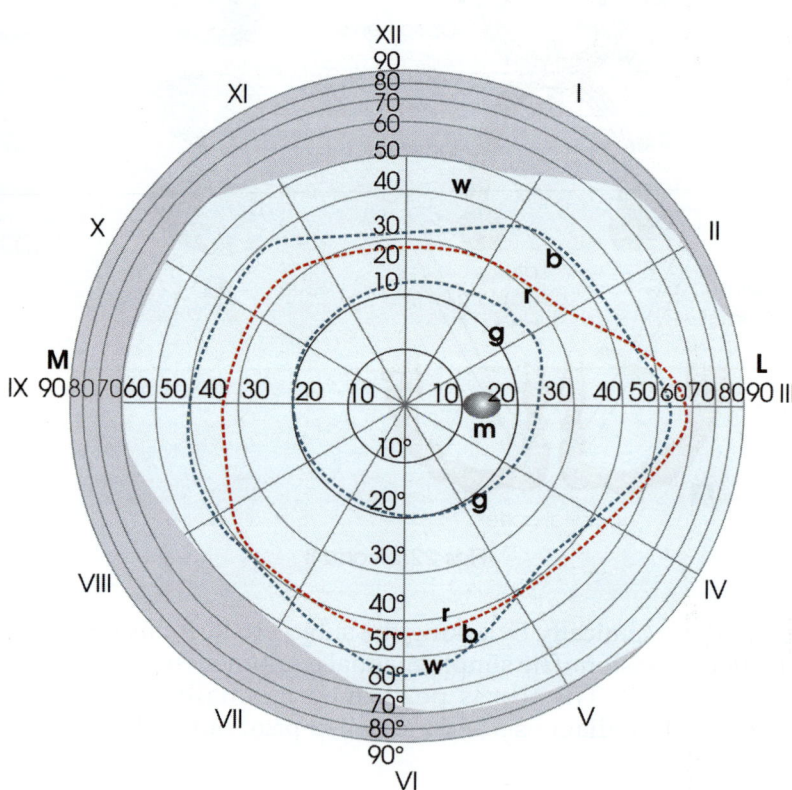

Fig. 22.4: Chart paper for plotting field of vision for right eye shows the plotted field

visual angle in the visual axis at the nodal point of the eye. Isopter is measured in degrees. The lines through the center of the circle, specify the various meridians in degrees. The chart is attached to the back of perimeter and it rotates with the arc as the perimeter charts the visual field.

Procedure

Recognition of the chart: It is physiological convention to chart the field as seen by individual self. Place the chart in front of your eyes so that temporal field is on outer side and blind spot in the temporal field in lower quadrant.

Place the metallic arc in the horizontal position on the right of the subject. The chart is fixed at the back of the perimeter taking care to fix central point and the 90 degree meridian to correspond with the arc.

1. Ask the subject to be seated on stool and rest his chin on one of the two chin rests. When the field of the left eye is to be plotted the subject rests his chin on the right chin rest and vice versa. This eye is brought in line with the fixation point as chin is placed on chin rest. The subject is asked to close the other eye which is not being tested with his hand (Fig. 22.5). Field is first mapped with a white object 5 mm in diameter.

2. Bring the object gradually from the periphery (90°) towards the centre (fixation point) after adjusting metal arc in one of the meridians. At least 8 meridians (preferably 16) are tested.

3. The subject is asked to keep the focus on the central fixation point, and asked to point at when first sees the moving object. Then still carry the object slowly towards the central point and while you ask the subject to report if he fails to see again at any point. This ensures to record any blind point/area in the field (scotoma).

4. The reading in degrees on the meridian when first sees the object also if at any point fails to see again is marked on the chart.

5. Repeat the procedure on the chart for various meridians till the field of vision is plotted in four quadrants. All points in different meridians joined together give the limit of field of vision.

6. Map the blind spot—fix the metallic arc in the horizontal meridian in the temporal quadrant. At a point the object disappears but reappears again when the object is moved further towards the fixation point. This marks the blind spot (physiological scotoma).

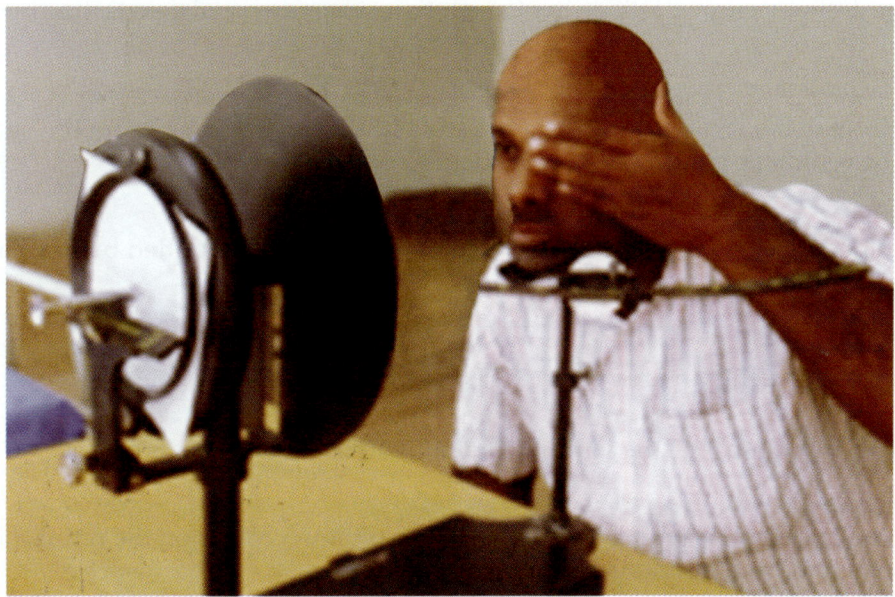

Figs 22.5: Field of vision being charted in the subject

Repeat the procedure: The first test is done with an object of white colour of size of 5 mm in diameter, then repeat the test with white objects of different sizes and then with objects of different colours, red green and blue in that order of colours.

Field of vision for coloured objects: Test the same way using different coloured objects and of similar size. The limit for the field of colour is the point which passing from periphery to centre, the colour first becomes evident. Peripheral to this colour of the object appears grey in ordinary illumination.

Limits of field of vision are affected by: Intensity of light, saturation of colour, size of object.

Precautions

1. Check that there is good illumination where test is performed.
2. The subject should maintain the focus of his eyes over central fixation point while testing the field of vision in different meridians.
3. The subject should immediately respond as he sees the test object.

4. The blind spot should be marked along the horizontal meridian in the temporal lower quadrant. Where optic nerve leaves the eye there are no photoreceptors and this is physiological blind spot, and it is in the temporal field of vision as the nerve leaves medial to the posterior pole of the retina.

5. Spectacles if being worn should be removed for testing as the frame may obstruct and interfere with the test.

6. Discard the first record if the subject is not cooperating.

Results: Fix the perimeter chart recording in your practical notebook and report on the field of vision for each eye of the subject. Mention the size and color of the object being used and report on the test with different colours of the object.

....

....

....

....

OSPE NON-SKILLED

Q1. What is the difference between visual acuity and visual field testing?

Ans. Visual acuity tests the eye's greatest power of resolution, whereas visual field testing measures the peripheral sensitivity.

Q2. Define visual field defect.

Ans. Visual field defect denotes a portion of the visual field that is not being seen, the subject is unable to see there. It may be central or peripheral field defect.

Q3. What is scotoma?

Ans. Scotoma is a type of visual field defect at particular site and is surrounded by normal visual field.

Q4. What are the types of scotoma?

Ans. Scotoma is of two types:

Relative scotoma represents an area where objects of low luminance cannot be seen but larger or brighter ones can.

Absolute scotoma—nothing can be visualized at all within that area.

Q5. What is physiological scotoma?

Ans. The spot where optic nerve leaves the eye there are no photoreceptors on the retina, hence it is a blind spot and corresponds to optic disc and is physiological scotoma.

Q6 What is hemianopia?

Hemianopia is a visual defect in eye's hemi-field.

- In bitemporal hemianopia the nasal fibres of both the eyes are affected and as a result the temporal fields of both sides are blind, two halves of outer field in each eye's peripheral vision.
- In homonymous hemianopia—the two halves lost are on the corresponding area of the visual field in both eyes (either the right or the left half of the visual field).
- Incomplete hemianopia referring to a quarter of visual field loss is known as quadrantanopia.
- An incomplete hemianopia is a sectorial defect.

Q7. Define optical axis, visual axis and nodal point.

Ans. The line which joins the anterior pole to the posterior pole of the eye is called optical axis.

The line which joins the fixation point to the fovea is called the visual axis.

Centre point of the lens is called nodal point.

Q8. What is isopter

Ans. All points in a particular concentric line subtend the same visual angle with the visual axis at nodal point of the eye.

Q9. Why is blind spot present in the eye?

Ans. It represents optic disc in the eye where there are no photoreceptors and so is physiological blind spot.

Q10. What is the size of blind spot?

Ans. Blind spot measures 7.5 degrees in height and 5.5 degrees in width.

OSPE SKILLED

Q1. Perform a confrontation visual field testing in the subject.

Ans.

1. Ask the patient to sit on the stool at approximately 1 metre distance facing towards you. Remove the subject's glasses if worn. (Yes/No)
2. Instruct the subject to look at your nose and you focus your vision towards subject nose. (Yes/No)
3. Test each eye separately. Ask the subject to cover the other eye which is not being tested. (Yes/No)
4. Ensure that the target is equidistant between you and the patient. (Yes/No)
5. Starting at the outer quadrant move the target object in from the side and ask the subject to tell you when he first sees the object and, as you move towards the centre, whether it disappears. (Yes/No)
6. The process is to be repeated in each quadrant and for each eye separately. If you detect a defect, that area needs to be reexamined and define it further. Also assess the blind spot. (Yes/No)

VIVA VOCE QUESTIONS

Q1. What is the advantage of binocular vision?

Ans. Two visual fields of each eye overlap in the medial part and form the area of binocular vision where an object is seen by both. Helps in appreciation of depth and distance and hence in the proportion of objects.

Q2. What is Donders test?

Ans. Donders test is the confrontation visual field exam. The examiner asks the patient to cover one eye and look straight towards his eyes. The examiner will move his hand out of the patient's visual field and then bring his hand. The examiner may use a slowly wagging finger or a hat pin. The patient signals towards the examiner as examiners hand comes back into view. This is simple and preliminary test carried out to have a view of status of field of vision of the patient.

Q3. What are the applications of automated perimeter?

Ans. Automated perimeters are employed in diagnosing disease, as part of medical screening during job selection, visual competence assessment, school or community screenings, military medical fitness screening, and disability classifications.

Q4. What is the normal field of vision in a healthy individual?

Ans. The normal eye can detect stimuli over a 120° range vertically and a nearly 160° range horizontally. From the point of fixation, stimuli can typically be detected 60° superiorly, 70° inferiorly, 60° nasally, and 100° temporally.

Q5. Enlist the advantages of automated perimetry.

Ans. Advantages of automated perimetry include:

1. The results are more sensitive and reproducible.
2. It provides quantitative information.
3. Results can be reported in a more timely manner.
4. Experienced perimetrist is not required.
5. With newer perimetric tests, early detection of glaucomatous damage is possible.

Q6. Explain how vision will be compromised due to lesion along the optic tract.

Ans.

1. Lesions at the level of the retina will affect one eye only.
2. Lesions before the chiasm will produce a field deficit in the ipsilateral eye.

3. Lesions at the chiasm produce a bitemporal hemianopia.

4. Lesions after the chiasm produce homonymous field defects; a lesion in the right optic tract produces a left visual field defect.

   A. Lesions in the main optic radiation cause complete (left or right) homonymous hemianopia without macular sparing.

   B. Lesions in the anterior visual cortex produce a contralateral homonymous hemianopia with macular sparing

   C. Lesions in the macular cortex produce congruous homonymous macular defect.

   D. Lesions of the intermediate visual cortex produce an homonymous arc scotoma, with sparing of both macula and periphery.

HISTORICAL UPDATE

1. The first record of a visual field defect is found in Hippocrates description of a hemianopia in the late fifth century BC.

2. Ptolemy first attempted to quantify the visual field and noted its circular form in 150 BC.

3. Galen was the first physician "to record a recognition of Extramacular fields." which was published in an article by Ulmus of Padua in 1602.

4. Leonardo da Vinci recognized that temporally the visual field reaches around more than 90 degrees from fixation in the year 1510.

5. Physiological blind spot was reported by Mariotte in the year 1668.

6. Thomas Young in 1801 made the first exact measurement of the visual field. He reported that the visual axis varies in different angle—upwards it extends to 50 degrees, inwards to 60 degrees and downwards to 70°.

7. In 1825 Purkinje refined Young's work and noted the lateral limits to be 100 degrees, upper 60 degrees, the nasal 60 degrees and lower 80 degrees.

8. Joesph Georg Beer of Vienna in 1817 used terms such as 'central scotoma' and 'paracentral scotomata', 'concentric contraction of the visual field' and 'half field loss'.

9. Boerhaave was first to describe scotomas in 1708.

10. Von Graefe (right) is credited with introducing perimetry into clinical medicine in the year 1855.

RECENT UPDATES

All perimeters measure sensitivity to stimuli at multiple locations in the visual field although multiple variables are defining the perimeter. Nowadays standard automated perimetry or white on white perimetry is the most common form of visual field testing. A white stimulus is projected on a white background to determine the threshold values.

Clinical Prospective

Tests are conducted to detect any defect in the central and peripheral vision. Such defects may occur in. Central field loss occurs with age related macular degeneration, optic neuropathy, Lebers optic atrophy, cone dystrophies, macular holes and a number of rare conditions like Best's disease, Stargardt's disease and achromatopsia. Peripheral field loss occurs with: glaucoma, retinal detachment, retinitis and chorioretinitis, stroke, glaucoma, brain tumours or other neurological deficits.

Method

Principle: Perimetry is systematic measurement of differential light sensitivity in the visual field by the detection of the presence of test targets on a defined background.

OBSERVATIONS: EXERCISE FOR STUDENTS

....

....

....

....

....

Electroencephalogram (EEG)

PY 10.12*

Brief Review

Electroencephalogram (EEG) is the recording of the electrical activity of the brain from the scalp. If the electrical activity is recorded from the exposed cortex it is called electrocorticogram. The recorded waveforms reflect the cortical electrical activities. Both the amplitude and pattern of electrical signals keep changing depending upon the state of brain activity. Most of the time the brain waves are irregular but still it is possible to distinguish certain discrete patterns of rhythmic activities.

The electroencephalogram is a record of oscillatory potential differences between two recordings. Electrodes placed on the head these oscillations differ in frequency and amplitude from place to place in different states of awareness. They persist in but in altered form during excitement, drowsiness, sleep, coma, anaesthesia, epileptic attack and during severe changes in blood gas or cerebral metabolic concentrations. They cease when massive cerebral catastrophy or impending or actual death. The recording and analysis of EEG is an important diagnostic tool because there is a constant association between certain brain wave pattern and states of altered brain function.

EEG recordings are ordinarily made from a large number of electrodes positioned on the surface of the head. The potential changes that occur are amplified by high gain differential capacity coupled amplifiers. The output signals are usually recorded by ink writing oscillographs writing on moving paper.

The normal EEG thus recorded shows in terms of rhythmic activity and transients four types of main waves. The EEG is typically the rhythmic activity divided into bands by frequency. EEG bandwidths are known as alpha, beta, theta, and delta. The signal intensity EEG activity is quite small and measured in microvolts (μV). The signal frequencies of the human EEG waves are:

Alpha waves have a frequency between 7.5 and 13 Hz. Amplitude 50 μV (20–100 μV), this posterior dominant rhythm is usually best seen in the posterior regions of the head on each side and is higher in amplitude on the dominant side. It appears with closing of the eyes and in relax state of mind and disappears on opening the eyes or mental alertness or mental exertion.

Beta wave has a frequency of 14 Hz and greater and amplitude 5–20 μV. It is closely linked to motor behaviour and is attenuated during active movements. It is usually seen on both sides in symmetrical distribution and prominently evident frontally. It is accentuated by sedative-hypnotic drugs such as benzodiazepines and the barbiturates. It may be reduced or not present in areas of cortical damage. It is regarded as a normal rhythm. It is the dominant rhythm in individual who are alert or anxious or have their eyes open.

Theta wave has a frequency of 3.5 to 7.5 Hz amplitude 10–100 μV. Theta is seen normally in young children up to 13 years and in sleep. It may be seen as a manifestation of focal subcortical lesions; after meditation; in generalized distribution with diffuse disorders such as metabolic encephalopathy or some instances of hydrocephalus.

*Competency achievement as per competency based Undergraduate Curriculum for the Indian Medical Graduate, 2018, 1; Medical Council of India.

Delta wave has a frequency of 0.5 to 4 Hz amplitude 20–200 µV. It is the highest in amplitude and the slowest waves. It is normal and the dominant rhythm in infants up to one year and in stages 3 and 4 of sleep. It may occur in general distribution with diffuse lesions, hydrocephalus, metabolic encephalopathy or deep midline lesions and focally with subcortical lesions.

Derivatives of the EEG technique are evoked potentials and event-related potential. The evoked potential (EP) involves averaging the EEG activity time-locked to the presentation of a visual auditory or somatosensory stimulus. The event-related potentials (ERPs) refer to averaged EEG responses that are time-locked to more complex processing of cognitive stimuli.

Aim of the Experiment

Record the EEG from the scalp.

Principal

It is based on the fact that nerve cells in aggregated produce spontaneous electrical currents which can be amplified and recorded. From the interpretation of the recorded pattern of electrical activity inferences can be drawn about the activity on the CNS.

Recording

1. As the patient reports for EEG recording; explain the procedure of recording to patient and allay his anxiety.
2. Prepare the scalp area by light abrasion to reduce impedance as due to dead skin cells.
3. The recording is obtained by placing disc electrodes 0.5 cm in diameter over the scalp with a conductive gel or paste. These electrodes are small metal discs usually made of stainless steel, tin, gold or silver covered with a silver chloride coating. Some recording systems use a cap into which electrodes are embedded; this facilitates recordings when high density arrays of electrodes are needed or when comparing recording sites.
4. Electrodes are placed on the scalp in special positions as specified under International 10/20 system. All electrode sites are labeled with a letter and a number. The letter refers to the area of brain underlying the electrode, e.g. O: Occipital lobe, F: Frontal lobe and T: Temporal lobe. Odd numbers denote the left side of the head and even numbers the right side of the head. In most clinical applications, 19 recording electrodes (plus ground and system reference) are used. Indifferent electrodes are placed over the ear lobes. (The electrodes applied are connected to the jack-box which in turn is connected to the EEG machine, which consists of preamplifier and ink writing device.)
5. Connect each electrode to one input of a differential amplifier (one amplifier per pair of electrodes); a common system reference electrode is connected to the other input of each differential amplifier. These amplifiers amplify the voltage between the active electrode and the reference electrode typically 1,000–100,000 times.

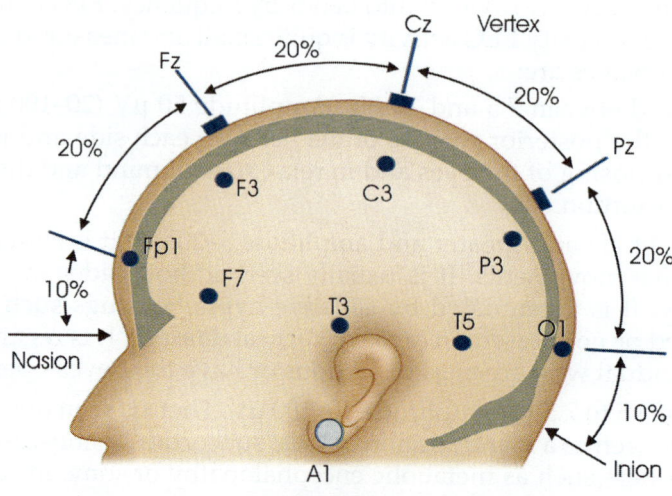

Fig. 23.1

In analog EEG, the signal is then filtered and the EEG signal is output as the deflection of pens as paper passes underneath. Most EEG systems these days are digital, and the amplified signal is digitized via analog-to-digital converter and its sampling typically occurs at 256–512 Hz in clinical scalp EEG.

During the recording, a series of activation procedures such as hyperventilation, photic stimulation (with a strobe light), eye closure, mental activity, are carried out.

Other procedures such as sleep and sleep deprivation could be carried out.

Precautions

1. Check main supply and ensure adequate voltage.
2. Place the electrodes in proper position.
3. Calibrate the different channels so that the deflection to a standard stimulus in each channel is the same (10 mm for 50 µV) so that voltage of different waves can be easily assessed. Move the paper at 25/mm sec for recording the EEG.
4. Turn the switch on for 15 minutes before use.

Q.1. Draw a well-labelled diagram of EEG waves. Explain them briefly.

Ans.

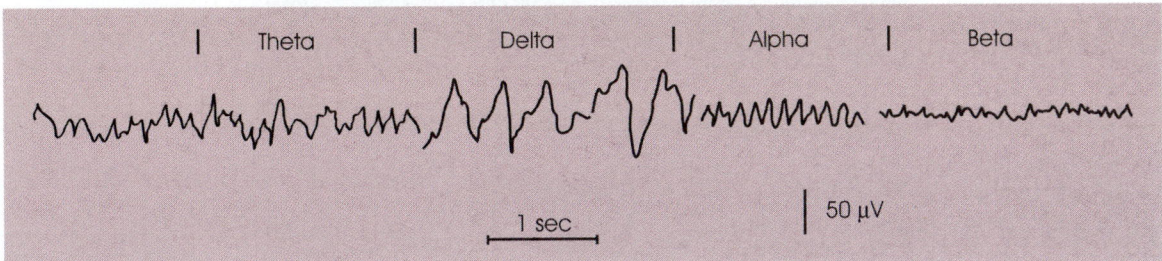

Alpha wave has a frequency between 7.5 and 13 Hz. This posterior dominant rhythm is usually best seen in the posterior regions of the head on each side and is higher in amplitude on the dominant side. It appears with closing of the eyes and in relax state of mind and disappears on opening the eyes or mental alertness or mental exertion.

Beta wave has a frequency of 14 and greater Hz. It is closely linked to motor behavior and is attenuated during active movements. It is usually seen on both sides in symmetrical distribution and prominently evident frontally. It is accentuated by sedative-hypnotic drugs such as benzodiazepines and the barbiturates. It may be reduced or not present in areas of cortical damage. It is regarded as a normal rhythm. It is the dominant rhythm in individual who are alert or anxious or have their eyes open.

Theta wave has a frequency of 3.5 to 7.5 Hz. Theta is seen normally in young children up to 13 years and in sleep but abnormal in awakened state in adults. It may be seen as a manifestation of focal subcortical lesions; after meditation; in generalized distribution with diffuse disorders such as metabolic encephalopathy or some instances of hydrocephalus.

Delta wave has a frequency of 4 Hz or below. It is highest in amplitude and the slowest waves. It is normal and the dominant rhythm in infants up to one year and in stages 3 and 4 of sleep. It may occur in general distribution with diffuse lesions, hydrocephalus, metabolic encephalopathy or deep midline lesions and focally with subcortical lesions.

Q1. Why is electrode gel applied while recording EEG?

Ans. Electrode gel acts as a malleable extension of the electrode, so that the movement of the electrodes cables does not have least chance of producing artifacts. The gel allows for a low-resistance recording through the skin and maximizes skin contact. It is injected into each cavity until a small amount comes out the hole in the mount.

Q2. Explain the electrode positioning (10/20 system).

Ans. The standardized placement of scalp electrodes for a classical EEG recording is the distance in percentages of the 10/20 range between Nasion-Inion and fixed points. These points are marked as the Frontal pole (Fp), Central (C), Parietal (P), Occipital (O), and Temporal (T). The midline electrodes are marked with a subscript z, which stands for zero. The odd numbers are used as subscript for points over the left hemisphere, and even numbers over the right.

Q3. Describe the EEG waves in various stages of slow wave sleep.

Ans. The normal EEG varies depending on stage of sleep:

Stage I sleep (equivalent to drowsiness in some systems) appears on the EEG as drop-out of the posterior basic rhythm. There could be increase in theta frequencies.

Stage II sleep is characterized by sleep spindles. These are transient runs of rhythmic activity in the 12–14 Hz range that have a frontal-central maximum. Most of the activity in Stage II is in the 3–6 Hz range.

Stages III and IV sleep are defined by the presence of delta frequencies and are often referred to collectively as "slow-wave sleep".

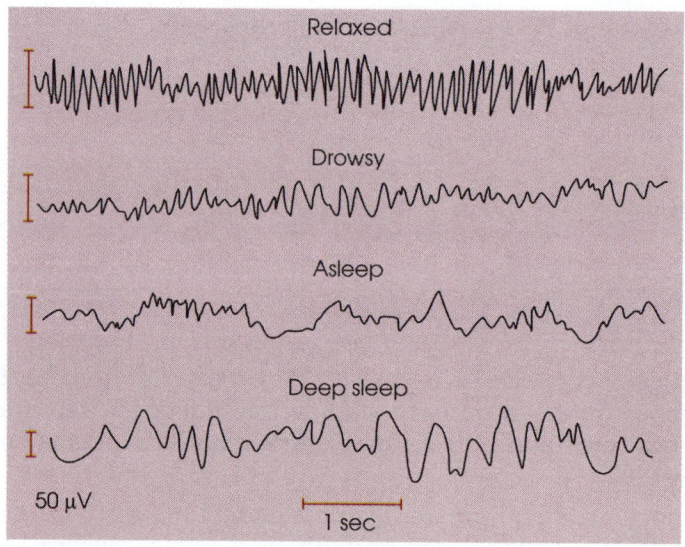

Q4. Describe the EEG in REM sleep. Why is it also called paradoxical sleep?

Ans. In REM sleep the EEG is low voltage fast activity. Since this type of sleep is considered deeper sleep but the EEG is of alert state, this type of sleep is called paradoxical sleep.

Q5. What is the effect of sensory stimulation on EEG pattern?

Ans. Sensory stimulation: Any type of sensory stimulation alters the EEG pattern. In full mental rest, there is appearance of alpha wave but with attempt of solving a mathematical problem it is abolished by fast and irregular low voltage activity.

Q6. Make a drawing to show the changes in EEG as person goes into sleep.

Sleep and EEG:

Alert	Drowsy	Slow wave sleep	Paradoxical sleep

Q7. What is the change in EEG alpha pattern if eyes are opened by the person in relaxed wake state? Make a drawing.

Ans. The recording is low voltage activity called desynchronization or alpha block.

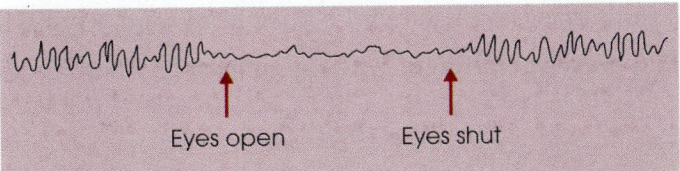

Q8. What is the difference in bipolar recording and monopolar recording of EEG?

Ans. Bipolar is the record of potential fluctuations between two cortical electrodes, whereas the unipolar is the record of potential differences between a cortical electrode and an indifferent electrode placed on some part of the body.

Q9. Delta activity in an awake adult person is not normal—comment.

Ans. Yes, the figure below shows the delta activity in EEG of a patient with tumour.

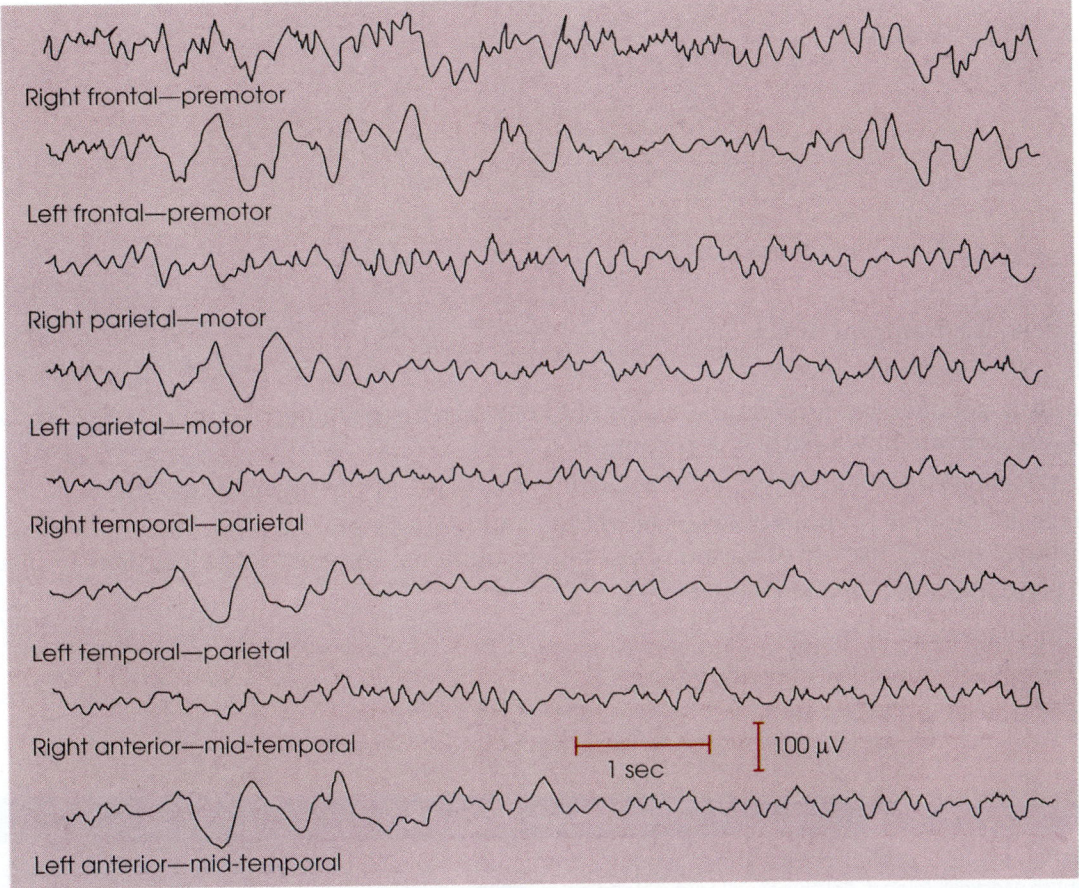

Electroencephalogram of brain tumour in left parietotemporal regions showing delta waver.

Q10. Name some clinical conditions where EEG is of help.

Ans. Electroencephalography is now widely accepted as a reliable method of studying the electrical changes occurring in the cerebral cortex during normal and abnormal conditions. It is helpful in localising the exact site of cerebral tumours, abscesses, etc. It is of special importance in investigating the presence of epilepsy and the types of fits that occur in the epileptic subjects. Besides, it is also helpful in the diagnosis and investigation of impaired cerebral functions in various diseases of cerebral cortex, head injury, brain death, etc.

Q11. Indicate a few conditions where ECG is useful for diagnosis.

Ans. Electroencephalography is a reliable method of studying the electrical changes occurring in the cerebral cortex during normal and abnormal conditions. It is helpful in localising the exact site of cerebral tumours, abscesses, etc. It is of special importance in investigating the presence of epilepsy and the types of fits that occur in the epileptic subjects. Besides, it is also helpful in the diagnosis and investigation of impaired cerebral functions in various diseases of cerebral cortex, head injury, brain death, etc.

Q12. What are the types of EEG waves in different types of epilepsy?

Ans.

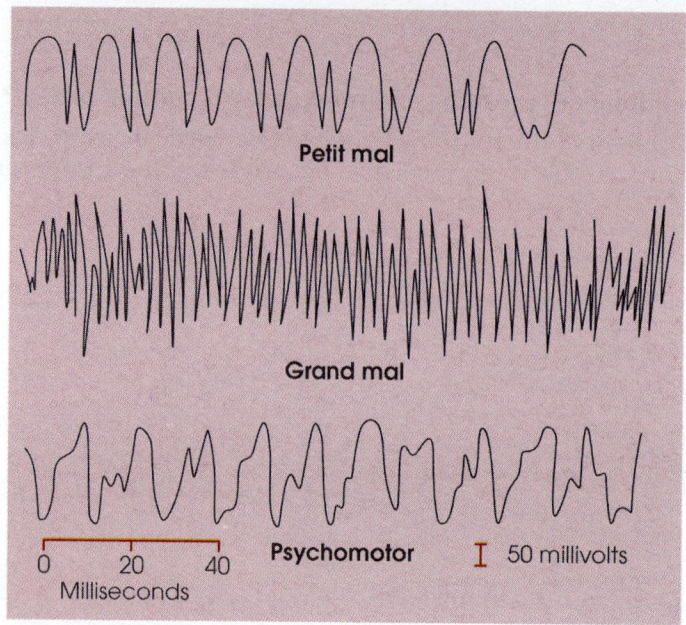

Q13. Enlist a few disadvantages of EEG.

Ans. *The few of the disadvantages are:*

A. It has low spatial resolution on the scalp. EEG requires intense interpretation just to hypothesize what areas are activated by a particular response.

B. EEG poorly measures neural activity occurring below the upper layers of the brain.

C. It takes a long time to connect a subject to EEG and requires precise placement of dozens of electrodes over the scalp and the use of various gels, saline solutions, and pastes to electrodes in place.

1. The placement of the electrodes
2. The placement of the gel
3. The placement of the amplifier
4. The placement of the filter.

HISTORICAL UPDATES

Richard Caton in the year 1875 published his findings about electrical phenomena of the exposed cerebral hemispheres of rabbits and monkeys in the British Medical Journal. Polish physiologist Adolf Beck in 1890 published an investigation of spontaneous electrical activity of rhythmic oscillations under influence of light in brain of rabbits and dogs. He placed electrodes directly on the surface of brain to test for sensory stimulation. Becks findings of fluctuating brain activity lead to the conclusion of brain waves.

Russian physiologist Vladimir Vladimirovich Pravdich Neminsky published the first animal EEG and evoked potential of mamallian dog in 1912. Jelenska-Macieszyna and Napolean Cybulski in 1914 photographed first EEG recordings of experimentally induced seizures in 1914.

German physiologist Hans Berger was first to record an EEG in 1924. He also invented the electroencephalogram (giving the device its name), and is one of the most surprising, remarkable, and momentous developments in the history of clinical neurology.

RECENT UPDATES

The long-term EEG recordings in epilepsy patients are still used today for seizure. EEG is being used quite extensively in the field of neuromarketing. Pharmaco Electroencephalography is developing newer methods to identify substances that alter brain functions for therapeutic and recreational use. Honda is in process of developing a system to enable an operator to control its robot using EEG, a technology it plans to incorporate into its automobiles. EEG is presently used as evidence in criminal trials in Maharashtra.

Clinical Perspective

Routine EEG is recommended in the following clinical circumstances:

1. To identify epileptic seizures and distinguish them from psychogenic non epileptic seizures and syncope. To characterize seizures for the purposes of treatment.
2. To differentiate "organic" encephalopathy from primary psychiatric syndromes like catonia.
3. To confirm brain death.
4. In order to determine whether to wean anti-epileptic medications.
5. Monitor for non-convulsive seizures and non-convulsive status epilepticus.
6. Monitor the effect of sedative/anaesthesia in patients in medically induced coma on treatment of refractory seizures or increased intra-cranial pressure.
7. To monitor for secondary brain damage in conditions such as subarachnoid haemorrhages.

OBSERVATIONS: EXERCISE FOR STUDENTS

Clinical Spotters
Section 1

Q1. **Transmembrane potential recorded with related ionic events.**

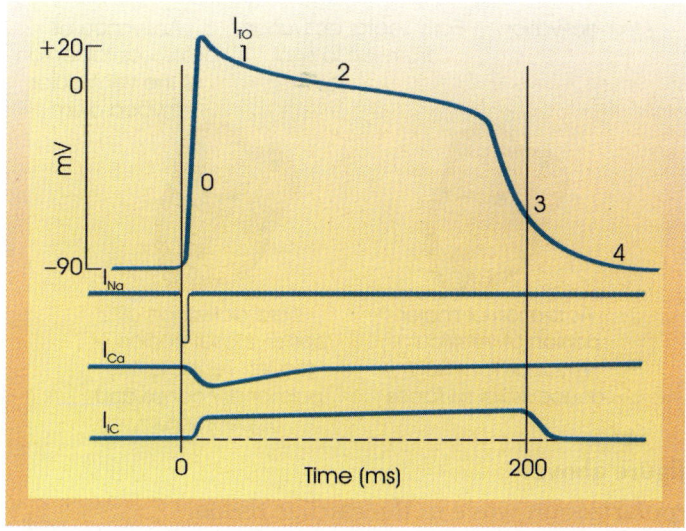

    a. Identify the muscle showing this type of membrane potential.
    b. What is the cause of long duration of action potential?
    c. Is there any advantage of such action potential?

Ans. It is a membrane potential of cardiac muscle with intracellular recording.
    There is a plateau phase in the action potential due to opening of late calcuim ion channels.
    Tetanus of the type in the skeletal muscle cannot be produced in the cardiac muscle due to long duration
    of action potential, when cardiac muscle is in refractory period.

Q2. **Identify the tissue that show this type of transmembrane potential. Give the function.**

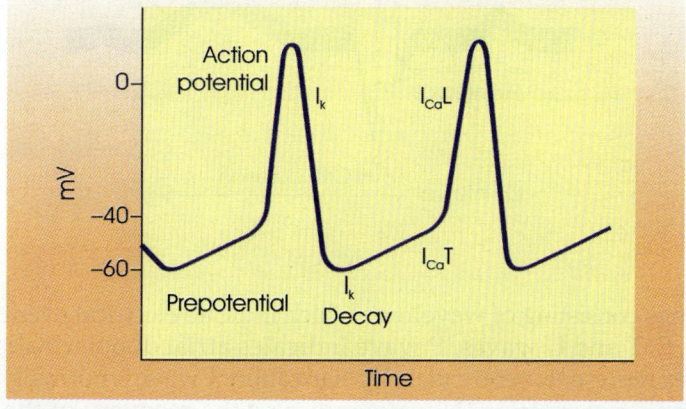

Ans. It is membrane potential of cardiac pacemaker. There is slow decline of resting membrane potential which
    when it reaches the firing level an action potential is produced. Hence tissue acts as a pacemaker that
    initiates cardiac impulse. SA node and AV node have this type of membrane potential.

Q3. What are the sites for recording body temperature?

Ans. **Recording of body temperature:** It can be measured by placing the thermometer (a) in the axilla (armpit), (b) rectally, (c) orally, (d) in the ear canal (the *otic* method), or (e) by placing against the forehead.

Q4. What is normal pulse rate? What are tachycardia and bradycardia?

Ans. The normal pulse rate ranges between 60 and 100/minute in an adult. Tachycardia is defined as a pulse rate more than 100/min and bradycardia as a rate less than 60/min.

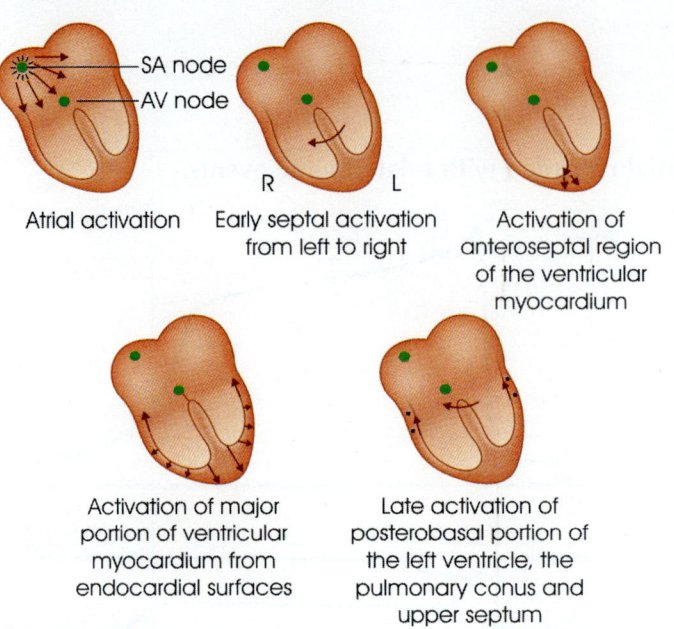

Atrial activation   Early septal activation from left to right   Activation of anteroseptal region of the ventricular myocardium

Activation of major portion of ventricular myocardium from endocardial surfaces   Late activation of posterobasal portion of the left ventricle, the pulmonary conus and upper septum

Q5. What is shown by the figure above?

Ans. The direction of the depolarization wave in the cardiac tissue.

Q6. Identify the figure below.

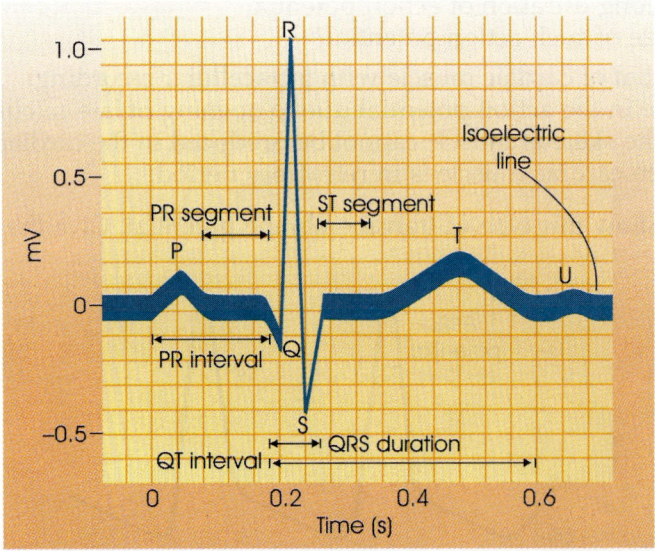

Ans. It is a normal ECG tracings consisting of waveform which indicate electrical events during one heart beat. These waveforms are P, Q, R, S, T and U waves. P wave indicates atrial depolarization. QRS complex follows the P wave. The QRS complex represents ventricular depolarization. T wave is normally a modest upwards waveform, representing ventricular repolarisation. U wave indicates the recovery of the Purkinje conduction fibres.

Q7. Name the event that produces P wave.

Ans. Atrial depolarization produces the 'P' wave in ECG.

Q8. What is the normal duration of PR interval? What does this interval represent?

Ans. PR interval ranges 0.12–0.20 sec (average 0.18 sec) represents atrial depolarization and conduction through AV node.

Q9. Identify the instrument below and give its parts.

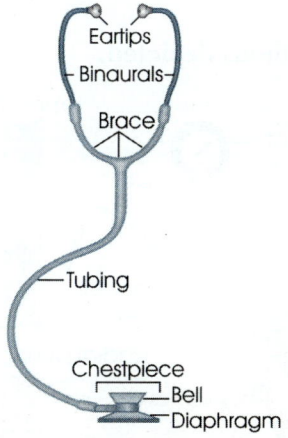

Ans. The instrument in the figure above is a stethoscope. The parts of stethoscope include:

a. The chest piece: It has the bell and diaphragm as two end pieces.

b. Ear frame: It has two curved metallic tubes (Binaural) approximated together to the y-shaped spring (braces). The y-shaped connector connects the metal tube to the chest piece. The plastic knobs are attached to the curved metallic tube at their open end and facilitate comfortable feeling in the ear.

Q10. Identify the figure.

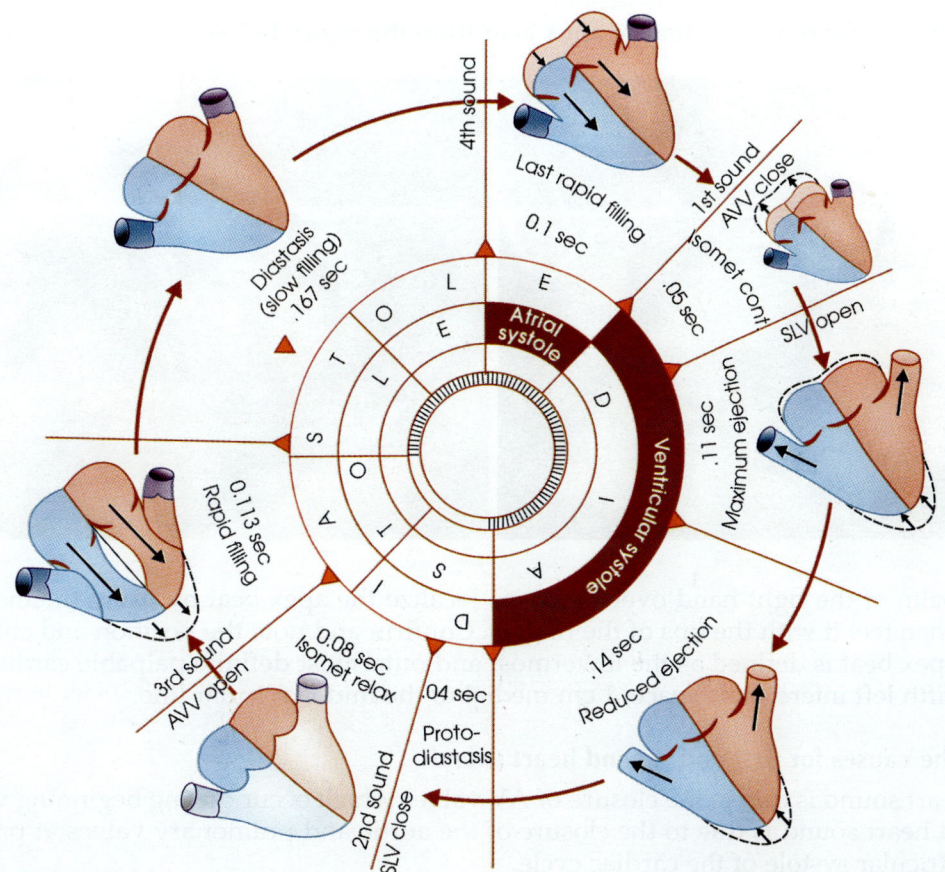

The figure represents the interrelations of the important events of the cardiac cycle. Condition of heart that corresponding to each important phase is also shown.

Ans. The figure depicts events of cardiac cycle. The total duration of cardiac cycle (average) is 0.8 seconds. It shows various events during atrial and ventricular systole and diastole. The total duration of atrial systole is 0.1 sec and atrial diastole is 0.7 sec and ventricular systole is 0.3 sec and ventricular diastole is 0.5 sec.

Q11. Identify the figure and the relevant methods depicted.

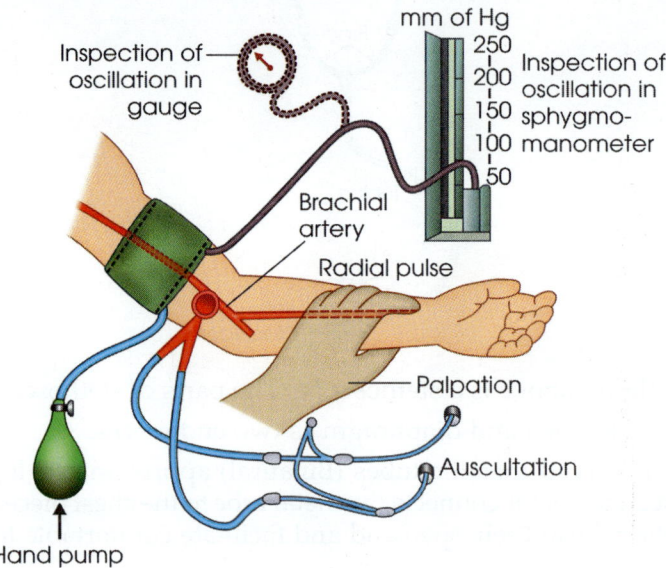

Ans. The figure shows measurements of arterial blood pressure by various methods in humans.

Q12. Explain the mechanism of palpation of apex beat from the figure below.

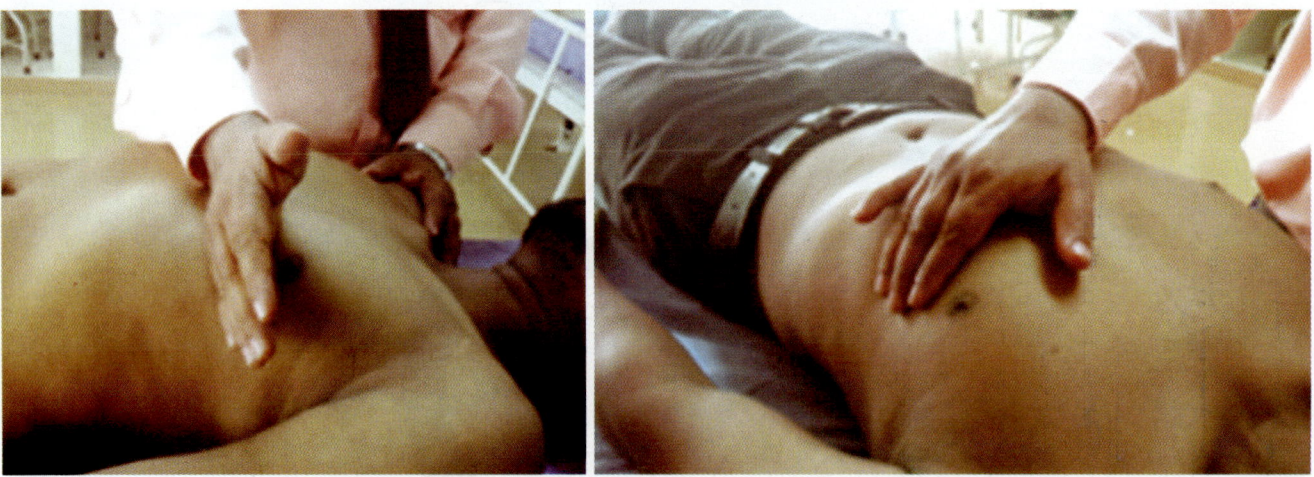

Ans. Place the palm of the right hand over the apex, localize the apex beat by using the medial border of the palm and then feel it with the tips of the fingers. Confirm and note the position and character of the apex beat. The apex beat is defined as the lowermost and outermost definite palpable cardiac impulse usually felt in the fifth left intercostals space, 1 cm medial to the mid-clavicular line.

Q13. What are the causes for first and second heart sound?

Ans. The first heart sound is due to the closure of AV valves which occur during beginning ventricular systole. The second heart sound is due to the closure of the aortic and pulmonary valves at protodiastolic phase end of ventricular systole of the cardiac cycle.

Q14. Define P-R interval.

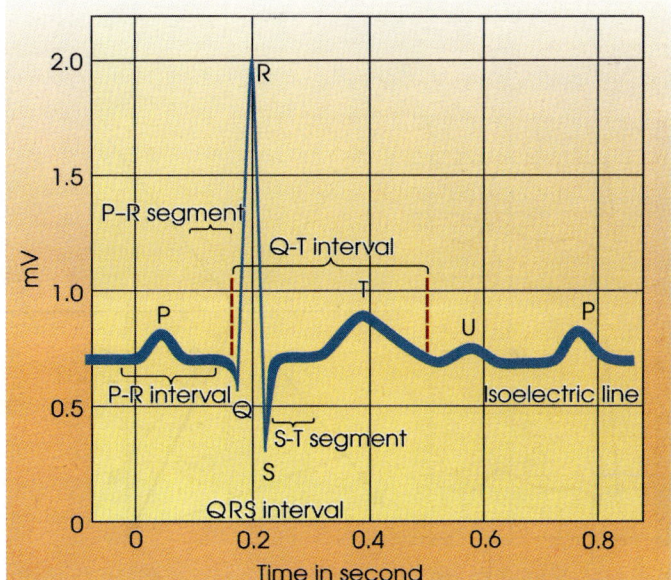

Ans. It is the interval from beginning of P to the beginning of ventricular complex. Since Q is often absent, it is called P-R interval.

Q15. What is the upper normal limit of P-R interval?

Ans. The upper normal limit of it is 0.2 sec. If it exceeds, it is called first degree heart block.

Q16. If the impulse arises in AV node, what would be the effect on PR interval?

Ans. PR interval would be shorter than normal.

Q17. What is the event that produces QRS complex?

Ans. QRS signifies ventricular depolarisation.

Q18. What is the significance of ST segment in ECG?

Ans. In normal ECG it is isoelectric segment. Any deviation of 2 mm or more in ECG is considered abnormal.

Q19. What is the event that produces T wave in ECG?

Ans. It signifies ventricular repolarisation.

Q20. What is the direction of T wave in standard limb leads?

Ans. It is upright in standard limb leads I and II and mostly in lead III. Its direction in normal ECG is the same as of the main ventricular deflection.

Q21. What are the normal limits for duration of QRS complex?

Ans. It ranges from 0.08 to 0.1 sec.

Q22. What is the direction of P wave in lead aVR?

Ans. Recorded as downward deflection.

Q23. How is atrial repolarisation recorded?

Ans. Atrial repolarisation gets merged with ventricular depolarisation as it occurs during that time.

Q 24. **How is mean electrical axis of ventricular complex plotted? What is its significance? What is normal average direction and its normal range? What are the causes of abnormal axis deviation of QRS complex?**

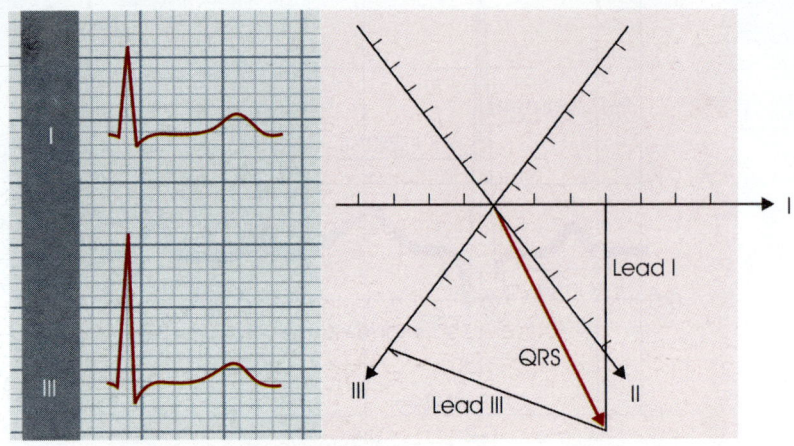

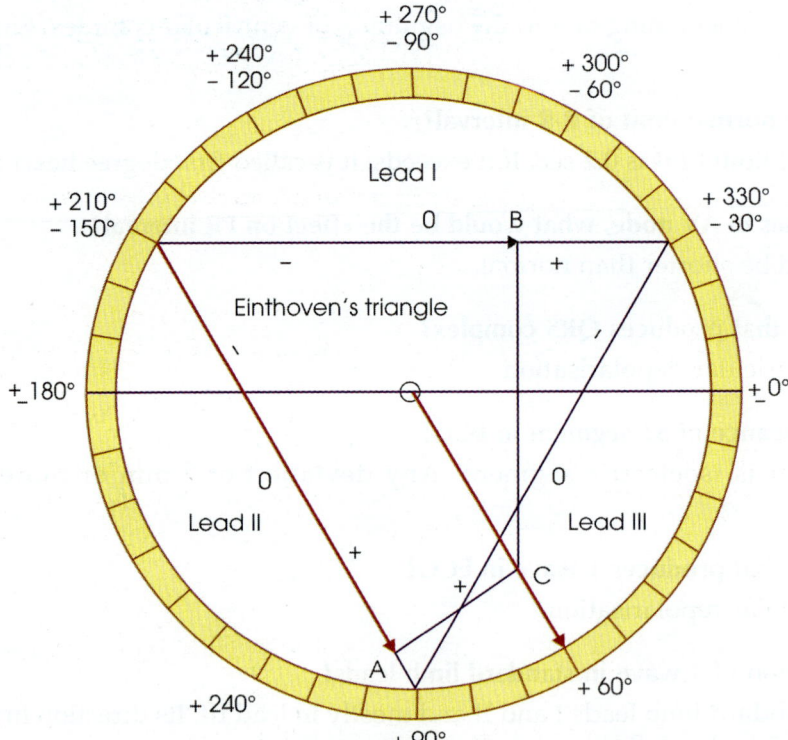

Ans. It can be plotted by measuring the net deflections of QRS complex (positive deflection minus negative deflection) in any two standard limb leads as in the two figures above, e.g. recordings in lead I and lead III values plotted along their electrical axes. Perpendicular lines from these points to intersect at a point, which is joined to the central point; this gives the direction of mean electrical axis of QRS complex.

Normal average mean electrical axis of QRS complex is 60 degrees, normal range as shown in the figure below.

Abnormal axis deviation is seen in hypertrophy of ventricles, bundle branch block. Normal variations around the mean are produced due to position of the heart (Figure below).

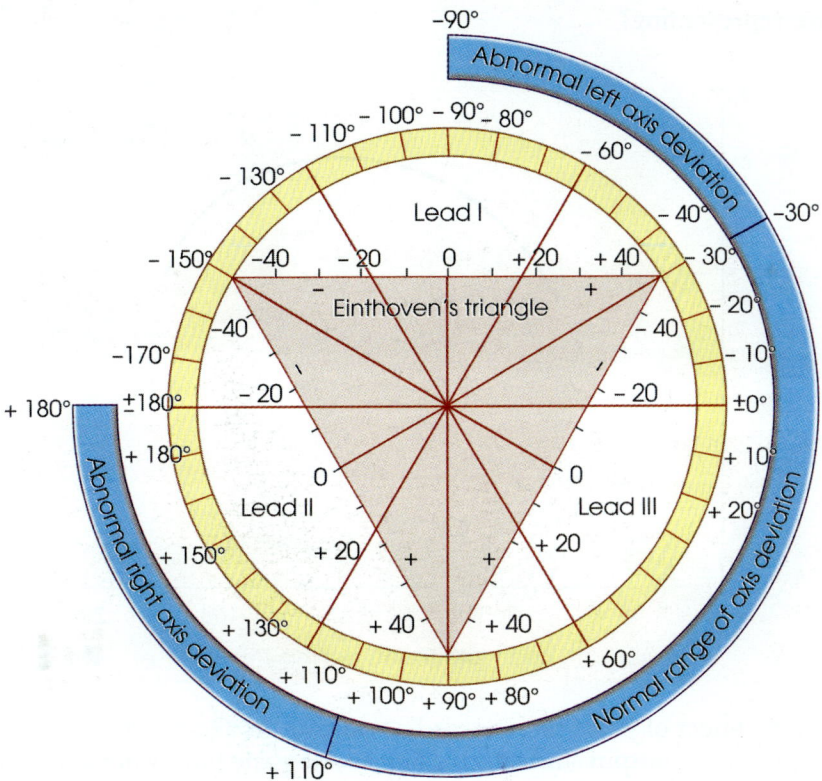

Q25. What is the figure representing? Define Starling Law of the heart.

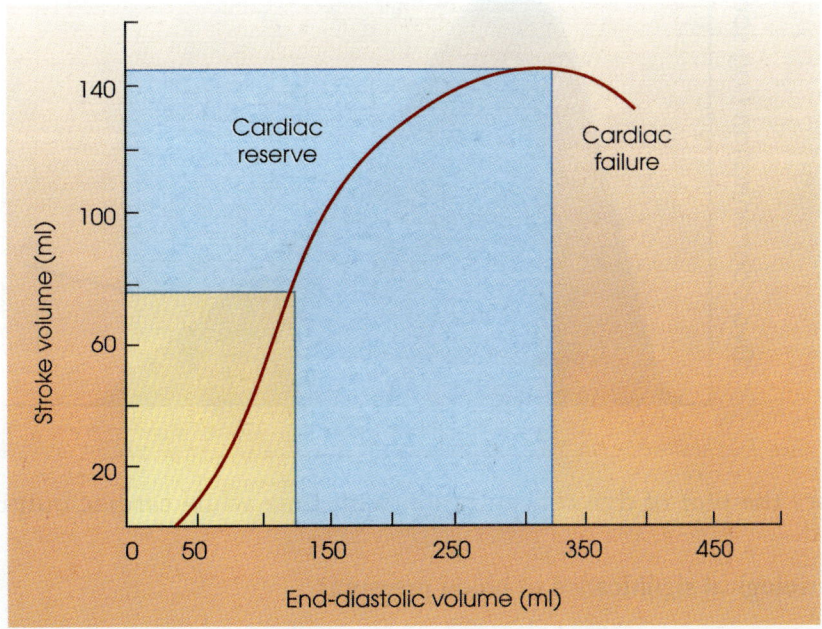

Ans. Figure shows when the end-diastolic volume increases, stroke volume increases, hence it is a graphic representation of Starling law of the heart. Starling law of the heart states that energy of contraction is proportional to the initial length of the muscle fibre within physiological limits. As end diastolic volume increases, stroke volume increase, as ventricles contract more vigorously.

Q26. What is the figure representing?

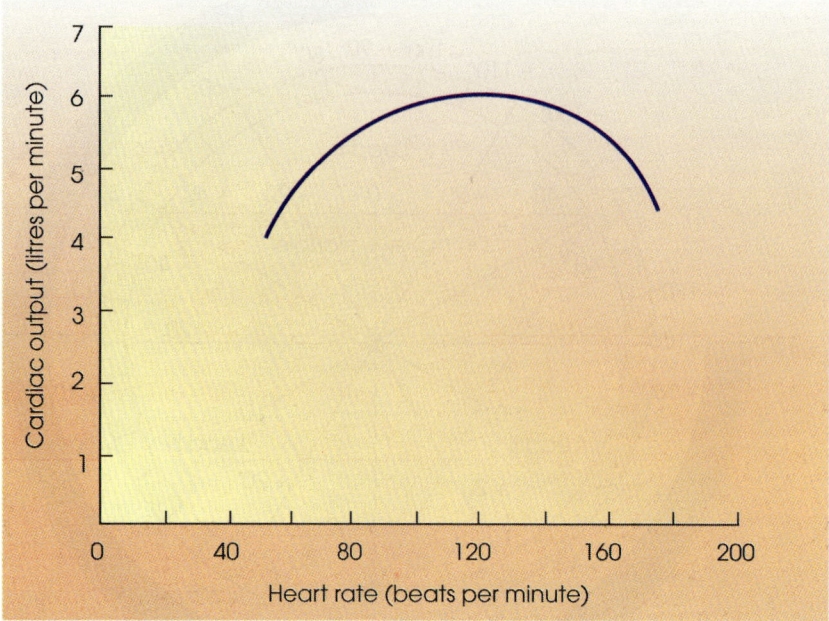

Ans. The figure shows the effect of heart rate on cardiac output. As the heart rate increases the cardiac output increases but beyond a limit output starts decreasing as adequate time is not available for filling of ventricles due to shortening of diastole.

Q27. Identify the graph.

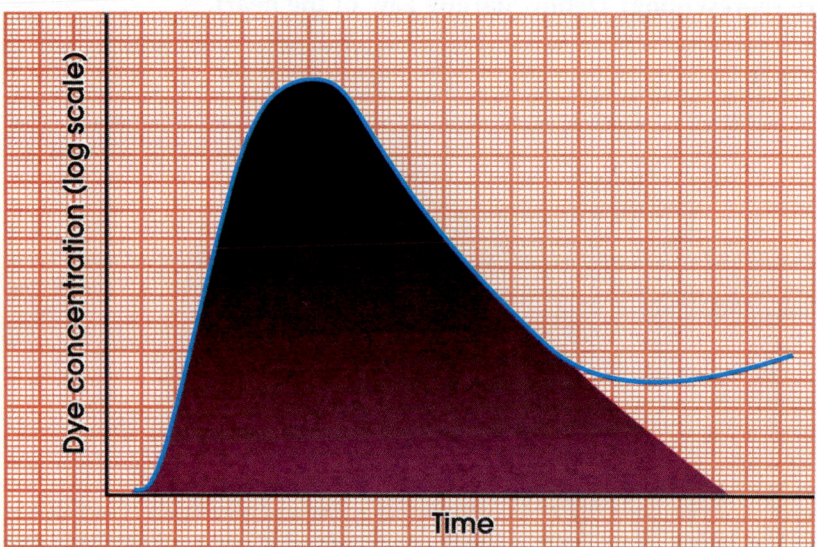

Ans. The figure shows the plot of dye concentration with time while cardiac output is measured by dye dilution method.

Q28. What is the physiological significance of blood pressure?

Ans.

1. Blood pressure maintains a sufficient pressure to keep the blood flowing.

2. Blood pressure provides motive force of filtration at the capillary bed, thus assuring nutrition to the tissue cells, formation of urine, lymph and so on. From these considerations, it is seen that, the range of blood pressure gives correct information about the state of the circulatory system as a whole and also about the functional condition of the tissue cells and organs.

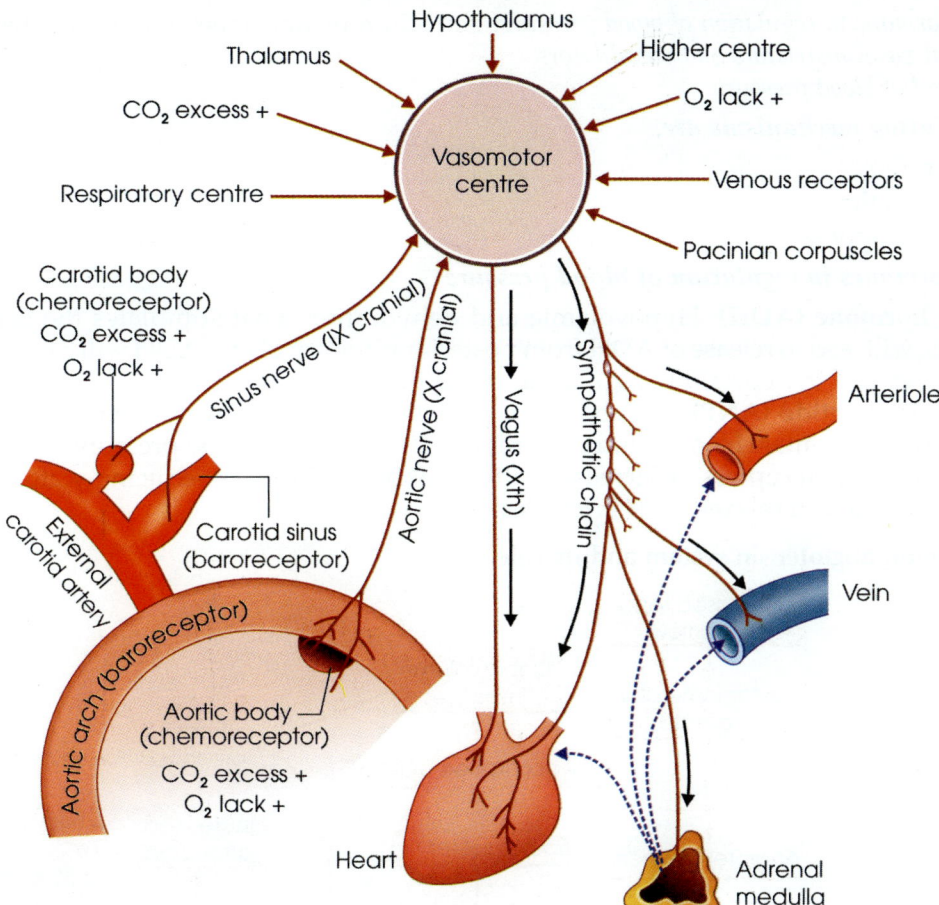

Q29. Identify the figure. What is it showing?

Ans. It shows all the factors which control blood pressure.

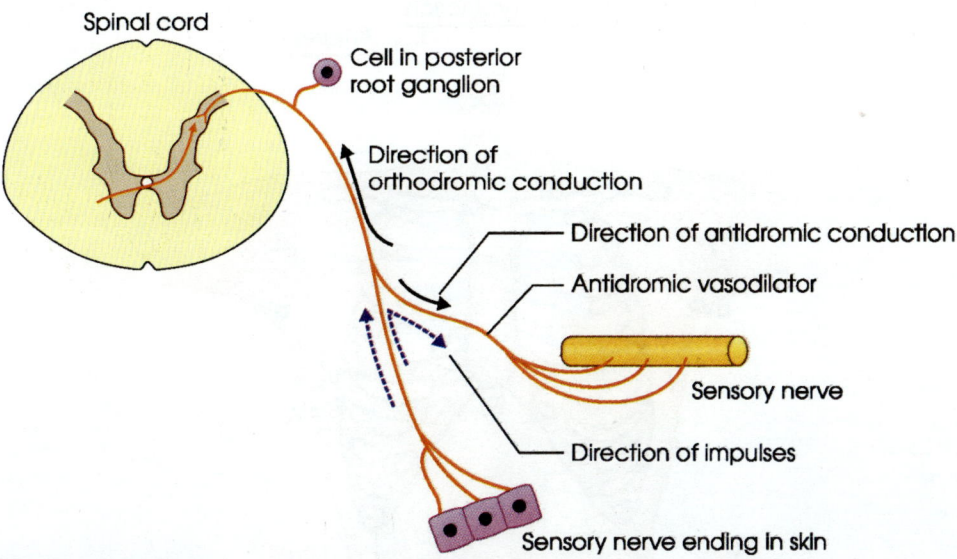

Q30. What is shown in the figure?

Ans. Figure shows the antidromic and orthodromic conduction in sensory nerves.

Q31. Describe the mechanisms for regulation of blood pressure.

Ans. Mechanism of regulation of blood pressure:

i. *Short-term regulating mechanisms*: Baroreceptor reflex, chemoreceptor reflex and CNS ischaemic response.

ii. *Intermediate mechanism of regulation*: Stress relaxation of vasculature and capillary fluid shift mechanism.

iii. *Long-term regulating mechanism*: Renin angiotensin aldosterone mechanism.

iv. Role of other hormone in regulation of blood pressure: Anti-diuretic hormone and atrial natriuretic peptides.

v. Role of humoral vasoconstrictors and vasodilators.

vi. Chemical control of blood pressure.

I. Short-term regulating mechanisms are:

1. Baroreceptor reflex.
2. Chemoreceptor reflex.
3. CNS ischaemic response.

II. Role of other hormones in regulation of blood pressure

- **Anti-diuretic hormone (ADH):** Hypovolemia and dehydration what stimulates the osmoreceptors in the hypothalamus, will lead to release of ADH from posterior pituitary gland. ADH will cause water reabsorption at kidney tubules and thereby aid in regulating blood pressure.

- **Atrial natriuretic peptide (ANP):** This hormone is secreted from the wall of right atrium to regulate Na^+ excretion in order to maintain blood volume, thereby aid in regulating blood pressure. It is released in response to stimulation of atrial receptors. It increases salt excretion via kidneys reducing water reabsorption in the collecting ducts, and also relaxes renal arterioles.

Q32. Describe rennin angiotensin system and its role.

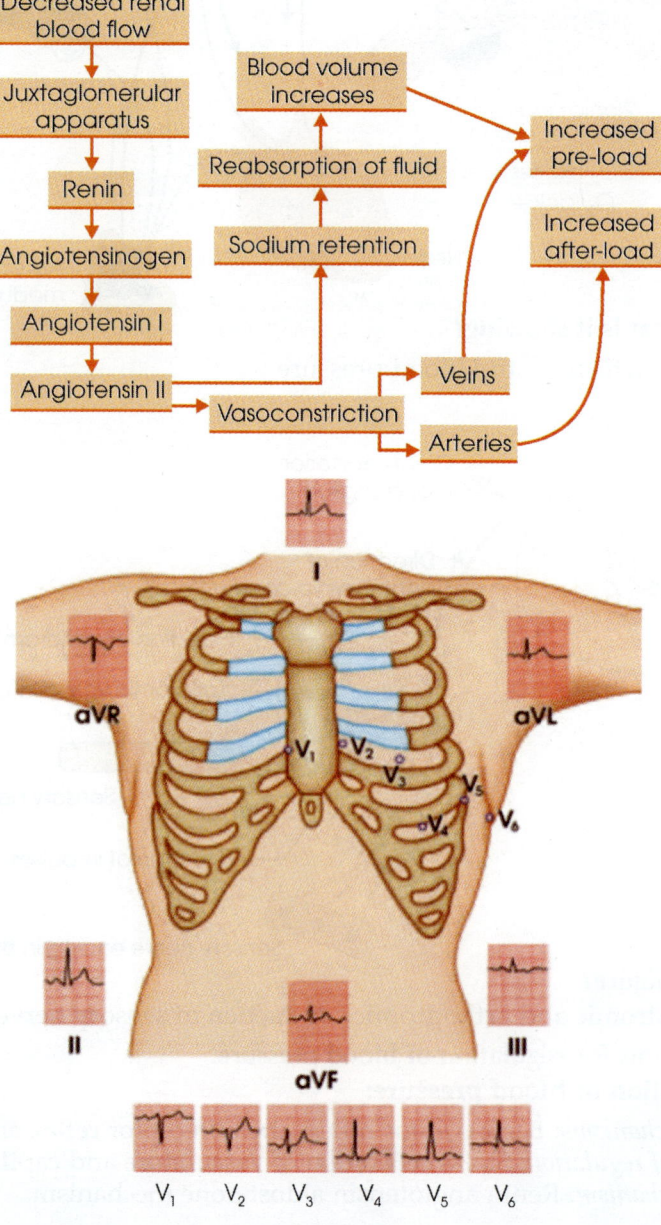

Renin angiotensin control mechanism to regulate blood pressure. Angiotensin II, stimulates aldosterone from adrenal cortex and hence enhances sodium reabsorption.

Q33. What does the figure show?

Ans. Figure shows the recording of ECG by placing electrodes at different positions. It shows bipolar lead recordings and unipolar chest and limb leads recordings. Position of leads are marked.

Short Notes:

1. Methods of recording of blood pressure.
2. Factors affecting blood pressure.
3. Physiological variation in blood pressure.
4. Sino-aortic mechanism.
5. Baroreceptors.
6. Chemoreceptors.
7. Renin-angiotensin system.
8. Humoral vasoconstrictors.
9. Humoral vasodilators.

Q34. Discuss the jugular venous pressure waves (JVP), its recording and interpretation of JVP waves.

Ans. Jugular venous pressure shows a, c and v waves. a wave is due to atrial systole because blood regurgitates into great veins when atria contract. The c wave is because of rise in atrial pressure because of bulging of tricuspid valve into the atria during isovolumetric ventricular contraction. The v wave is due to rise of atrial pressure before tricuspid valve open during diastole.

A fairly accurate estimate of central venous pressure can be made by noting the height to which the external jugular veins are distended. When the subject lies with the head slightly above the heart, the vertical distance between the right atrium and the place of collapse (where the pressure is zero) is the venous pressure in mm of blood. Venous pressure falls during inspiration and rises during expiration.

Q35. What is the clinical significance of bed side inspection of pulsations of jugular veins?

Ans. Central venous pressure is decreased during negative pressure breathing and shock. It is increased during positive pressure breathing. Straining, expansion of blood volume and heart failure.

Clinical Spotters
Section 2

Q1. Identify Figure 1.

Ans. Figure 1: Alveolar lining of lungs.

Q2. What is the important function of type II alveolar lining cells?

Ans. The cells form surfactant.

Q3. What is the function of surfactant?

Ans. It is surface tension lowering substance which prevents collapse of alveoli and lowers the effort to expand the lungs. During expiration the smaller alveoli would collapse into larger alveoli, which is prevented as the concentration of surfactant increases in these alveoli, preventing their collapse.

Q4. Identify Figure 2.

Ans. The lining of bronchial wall, which is ciliated epithelium.

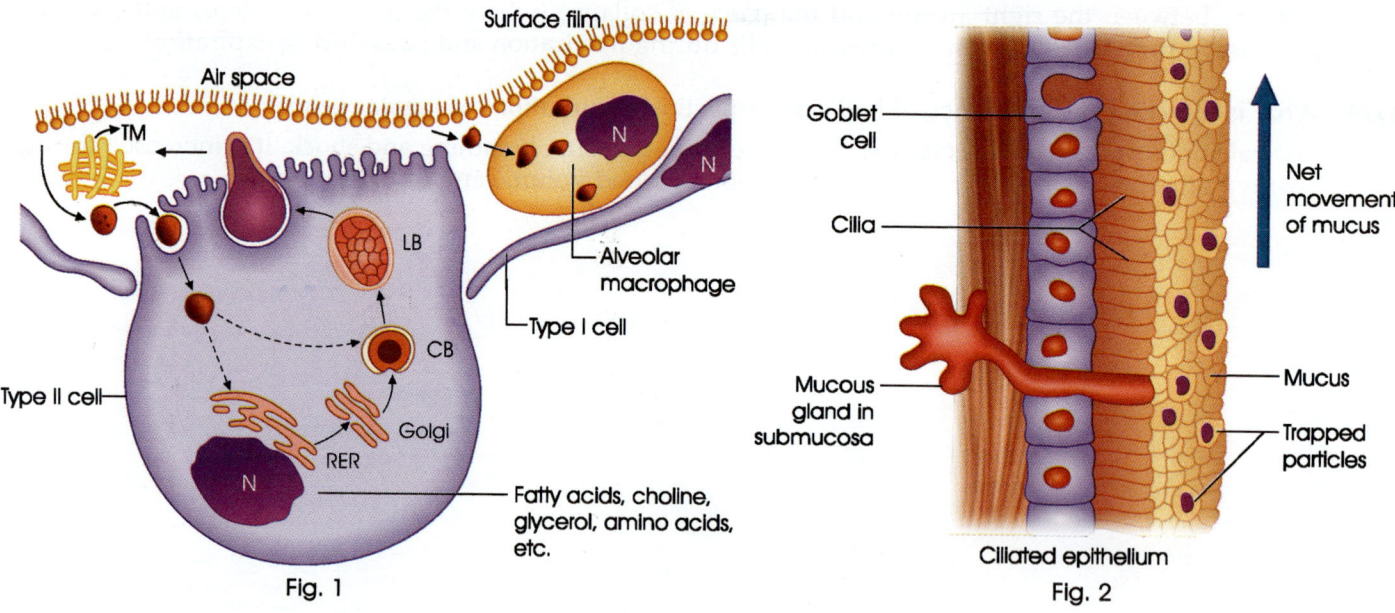

Fig. 1   Fig. 2

Q5. What is the function of cilia?

Ans. The inhaled particulate matter is trapped by mucus secreted in the lumen and cilia with their movement, move the mucus towards oral cavity to be expelled or swallowed.

Q6. Name some conditions when cilia function is defective.

Ans. Function of cilia can be paralysed with nicotine use. The function can be affected as a congenital condition.

Q7. Identify the figure. What does it indicate?

Ans. The figure shows passage of air through lungs, the space where no gas exchange takes place and also the gas exchange area.

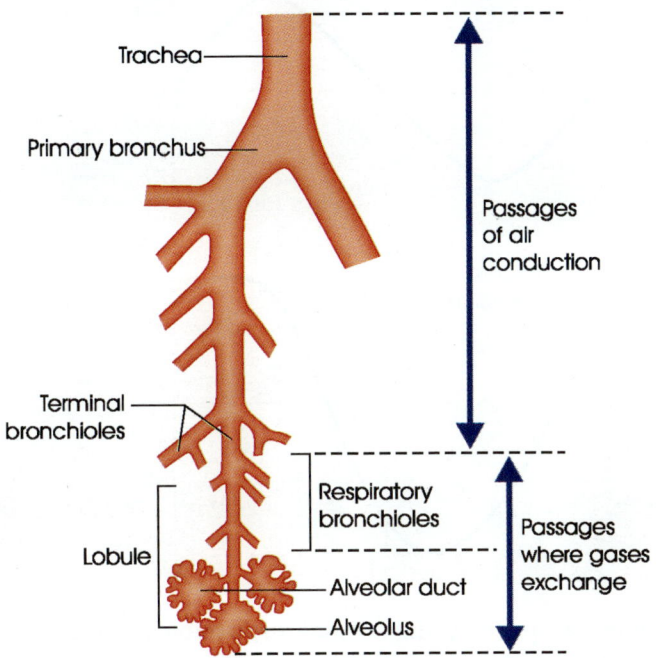

Q8. Define anatomical dead space.

Ans. It is the space where no exchange of gases takes place.

Q9. What is the function served by anatomical dead space?

Ans. Air gets warmed up and humidified in its passage through this space and particulate matter except those smaller than 2 μm get removed from the air while passing through this space.

Q10. What is the difference in the two figures of the thoracic cavity?

Ans. The figures show the effect of expansion of thoracic cavity during inspiration with increase of vertical and transverse diameters and the muscles of inspiration which are the diaphragm and eternal intercostals, also show the muscles of expiration the internal intercostals which work in forced expiration, normal expiration is by relaxation of inspiratory muscles.

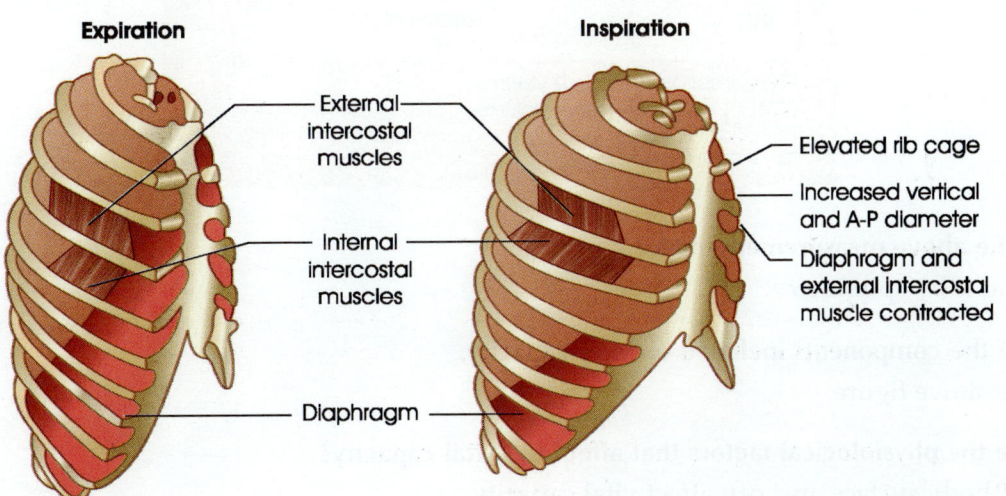

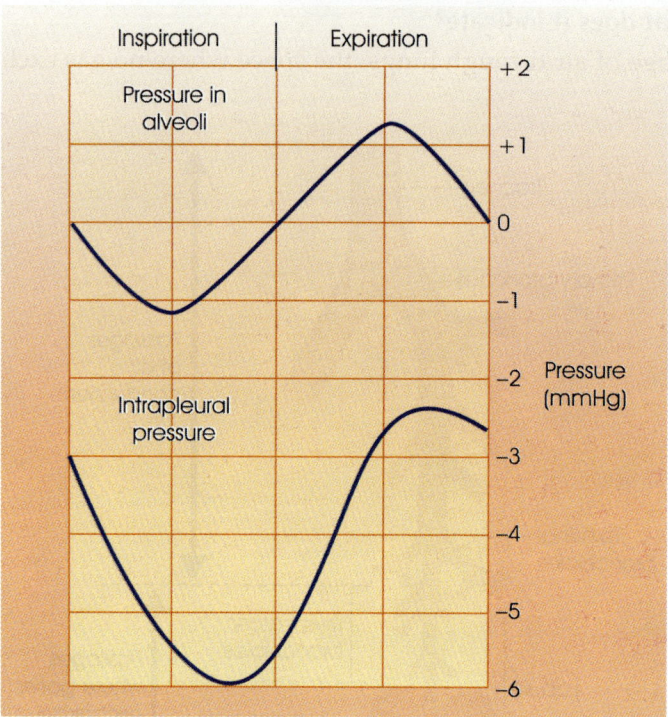

Q11. **The pressures in the intrapleural space during normal respiration are negative shown above. Do the pressures become more negative during forced inspiration?**

Ans. In forceful inspiration the pressures in the pleural cavity may reach –30 mmHg.

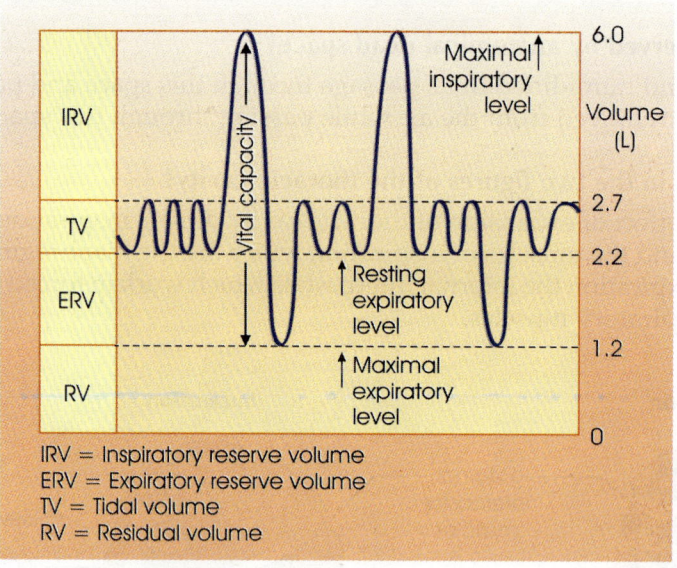

IRV = Inspiratory reserve volume
ERV = Expiratory reserve volume
TV = Tidal volume
RV = Residual volume

Q12. **How is the above measurement made?**

Ans. Recording is by spirometry.

Q13. **Name all the components included on vital capacity.**

Ans. From the above figure.

Q14. **What are the physiological factors that affect the vital capacity?**

Ans. Age, sex, body surface area can affect vital capacity.

Q15. Can residual volume be measured by spirometry?

Ans. No residual volume cannot be measured by spirometry.

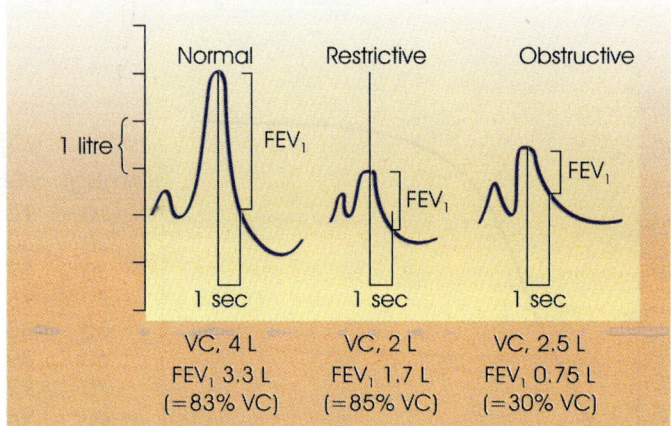

Q16. What are the changes seen in the recording of vital capacity in obstructive lung disease and how do these differ from those in restrictive lung diseases?

Ans. FEV_1 in obstructive lung disease as a percentage of FEV is greatly decreased in obstructive lung disease, whereas FEV_1 as the percent change is not decreased in restrictive lung diseases.

Q17. What are the restrictive lung diseases?

Ans. Asthma, emphysema are obstructive lung diseases.

Q18. Give one example of restrictive lung disease.

Ans. Fibrosis is a restrictive lung disease.

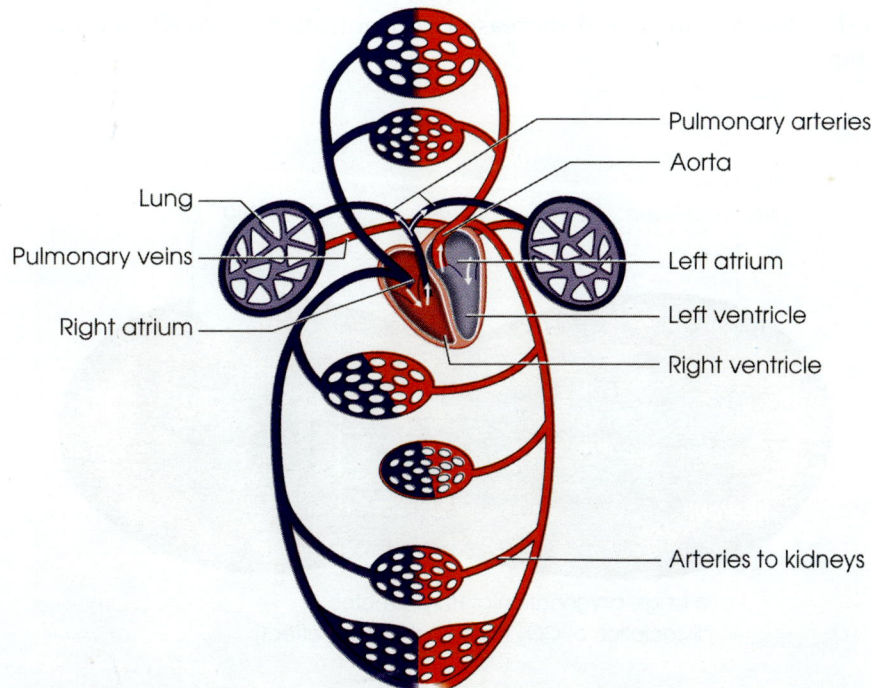

Q19. What are pressures in the pulmonary circuit and are they lower than in the systemic circuit? Give normal values.

Ans. Pressures in the pulmonary circuit are lower than in the systemic circuit. Systolic pressures on average 25 mmHg, average diastolic is 10 mmHg.

Q20. What is the advantage of lower pressures?

Ans. It prevents exudation of fluid in the alveoli of lungs. The lower pressures result in lower work load for right ventricle.

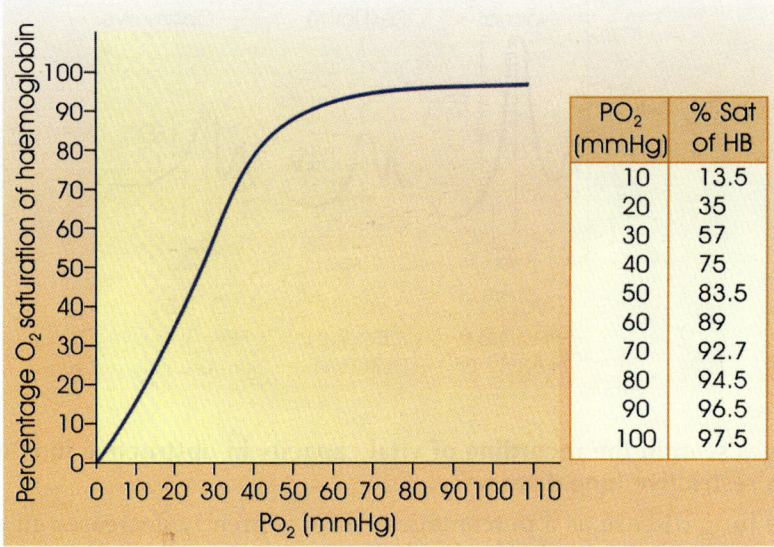

Q21. The oxygen dissociation curve of haemoglobin is S-shaped. What is the advantage?

Ans. The advantage at the upper end of the curve is that if the oxygen tension in the lungs decreases below 60 mm of Hg, the haemoglobin still gets adequately saturated in the lungs, and in the lower end the advantage is that if the oxygen tension decreases very low in the tissues, the release of oxygen is further facilitated.

Q22. Name the factors which influence the curve.

Ans. CO_2 tension, higher temperature, and increased concentration of ADP facilitates unloading of oxygen from haemoglobin.

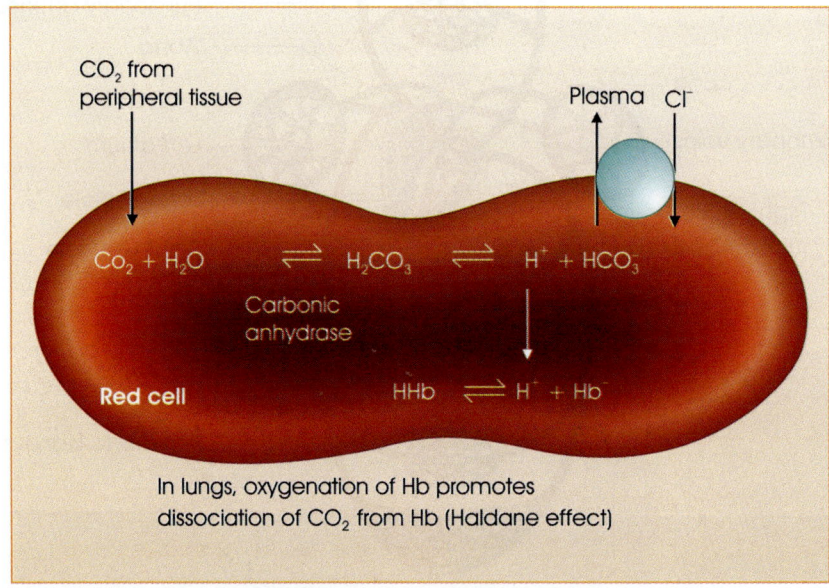

Q23. Name the different mechanisms by which CO_2 is transported in the blood. Does the above figure show any of the mechanism?

Ans. It is transported as carbonic acid, as bicarbonate ion and as carbamino compounds. The figure shows the formation of bicarbonate in the red cells and transport in plasma.

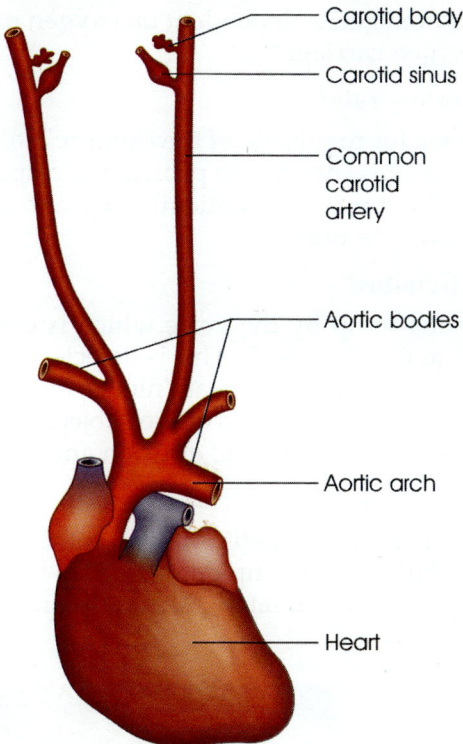

Q24. What is the function of aortic and carotid bodies? What do these structures sense to regulate respiration?

Ans. They have a role in chemical regulation of respiration. Decrease of oxygen pressure, increase of carbon dioxide pressure and decrease of pH of blood are stimuli to which they respond.

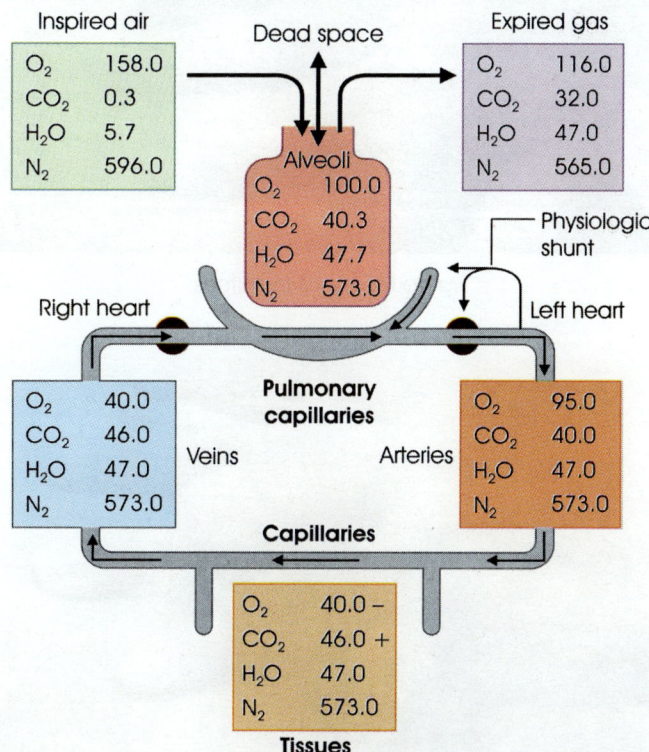

Q25. The above figure shows gas pressures in the pulmonary circuit and blood vessels. Name the type of hypoxia when oxygen pressure decreases in arterial blood?

Ans. It is hypoxic hypoxia.

The saturation of haemoglobin by oxygen is dependent on oxygen pressure and hence there is decrease in oxygen saturation and hence oxygen carriage.

Q26. How do you calculate the respiratory rate?

Ans. Count the respiratory rate and look for regularity of the rhythm. Holding the patient hand and continuing conversation with patient enquiring his/her health profile, the respiratory moments can be observed and respiratory rate counted. This will not make the patient aware and conscious, otherwise voluntary efforts by patient in nervousness may alter the rate.

Q27. How do you examine for vocal fremitus?

Ans. Vocal Fremitus refers to vibrations setup by the voice which is conducted from the larynx through the trachea, bronchi and lung tissue to the chest wall. This is detected by placing the hand of the examiner on the chest. The patient/individual are asked to repeat "ninety-nine" continuously. Place the ulnar border of your palm on corresponding areas on both sides of the subject's chest and compare the vibration set up by the voice. Vocal fremitus is decreased in pleural effusion and increased in consolidation.

Q28. Demonstrate the procedure of percussion.

Ans. Place the middle finger of the left hand (pleximeter) firmly on the part to be percussed and strike the back of its middle phalanx perpendicularly with the tip of the middle finger of your right hand. The percussing finger needs to be bent so that its terminal phalanx is at right angles and it strikes the pleximeter finger exactly perpendicular.

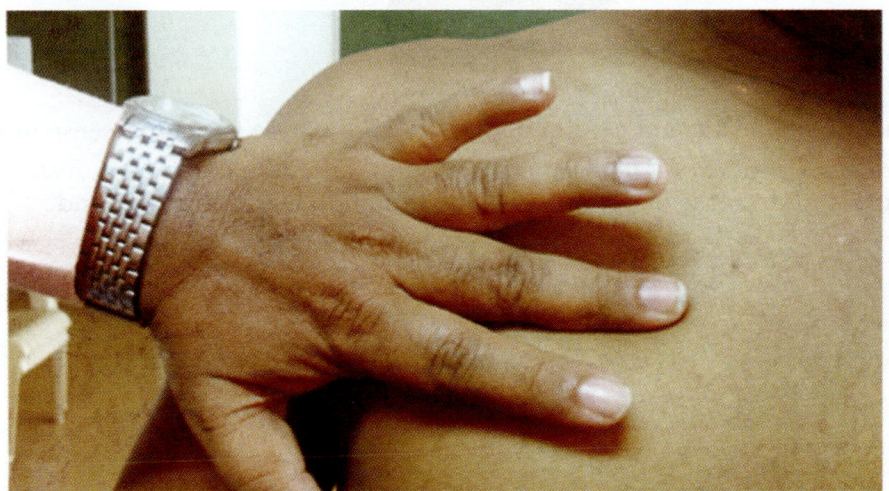

Figure for vocal fremitens

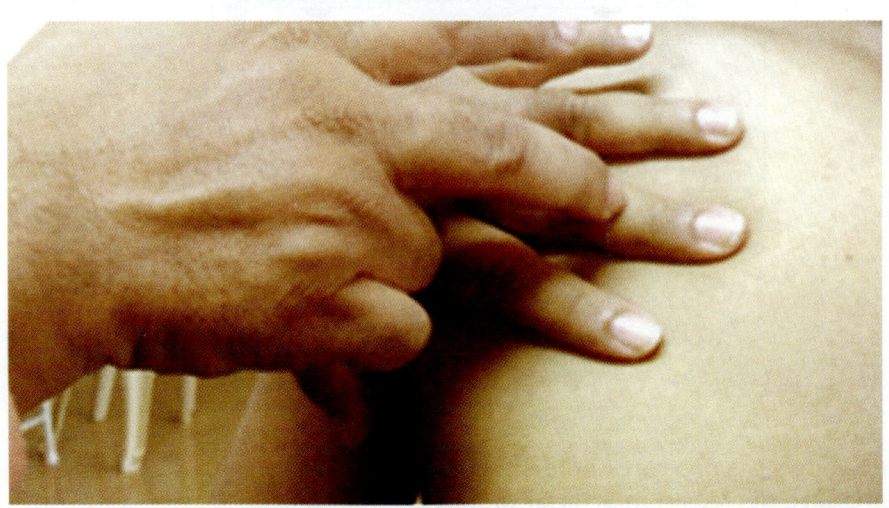

Figure for percussion

Q29. Discuss the characters of normal breath sound.

Ans. Character of the breath sounds: There are two typical types of breath sounds, vesicular and bronchial. Vesicular breath sounds are produced by the passage of air in and out of normal lung tissue and are heard all over the chest under normal conditions. The vesicular breathing is low pitched and rustling in character. The inspiratory sound is intense and audible during the whole of inspiration. The expiratory sound follows the inspiration without a distinct pause. The inspiratory sound is heard for a time twice as long as the expiratory sound. Bronchial breath sounds are produced by the passage of air through the trachea and large bronchi. This inspiratory sound is moderately intense and becomes inaudible before the end of inspiration. The expiratory sound is more intense and the duration extends through the greater part of expiration.

Q30. Describe the figure below.

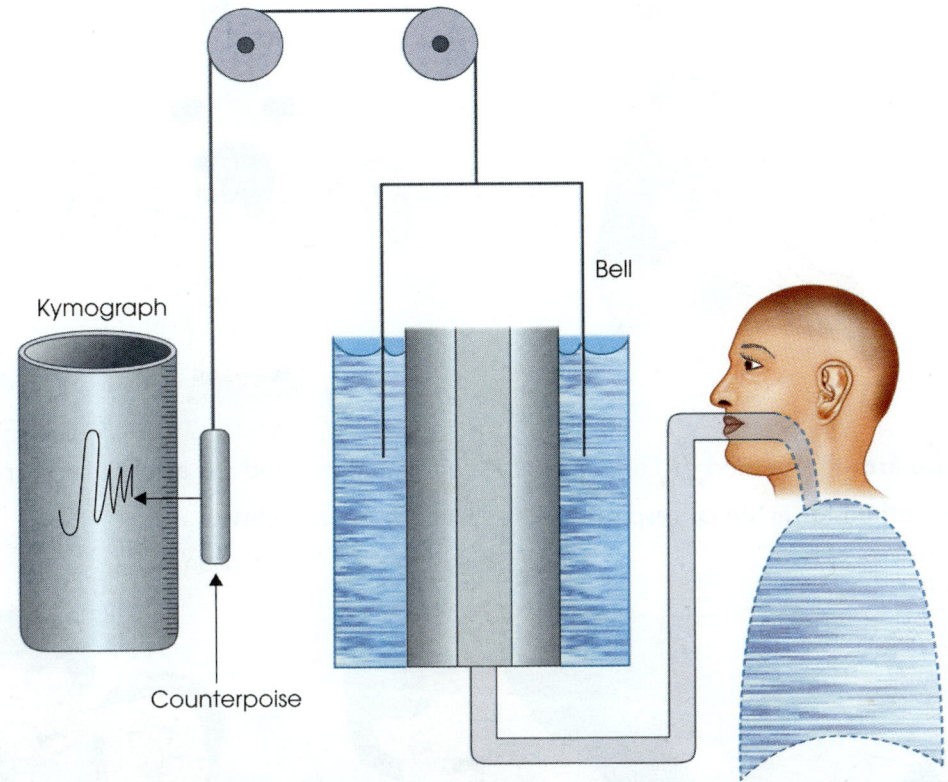

Ans. The instrument is vitalometer. It is used for recording the vital capacity of lung in the subject. Inspiration causes the spirometer bell to descend and the writing lever to move upwards on the chart. The chart is calibrated so that measurements of lung volume change can be made.

Q31. Identify the method for artificial respiration from the figure below.

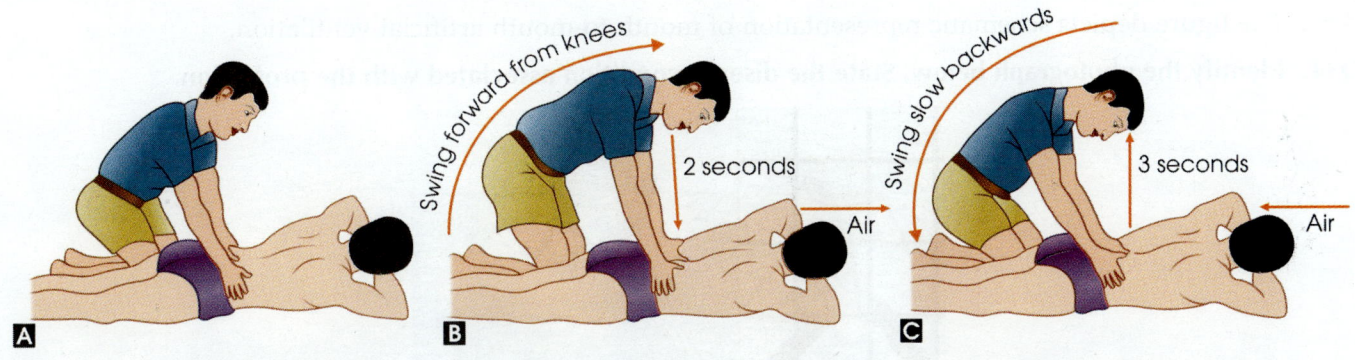

Ans. Schafer's manual method for artificial respiration.

Q32. Identify the method for artificial respiration from the figure below.

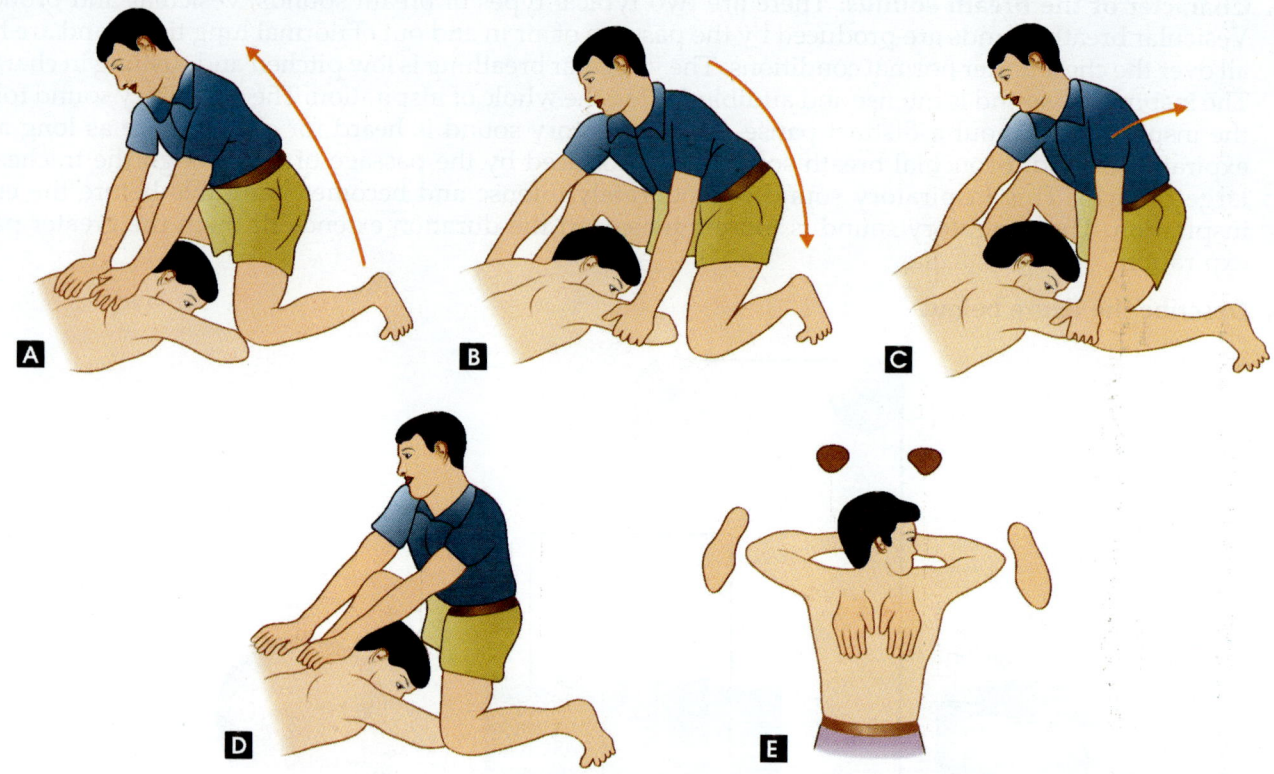

Ans. Back-pressure-arm-lift method or Holger-Nielsen's manual method for artificial respiration.

Q33. Identify the method for artificial respiration the from the figure below.

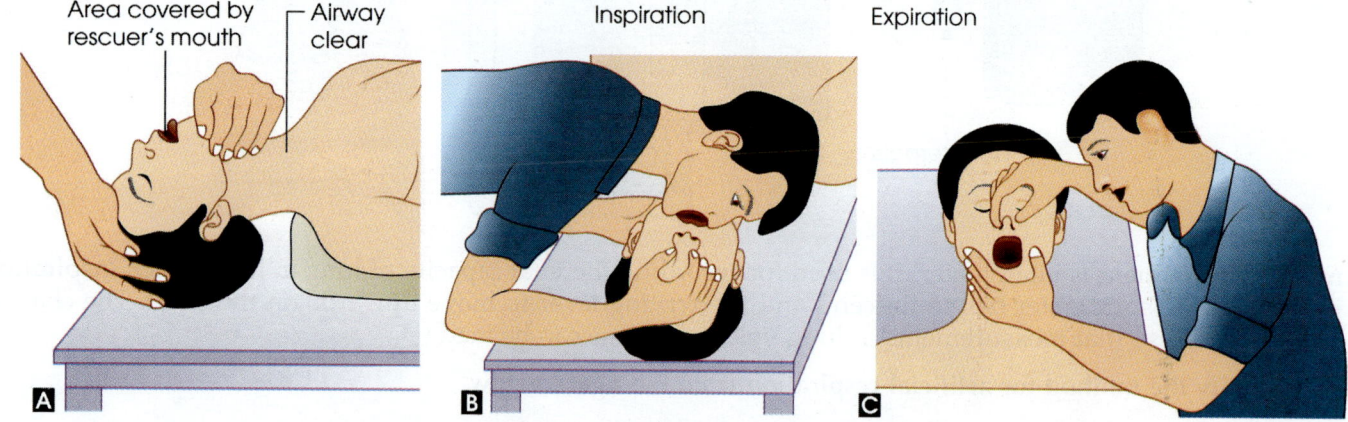

Ans. The figure depicts schematic representation of mouth-to-mouth artificial ventilation.

Q34. Identify the photograph below. State the disease condition associated with the profession.

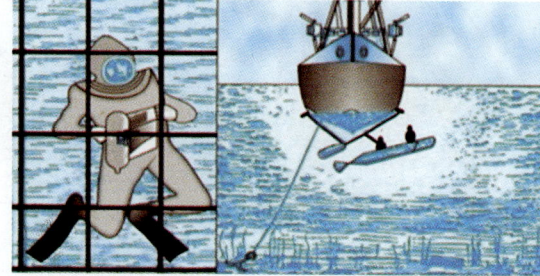

Ans. Deep sea diving: The disease condition associated with the profession is caisson disease.

Q35. Give the function of each of the glial cells shown below.

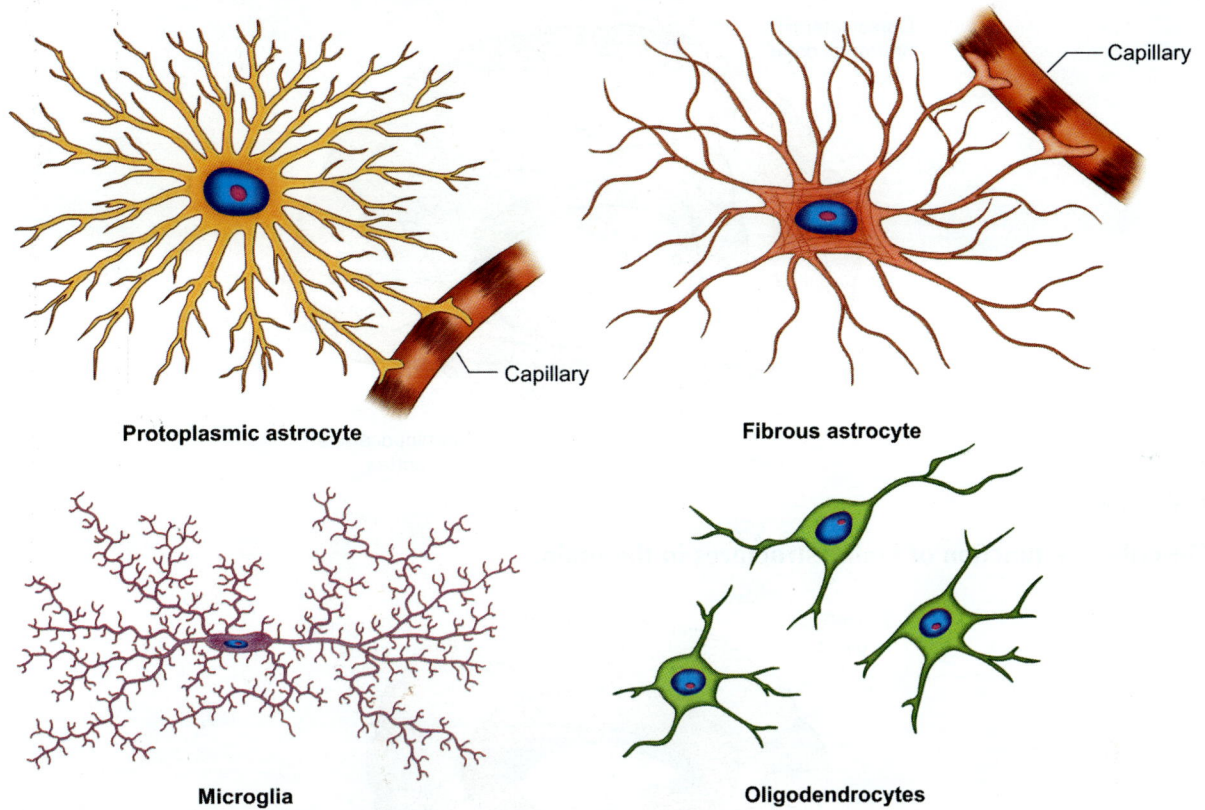

Protoplasmic astrocyte

Fibrous astrocyte

Capillary

Capillary

Microglia

Oligodendrocytes

Ans. Astrocytes: They are found throughout the brain.

Astrocytes form the *supporting tissue* of the CNS. They produce *substances that are trophic to neurons.* They maintain the **appropriate** *concentration of ions and neurotransmitters in the environment* surrounding the neurons as they can take up K$^+$ and neurotransmitters substances, glutamate and gamma aminobutyric acid (GABA) and metabolize them. They send processes to *isolate synapses.* They *induce capillaries to form tight junctions* that form blood–brain barrier. They are of protoplasmic and fibrous types.

Microglia: Which are scavenger cells that resemble tissue macrophages. When CNS is damaged they help to remove the products of damaged cells. Hence, they are latent phagocytes.

Oligodendrocytes: These are the glial cells which form myelin sheath on the nerve fibers which are inside the CNS providing insulation to the nerve impulses.

Q36a. Mention the sensations that are relayed in ventral posterior nucleus of thalamus.

b. Mention the connections of ventral lateral nucleus and ventral anterior nucleus of thalamus.

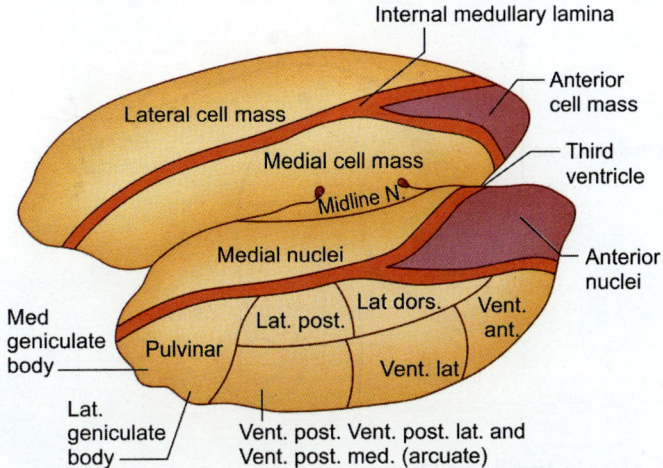

Ans. Impulses from somatic sensory pathways from the contralateral side of body.

Q37. Mention the role of hippocampus in the brain.

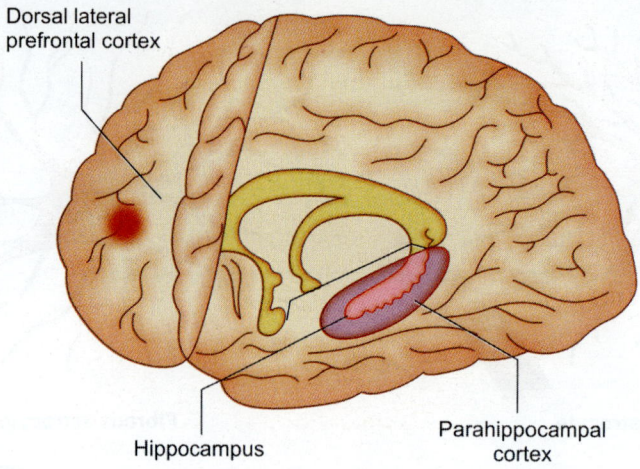

Ans. Role in memory.

Q38. Describe the function of limbic structures in the brain.

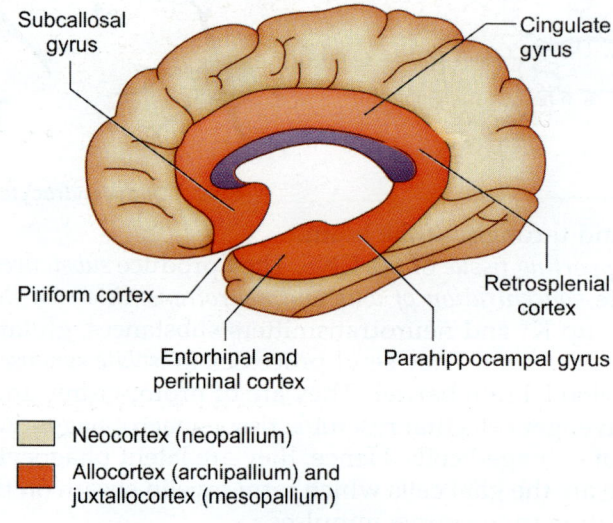

Ans. Limbic system has role in emotions generation and affects of emotions.

Q39. How does the figure below explain the basis of referred pain?

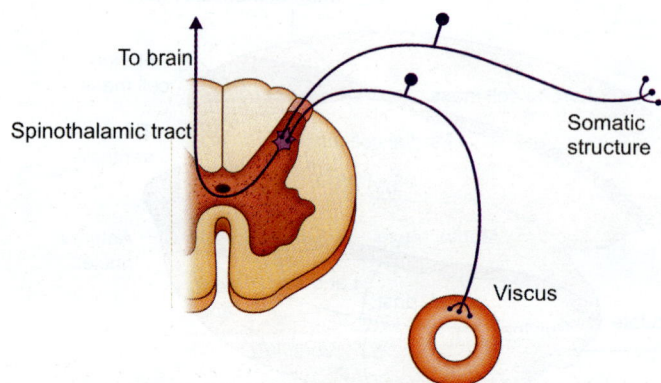

Ans. Figure explains that neurons in the dorsal horn are receiving impulses from superficial and deeper regions, and the pain from deeper regions may be interpreted as coming from superficial region.

Q40. Explain how pain sensation is influenced by descending connections from higher centres.

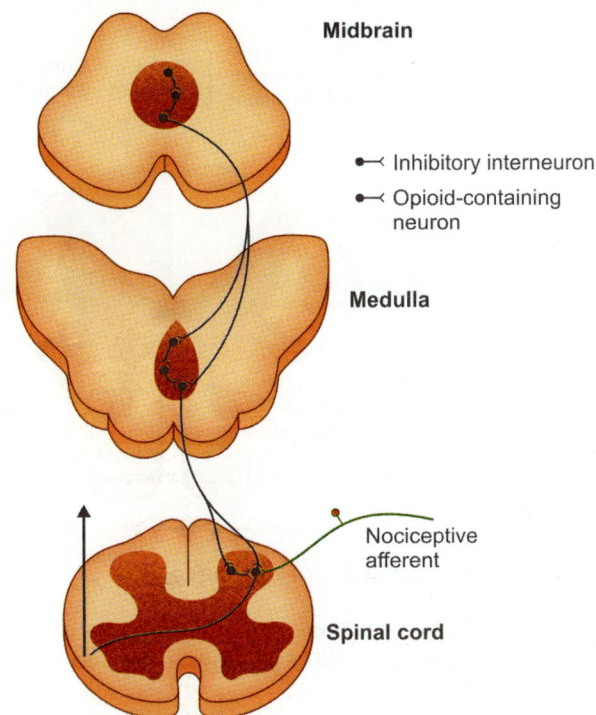

Midbrain

•—< Inhibitory interneuron

•—< Opioid-containing neuron

Medulla

Nociceptive afferent

Spinal cord

Ans. There is an inhibitory descending pathway from the brain that modifies transmission of pain in the spinal cord.

Q41. Mention the synaptic transmitter released at myoneural function.

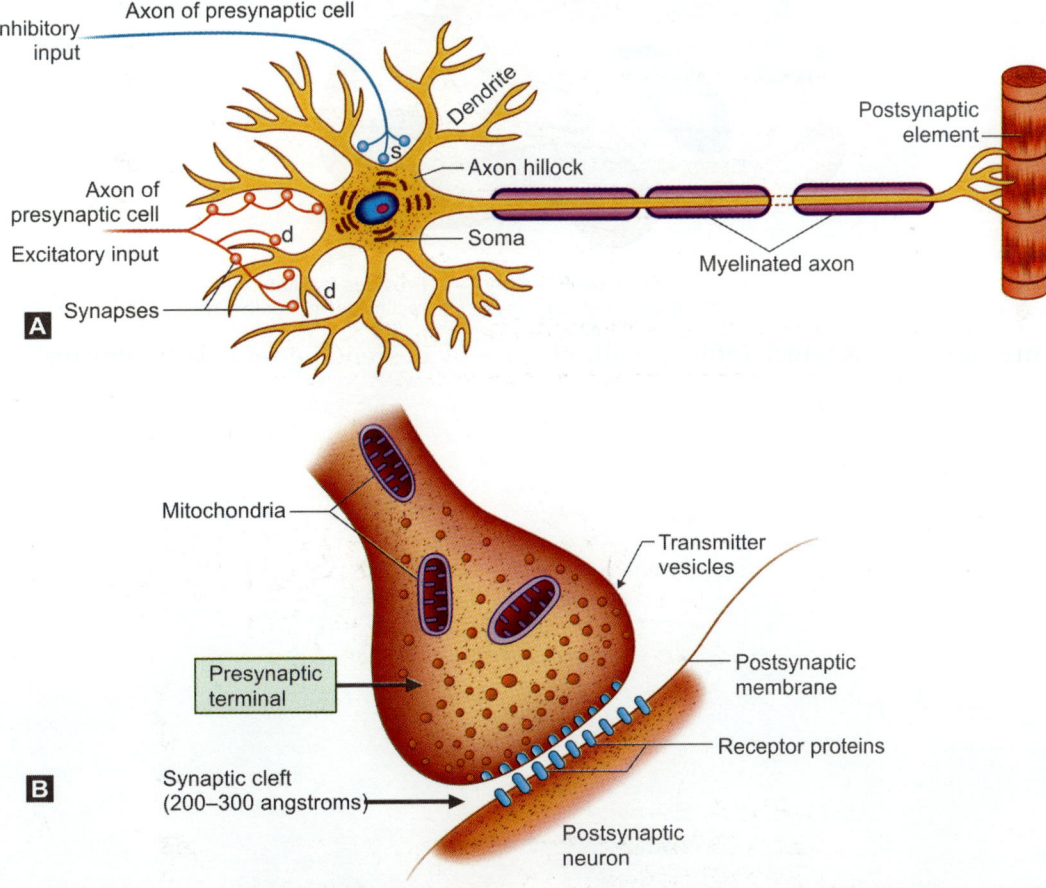

Axon of presynaptic cell

Inhibitory input

Dendrite

Postsynaptic element

Axon hillock

Axon of presynaptic cell

Soma

Excitatory input

Myelinated axon

A Synapses

Mitochondria

Transmitter vesicles

Presynaptic terminal

Postsynaptic membrane

Receptor proteins

B Synaptic cleft (200–300 angstroms)

Postsynaptic neuron

Ans. Acetylcholine is the neurotransmitter.

Q42. Describe how the touch sensation transmitted in dorsal column differs from that transmitted in spinothalamic tract.

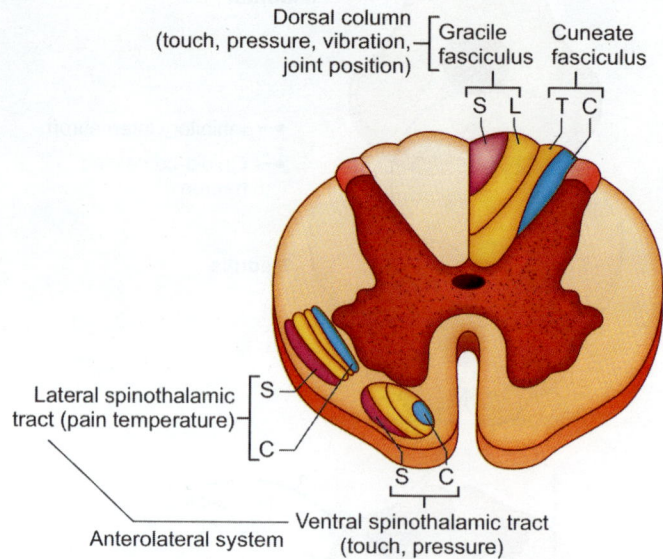

Ans. Touch sensation in the dorsal column carries impulses for fine touch, tactile localization, tactile discrimination and stereognosis, whereas tactile sensations carried by spinothalamic tract are for crude touch.

Q43. Comment on the figure below.

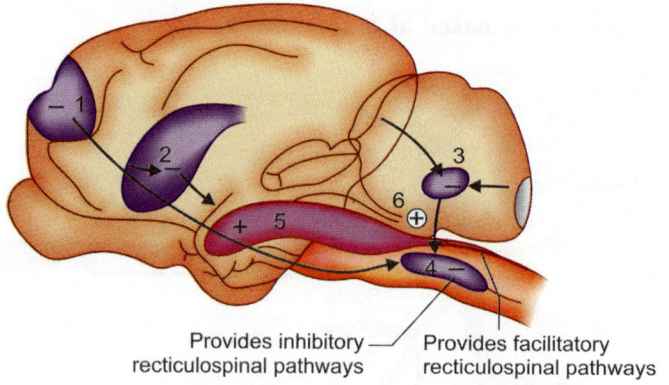

Ans. The figure shows areas which influence muscle tone by descending reticular pathways.

Unit

3

Amphibian Practicals with Spotters

PY 3.18*

1. Introduction to Amphibian Experiments

2. Apparatus for Amphibian Experiments

3. Nerve Muscle Preparation

4. Simple Muscle Twitch

5. Effect of Temperature on Simple Muscle Twitch

6. Velocity of Nerve Impulse

7. Effects of Two Successive Stimuli

8. Genesis of Fatigue in the Isolated Nerve Muscle Preparation

9. Effect of Increasing the Strength of Stimulus

10. Genesis of Tetanus

11. Effect of After Load and Free Load on Muscle Contraction and Calculation of Work Done

12. Recording of Normal Cardiogram

13. Effect of Temperature on Frog's Heart

14. Properties of Cardiac Muscle

15. Properties of Cardiac Muscle II

16. Effects of Various Drugs on the Frog Heart Muscle

Spotters

*Competency achievement as per competency based Undergraduate Curriculum for the Indian Medical Graduate, 2018, 1; Medical Council of India.

1

Introduction to Amphibian Experiments

Amphibian experiments provide better understanding of motor nervous system which is concerned with response of body to change in environment . The response of the nervous system is studied on skeletal and cardiac muscles of frog.

In the lab, for the study of response of living tissue to a stimulus, three things are required.

1. Living tissue preparation.
2. Stimulus providing device.
3. Recording system.

The living tissue includes the nerve muscle preparation and cardiac muscles of frog. There are various reasons for the selection of frog for experiments in the labs:

1. To great extent, the mechanisms of physiological activity of human beings resemble with that of lower animals like frog.
2. Frogs were easily available throughout the year, absolutely harmless and easy to handle.
3. Frogs are cold-blooded animals and their survival in the labs are better than the warm-blooded animals.
4. Tissues can be isolated from body which have better survival without oxygenation and temperature control. Their muscles can absorb oxygen from the atmosphere.

NERVE MUSCLE PREPARATION FROM FROG

For the experiments of nerve and muscles, the sciatic nerve along with spinal segment and gastrocnemius muscle of leg is isolated. In the isolated preparation, muscle can be made to contract by stimulating nerve or by directly stimulating its belly.

FROG HEART

Frog heart is exposed and most of the properties are studied with intact heart.

Stimulating System

Transformer is setup in the lab which convert alternating current (AC) into low voltage direct current (DC) which is connected with Du Bois-Reymond induction coil and induced current generated and used to give electrical stimulus.

STIMULUS

A stimulus is a change in the environment to which tissue respond. This change may be in external or internal environment.

Types of Stimulus

The different types of stimuli are:

Physical: Drying. Cooling and warming.

Mechanical: Tapping, pinching, cutting and crushing.

Chemical: Acids, alkalis and other chemicals.

Osmotic: Strong salt solution, glycerine.

Electrical: Various types of electrical stimulus are Galvanic current (galvanic or direct current, DC), Faradic or induced current, rectilinear (rectangular), and sine wave (AC or alternating current).

Preference of Electrical Stimulus

In all these stimuli, electrical stimulus is preferred for experimental work due to the following reasons:
1. Strength and duration of electrical stimulus can be easily controlled.
2. Electrical stimuli are of short duration and do not damage the tissues and can be applied repeatedly, if required, without producing any harmful effects.
3. Application of electrical stimuli resemble with natural way of working of tissues as resting membrane potential and action potential are electrical in nature.
4. This can be easily provided in the labs, by using induction coil or electronic stimulator

Stimulus can also be Classified on Basis of Strength of Stimuli

1. **Threshold stimulus**—is the minimum strength of stimulus that is required to produce a response.
2. **Sub-threshold**—(sub-minimal, or subliminal) **stimulus** is weaker than a threshold stimulus and is unable to produce a response.
3. **A maximal stimulus**—which results in giving a maximum response.
4. **Sub-maximal stimulus**—has strength more than threshold stimuli but less than the maximal. Here as the strength of stimulus increases, the magnitude of response also undergoes enhancement.
5. **Supra-maximal**—stimuli has more strength than a maximal stimulus but response does not hike.

On the Basis of Number of Times Stimulus Given, it may be

a. **Single**—single electric shock is given.
b. **Two successive stimuli**—two electric shocks (one after other) are given.
c. **Multiple successive stimuli**—many electric shocks are given.

Recording System

Recording of response of tissues is performed by writing lever attached to ink pointer which writes on white paper pasted on kymograph drum or on physiograph. Alternatively a triangular pointer which writes on smoked paper can be used.

OBSERVATIONS: EXERCISE FOR STUDENTS

....

....

....

....

....

....

....

....

....

....

2

Apparatus for Amphibian Experiments

HIGH VOLTAGE MAINS

It is routine domestic electrical supply of alternating current of 220 volts which is used only for kymograph. No other electrical appliance used in amphibian experiment is connected to it.

1. Low Voltage Mains

By using step-down transformer, main alternating current is converted into low voltage direct current having strength between 4 and 10 volts which is used in the primary circuit. Two terminals of primary coil of induction coil are connected with low voltage main.

Du Bois-Reymond Induction Coil

This is a device which converts low voltage, high ampere, direct continuous current into induced current which is always of short duration. Induced current is of high voltage low ampere and phasic current and produced at make and break of electrical circuit. It is named after the inventor Emil Du Bois-Reymond (1818–96), a German electro-physiologist.

Various Parts of Induction Coil

Du-bois Reymond Induction Coil has the various parts: Wooden or metallic platform, primary and secondary coil, terminals of primary and secondary coil and assembly of Neef's hammer.

1. Wooden or metallic platform on which various parts are fixed and a graduated measuring scale is attached on it which is used to measure the distance between primary and secondary coil.
2. Primary and secondary coils are composed of insulated copper wire wound round the iron core. Primary coil has 2500–3000 turns of relatively thick, cotton-covered, copper wire wound round a wooden reel which contains an iron core. The secondary coil has 7000 to 8000 turns of thin enameled, copper wire. The primary coil is fixed but secondary coil can move toward or away to primary coil to alter the strength of stimulus.
3. Terminals of primary coil are connected to the low voltage main to pass direct current in the primary coil and terminals of secondary coil are connected to stimulating electrodes.
4. Assembly of Neef's hammer is lying on the opposite side of primary coil and composed of Neef's hammer, electromagnet and terminals of Neef's hammer. Neef's hammer is a horizontally placed T-shaped iron bar

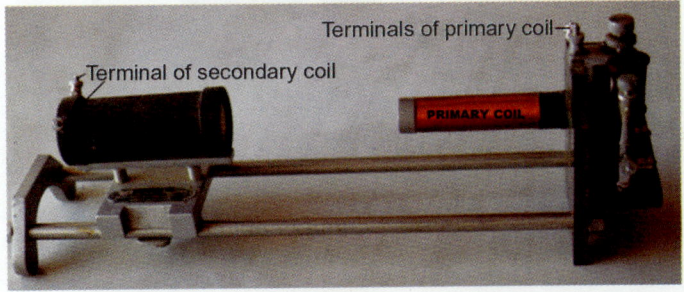

Fig. 2.1: Du Bois-Reymond induction coil

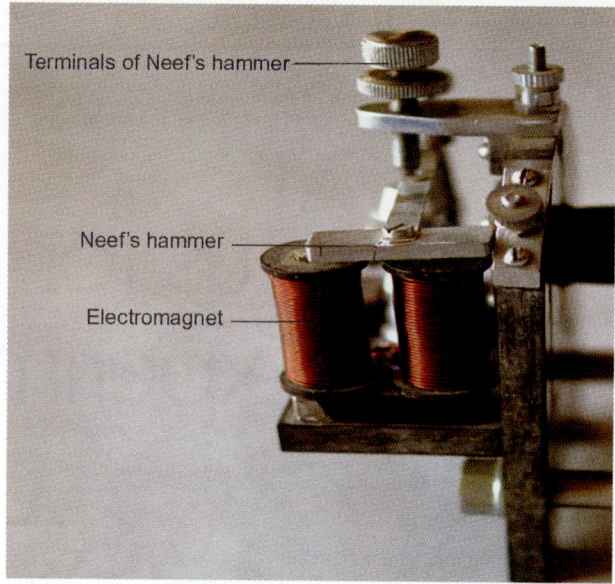

Terminals of Neef's hammer

Neef's hammer

Electromagnet

Fig. 2.2: Du Bois-Reymond induction coil showing Neef's Assembly

fitted with a spring and located over an electromagnet. Terminals of Neef's hammer are connected in the primary circuit when multiple, repeated stimuli are required.

Functioning of Device

On flowing the direct current from main to the primary coil through wires, induced current is generated in the secondary coil which is used to stimulate the tissues by connecting terminal of secondary coil to stimulating electrode. The induced current is generated only at make and break of primary circuit and it is stronger at the break.

The strength of stimulus can be modulated as strength of stimulus is minimum when secondary coil is at extreme far position and it increases on moving the secondary coil toward the primary coil. It is maximum when secondary coil is completely covering the primary coil.

Neef's hammer works on the principle of electric bell. On passing the current, the iron bar vibrates up and down and causes make and break of the primary circuit continuously at a rate of 30–40 to over 100 per second.

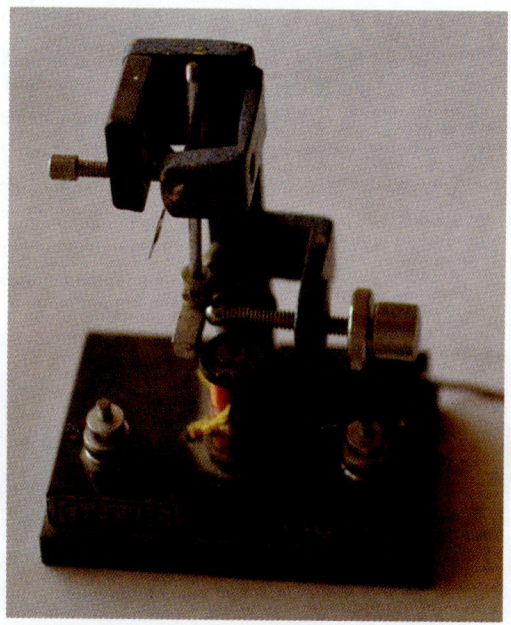

Fig. 2.3: Vibrating variable interrupter

2. Vibrating Variable Interrupter

It works on the principle of electric bell similar to that of Neef's hammer and enables more accurate interruption of the primary circuit at a much lower frequency (up to 25/sec) as that of Neef's hammer. It is connected in series with the induction coil and used to give multiple stimuli.

3. Electric Kymograph (Drum)

The Sherrington-Starling kymograph is a machine which records the movement of the tissue (i.e. muscle contractions) on the moving surface and runs on the mains 220 volts AC current. It records magnitude of contraction along vertical axis and time duration along the horizontal axis.

Various parts of kymograph: (1) Kymograph body containing electric motor and gear system, (2) Leveling screw, (3) On-off switch for mains current, (4) Calibrated speed setting system, (5) Clutch lever, (6) Electric contact block (7) Spindle, (8) Dual electric contact arms, (9) Cylinder, (10) Screw lift for cylinder, (11) Lever for fixing cylinder on the spindle.

1. Kymograph body containing electric motor and gear system is the main part of body which operates with AC current at 220 volts. With working of electric motor, drum fixed on shaft rotate on which movement of tissues is recorded. For the purpose of easy understanding and reference, the body can be divided into four surfaces: Anterior (front), posterior (behind), right and left lateral.

2. Leveling screw is located on base towards the front surface facing the observer and used to adjust the proper position of drum, otherwise working lever will not remain in contact during whole period of movement.

3. On-off switch for mains current is located on right lateral surface.

4. **Calibrated speed setting system:** The speed of rotating drum is selected by means of a calibrated speed setting lever.

   The two prongs of this lever have to be pressed together to move it up or down for engaging at a particular speed slot. There is one slot marked "N" (neutral) where the gears get disengaged from the motor. A variable speed lever permits speeds (fast and slow) between 0.12/0.25 mm/sec and 320/640 mm/sec (not revolutions per minute, RPM).

5. **Clutch lever:** It is placed on the left lateral surface of main body which is used to engage and disengage the gear and prevents the damage of gear. For changing the recording drum, the position of clutch must be kept at neutral position.

6. **Electric contact block:** Electric contact block is fitted on the top of the kymograph body, at the level of the striker. It performs the function of key. It has two electrical terminals and one terminal bears a plastic button having spring contact. When these terminals are included in the primary circuit, circuit is only completed when striker comes in contact with electric contact block. It is also used to mark the point of stimulus on the baseline of rotating drum.

7. **Spindle or shaft:** It is solid thick circular iron rod, attached with electric motor and rotate with different speeds (2.5 mm as slow speed and 640 mm as fastest speed).

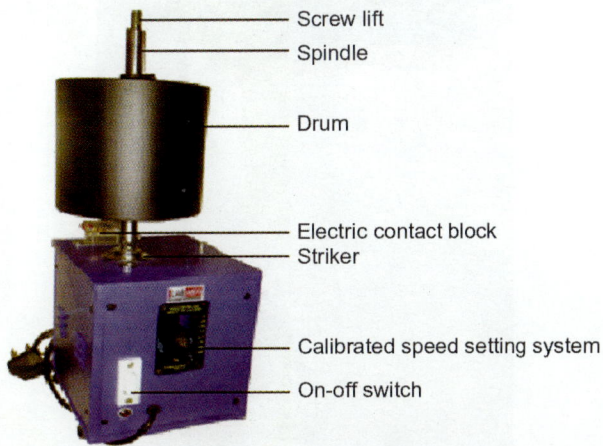

Fig. 2.4: Kymograph

It has vertical groove on one side with which drum is fixed and at the top, a screw lift has been setup by which drum can move up and down.

At the lower end, it is fitted with dual electric contact arms which rotate along with movement of shaft.

8. **Dual electric contact arms:** Dual electric contact arms (also called the **"striker"**) are fitted, one over the other, at the base of the spindle and rotate along with it and stimulus is produced on coming in contact with electric contact block. Two arms of striker can be separated when two successive stimuli (one after the other) are required.

9. **Cylinder or drum:** It is cylinder of 6″ × 6″ which is mounted on the shaft of kymograph and fixed to the axle with the help of drum grip latch located at the top of drum. A white paper is pasted on the drum which is smoked in case triangular object is used as pointer of writing lever for recording of response.

10. **Screw lift for cylinder:** It is used to move the recording drum up and down for adjusting the appropriate position.

Functioning of Kymograph

With working of electric motor, drum fixed on shaft rotate and pointer of isotonic writing lever having fixed gastrocnemius tendon is placed in contact with moving drum so that drum slides under the pen. When gastrocnemius muscle contracts, lever moves upward and in moving drum it gets recorded in the form of graph.

Effective stimulus: As the shaft rotates at a fast speed, each time the striker touches contact spring of electric contact block, the primary circuit is completed and called make followed by immediate break of the circuit. The induced current is generated at make and break but induced current of make becomes stimulus. As induced current of break is ineffective in the refractory phase of muscle.

The two arms of the strikers can be separated and can be kept at any angle and used to deliver two stimuli at a desirable interval of time.

4. Muscle Trough

It is made of Perspex or plastic. The trough holds the isolated nerve- muscle preparation as it is kept immersed in a nutritive solution. It carries the stimulating electrode on one side and a writing lever on the other side. The floor of the trough has a cork to which the nerve muscle preparation can be fixed. A drainage tube is attached to the floor of the muscle trough.

5. Myograph Board

Myograph board is a rectangular wooden board having clips each on the short side. By one clip, it is fixed with myograph stand and by another clip, writing lever is attached. The position of myograph board can be adjusted by moving vertically along rod of myograph stand.

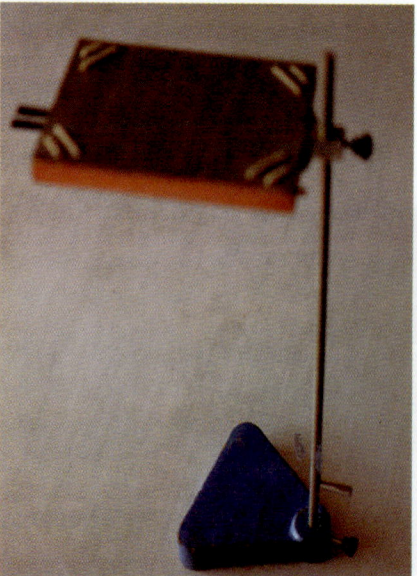

Fig. 2.5: Myograph board and myograph stand

6. Myograph Stand

It is made of a heavy base to which a vertical rod is attached. The muscle trough or myograph board is fixed to the vertical rod of the myograph stand.

7. Isotonic Muscle Lever

In amphibian experiments, two types of writing levers are used—one is isotonic muscle lever and the other is Starling heart lever.

Various parts of isotonic muscle lever: Metallic plate, wire, pointer, fulcrum, hook after loaded screw and supporting rod.

Isotonic muscle lever is attached to the myograph board. It records as well as magnifies the skeletal muscle contraction on the drum of kymograph.

It consists of a narrow metallic plate to which a long thin metal wire carrying a writing pen or triangular piece of photographic film is attached at one end. The narrow plate is attached to a metallic fulcrum rod at other end and this carries a hook. A screw support the hook and prevent the downward movement of the lever on applying weight and it is called the after loading screw. The writing lever mounts on one side of the muscle trough or myograph board. A small weight (10 g) is suspended from the holes of metallic plate about 2 cm from the fulcrum.

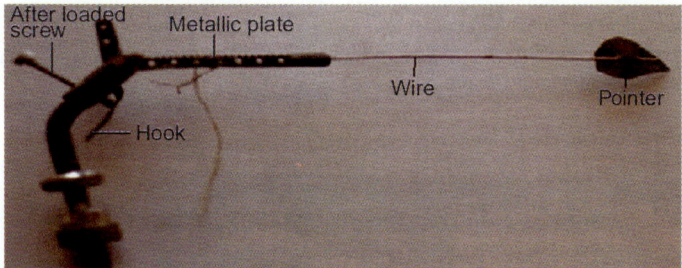

Fig. 2.6: Isotonic lever

Ink-writing lever: An ink-writing stylus (filled with ink) can be fitted on the writing lever. It can then directly inscribe on the glazed paper without the need of smoking of paper.

8. Starling Heart Lever

It is a writing lever used for recording the mechanical events of the frog's heart.

Various parts of lever: Lever frame/metallic stand, writing lever (composed of flat lever arm, wire and pointer), spring and supporting arm.

The frame of the lever or metallic stand has metallic rod in the centre on which supporting arm can be fixed at desirable position to alter the magnification of cardiac systole and diastole on recording drum. One end of metallic stand bears hole for mounting on myograph stand and other end has attachment for writing lever.

Writing lever carries a light, flat lever arm with a finely-adjustable tension spring which supports the writing lever in the horizontal position. A piece of thread tied to the writing lever carries a bent pin which can be hooked through the apex of the ventricle when its contractions are to be recorded.

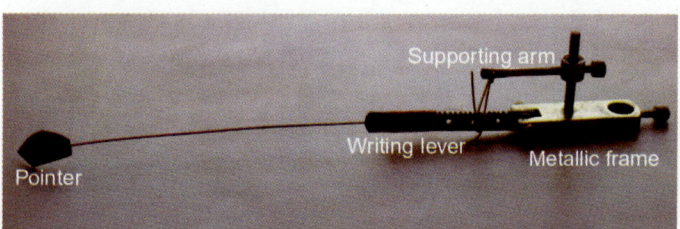

Fig. 2.7: Starling lever of heart

9. Tuning fork (100 Hz)

The tuning fork with a frequency of 100 vibrations per second is used for measuring the time interval for the nerve muscle experiments.

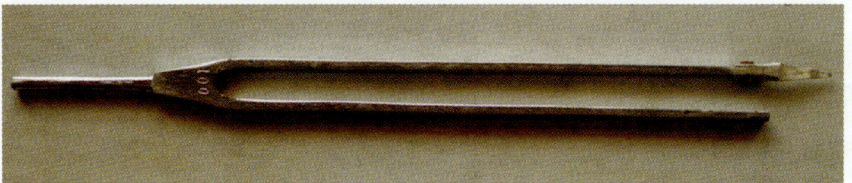

Fig. 2.8: Tuning fork

10. Keys

A key is used as a switch to make and break an electrical circuit. The different types of keys are used in amphibian experiments

   i. Simple key: It is an ordinary on-off switch fixed on a wooden or vulcanite base and is connected in primary circuit. The two poles of the switch are connected to two adjustable screw terminals. Other types of simple keys include metal blocks, morse key and unspillable mercury key.

  ii. Short-circuiting key: It is connected in the secondary circuit to prevent accidental passage of current into the tissues. It also prevents unipolar induction. It has 4 terminals, the two left and the two right hand terminals are permanently connected. The two poles of the switch are connected to the two inner terminals. When the switch is off, induced current will not be transmitted to stimulating electrode.

 iii. Tap key: It is used in primary circuit to make or break the primary circuit. The circuit is made by pressing the key.

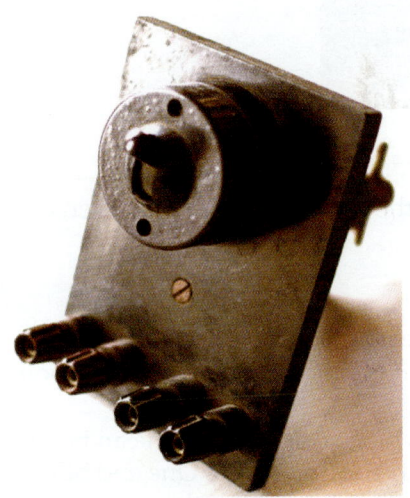

Fig. 2.9: Short circuiting key

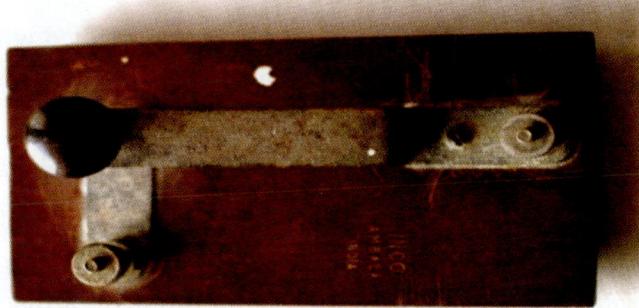

Fig. 2.10: Tap key

11. Stimulating Electrode

It consists of two insulated metallic wires which are exposed about 6–8 cm from insulated coating at their terminal ends. The exposed wires are passed through perspex block (plastic body) and the ends of wires emerging from this block are touched to tissues for stimulation. The perspex block has a hole in the centre for fixing it on myograph board with the pin.

12. Stimulus Marker (Signal Marker)

It consists of an electromagnet and a writing lever. Whenever the stimulus is applied to the tissue, the electromagnet gets magnetized and pulls the writing lever down. Thus, the time of the application of the stimulus is marked.

13. Weights

It consists of a metallic hook of 10 grams weight and metallic discs each having 10 grams weight.

Electric Circuit

For providing an electric stimulus to live tissues, two electric circuits primary and secondary are framed.

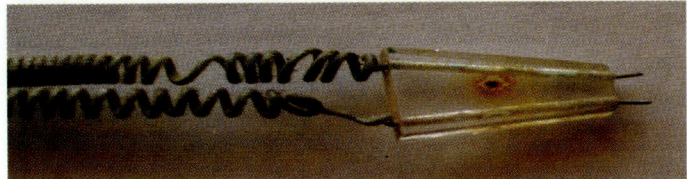

Fig. 2.11: Stimulating electrode

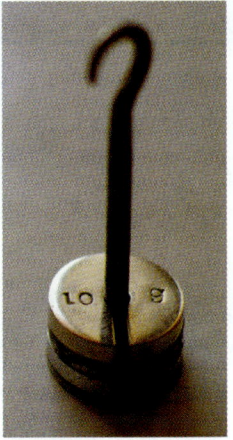

Fig. 2.12: Weights

Primary Circuit

1. Primary circuit is the circuit of low voltage main, primary coil, kymograph and keys which are connected in series with each other.
2. With wires, one knob of low voltage DC source is connected to the one terminal of primary coil through primary key and tap key. Other knob of source is connected to other terminal of coil through kymograph.

3.

```
                    ┌──→ (Primary key) ──→ (Tap key) ──→┐  Primary
         Source ────┤                                    │  coil
                    └──← (Kymograph) ←───────────────────┘
```

4. In some experiments where rotation of drum is not required. Drum is excluded and rest of the circuit is the same

Secondary Circuit

1. Secondary circuit is a parallel connection of secondary coil, short circuit key and stimulating electrode.
2. Terminals of secondary coils are connected with stimulating electrodes through short circuiting key.
3. When switch of secondary key is made to off position, no current passes to electrode and used to avoid the any extra stimulation.
4. Terminals of secondary coil ⇉ (short circuiting key) ⇉ (Stimulating electrode).

Shake down Test

Before performing experiments both primary and secondary circuits should be checked.

Primary circuit: After completing the primary circuit kymograph is switched on, primary key is closed and tapping key is pressed. When ever projecting striker of rotating drum come in contact with contact button of kymograph, primary circuit is completed and electric sparks are produced.

Secondary circuit: After completing both circuits, stimulating electrode is placed on muscles of frog, switch on the kymograph and press the tapping key, if circuit is correct, muscles will contract.

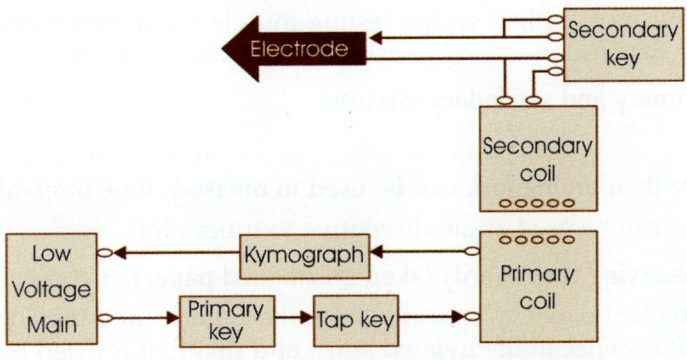

Fig. 2.13: Electric circuit

QUESTIONS AND ANSWERS

Q1. **What is the use of induction coil?**

Q2. **What is the principle on which Neef's hammer work?**

Ans. 1 and 2 see text

Q3. **What other appliances works on the same principle?**

Ans. Neef's hammer, vibrator variable interrupter and electromagnetic signal marker.

Q4. **What is the use of Neef's hammer?**

Ans. It is used to give multiple repeated stimuli as in experiment of genesis of tetanus.

Q5. **How much is the slow and fast speed of kymograph?**

Ans. Kymograph rotates as 2.5 mm as slow speed and 640 mm as fastest speed.

Q6. **What is use of electric contact block of kymograph?**

Ans. It is used for an instant make and break of electric circuit.

Q7. **What is the use of primary and secondary key?**

Ans. Primary key is just like an on and off switch which opens and closes the circuit and used in primary circuit. Secondary key is used in secondary circuit and kept closed for short circuiting the current.

Q8. **Why does induced current is preferred for giving stimulus?**

Ans. Induced current is of short duration which is produced at the make and break of circuit. It causes minimum damage to the tissue due to short duration and its strength can be modified.

Q9. **What is difference between primary coil and secondary coil?**

Ans.

Primary coil	Secondary coil
Has less turns (3000)	More number of turns (7000)
Made of thick copper wire	Made of thin insulated copperwire
Component of primary circuit	Component of secondary circuit
Primary coil is connected to main DC source	It is connected to stimulating electrode
Used to generate induced current in secondary circuit	Used to provide induced current to stimulating electrode

Q10. **Which current will be stronger out of these two currents, generated at make or current generated at break?**

Ans. The current generated at break will be stronger. At make of primary circuit, magnetic flux increases slowly from zero to maximum on the contrary at break of primary circuit magnetic flux rapidly change from maximum to zero so induced current is stronger.

Q11. **What is the function of writing lever?**

Ans. It records and magnify the muscle contraction.

Q12. **Give reason that a screw on hook of writing lever is called after loaded screw.**

Ans. The suspended weight is not applied on the resting muscle but it comes into play after the muscle starts contracting it (a screw which causes load to act only after the contraction begins).

Q13. **How will you form primary and secondary circuits?**

Ans. See text.

Q14. **Which appliance other than tuning fork can be used to measure time intervals?**

Ans. Electronic time marker can be used as an alternative to tuning fork.

Q15. **What is method of preserving the records taken on smoked paper?**

Ans. After taking record, smoked paper is separated from the cylinder and then dipped in a solution of fixative which contain resin and shellac in methylated spirit and finally it is dried by hanging.

Nerve Muscle Preparation

Aim: To isolate a gastrocnemius muscle and sciatic nerve of frog.

1. INSTRUMENTS AND CHEMICALS

Stunning rod, pithing needle, scissors, forceps, glass rod and amphibian Ringer's solution

Animal species: Frog.

Composition of Amphibian Ringer Solution

Sodium chloride: 0.6% (maintains isotonicity)

Potassium chloride: 0.014% (maintains the membrane potential)

Calcium chloride: 0.012% (maintains the muscle excitability and stimulate ATPase activity)

Sodium bicarbonate: 0.02% (maintains pH)

Sodium biophosphate: 0.001% (maintains pH)

2. PROCEDURE

After stunning and pithing, the frog is dissected to isolate the gastrocnemius muscle and sciatic nerve along the spinal segment of frog. Gastrocnemius muscle is isolated from leg, sciatic nerve from thigh and spinal cord segment from vertebral column.

a. Stunning of Frog

Hold the frog from trunk with cotton cloth and give a firm blow on the head of the frog with the stunning rod, the frog becomes unconscious and becomes easy to handle.

b. Pithing

i. Hold the frog in your left hand and keep index finger on external nares and thumb below neck on the dorsal surface of frog and rest of the fingers are kept on ventral surface below the level of forelimbs.

ii. Press the head with left index finger and feel a depression in the midline of dorsal surface of neck with right index finger. Through this depression, insert the pithing needle inside the cranial cavity and destroy the brain by rotating pithing needle.

iii. Remove the needle from cranial cavity and now insert pithing needle in downward direction in vertebral canal so as to destroy the spinal cord. On entering the vertebral canal, legs are straightened and urine is passed and on subsequent destruction of spinal cord, muscles of hindlimb become flaccid.

c. Dissection of Sciatic Nerve

1. Place the frog on its ventral surface on a dissection board as dissection is done on dorsal surface.

2. Take a scissor and cut the skin of the frog around its middle of the lower limbs using toothed forceps.

3. Lift the urostyle with blunt end forceps and cut the pelvic girdle on either side and take precaution that the underlying sciatic nerves are not damaged. Identify the insertion roots of the sciatic nerves.

4. Incise the vertebral column above and below the roots of the sciatic nerves. Cautiously separate the isolated segment of the vertebral column by cutting longitudinally into two halves.
5. The sciatic nerve is to be isolated and exposed with a blunt glass rod.
6. Trace the sciatic nerve from the thigh muscles up to knee joint by just separating the muscle bellies and remove all adhesions.

Dissection of Gastrocnemius Muscle

1. Identify the gastrocnemius muscle and free the muscle from the tibia. Separate its tendon from the ankle joint and tie a piece of thread to the tendon.
2. Cut the tibia below the knee joint and the femur above the knee joint taking care not to cut the sciatic nerve.
3. Isolate the nerve muscle preparation. Keep the nerve muscle preparation immersed in the amphibian Ringer's solution till it is used for the experiment.

PRECAUTIONS

1. During the dissection, pour Ringer solution continuously to prevent drying of tissues.
2. To avoid injury of nerve and undue stimulation of muscle, do not use any metal object rather use glass seeker for holding the nerve.
3. Do not try to dissect out the sciatic nerve at the knee joint . This will cause injury of nerve and is time consuming.

QUESTIONS AND ANSWERS

Q1. What is the composition of Ringer solution?

Q2. What is the function of each component?

Ans. 1 and 2—see the text.

Q3. Is there any other solution which can replace Ringer solution?

Ans. Yes, frog saline solution which is 0.6% solution of NaCl can replace Ringer solution.

Q4. What is the purpose of pithing?

Ans. Pithing is done to destroy the brain and the spinal cord so that the animal neither feels pain, nor there is any hindrance due to reflex or voluntary movements during the dissection.

Q5. How will you identify that pithing needle is in vertebral canal and not elsewhere?

Ans. On moving the needle in right and left direction, vertebral column also move along with needle.

Q6. What are the signs of proper pithing?

Ans.
a. Neither pain nor any movement is felt
b. Complete flaccidity is felt in the muscles of limbs
c. Corneal and conjuctival reflexes are lost.

Q7. What is the purpose of dissecting the segment of vertebral column?

Ans. With vertebral segment, nerve is not injured and can be used for a long time. Moreover, it is easier to handle the nerve by holding the vertebral piece.

Q8. Can other side of nerve preparation which is not dissected be utilized?

Ans. Yes, other side of nerve preparation can be used and for this reason segment of vertebral column is cut longitudinally so that both nerve muscle preparation have spinal segment.

Q9. Why is glass seeker/rod preferred for handling the nerve?

Ans. If nerve is handled with metal object, it can stimulate the nerve and cause muscle contraction. Muscle fatigue may occur by touching again and again.

Q10. What are the reasons for the selection of gastrocnemius muscle for amphibian experiments?

Ans. *Gastrocnemius muscle is selected due to various useful features:*
a. Easy to dissect with its nerve
b. Has long tendon for applying thread and fixing with lever
c. Easy to fix with knee joint
d. Has a sufficient belly to give stronger and recordable contraction.

Simple Muscle Twitch

Aim: To record the simple muscle twitch in an isolated skeletal muscle by giving a single electrical stimulus to the nerve supplying the muscle.

Instruments and chemicals: Stunning rod, pithing needle, scissors, forceps, muscle trough, writing lever, stimulating electrode, kymograph with recording drum, tuning fork (100 Hz) and amphibian Ringer's solution.

Simple muscle twitch (also called simple muscle curve) is a graphical representation of response of isolated skeletal muscle to single stimulus.

PROCEDURE

1. Isolate and make a gastrocnemius muscle and sciatic nerve preparation ready as described in Chapter 3.
2. Place it in the muscle trough (myograph board can also be used in the place of muscle trough). Pour the amphibian Ringer solution into the muscle trough.
3. Fix the knee joint with a pin to the cork base of the muscle trough.
4. Pull and attach the thread from the tendon to the hook of the writing lever.
5. Check whether the after loading screw touches the hook. Ideally a 10 g weight can be suspended from the hole of the writing lever around 2 cm from the fulcrum.
6. Complete the circuit as shown in Fig. 2.13.
7. Hold the vertebral piece with forcep and place the nerve on the stimulating electrode.
8. Switch on the primary and secondary circuit. Rotate the vertical rod of the myograph stand, ensuring that the writing lever does not touch the drum.

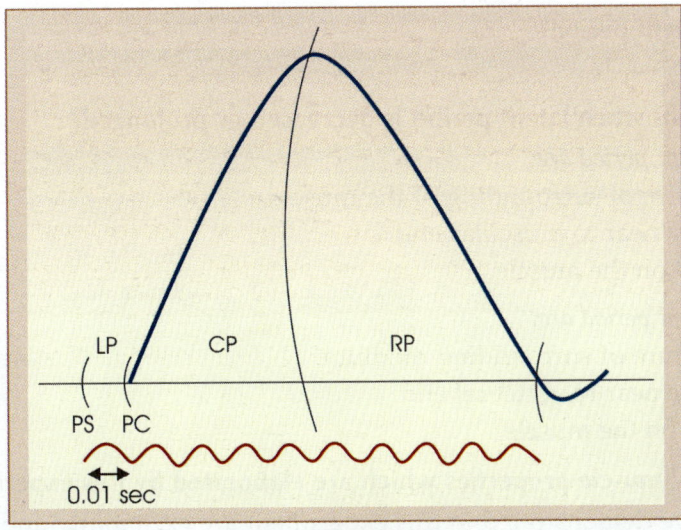

Fig. 4.1: Simple muscle twitch

9. Switch on the kymograph and allow it to rotate at the fastest speed (640 mm/sec), by turning the clutch to the vertical position. Increase the strength of stimulus gradually till a muscle twitch of 3–4 cm height is observed. Stop the kymograph by turning the clutch to horizontal position.

10. Rotate the vertical rod of the myograph stand and make the writing lever, now touch the drum and draw a base line.

11. Rotate the drum manually and make the contact arms touch the contact knob of the contact block. At this position, mark a vertical line on drum in order to indicate the point of stimulation.

12. Start the kymograph and record a simple muscle curve.

13. Label the point of stimulus (PS) and point of onset of contraction, the latent period (LP), contraction period (CP) and relaxation period (RP) on the simple muscle curve.

14. Allow the kymograph to rotate at the same speed (640 mm/sec). Using a tuning fork of 100 Hz, take a time tracing below the simple muscle curve.

15. Calculate the duration of the latent period, the contraction period and the relaxation period from the simple muscle curve.

OBSERVATION AND RESULTS

Simple muscle twitch is the contraction and relaxation of muscle following a single stimulus. The different phases of the simple muscle curve are: Latent period (LP), contraction period (CP) and relaxation period (RP).

Latent period (LP): It represents the period from the point of stimulus to the onset of contraction. The normal duration of latent period is 0.01–0.012 second. The latent period is due to the time taken for the transmission of an impulse along the nerve fiber to the muscle, neuromuscular delay, time taken for excitation contraction coupling and also due to inertia of lever. Time taken by nerve for impulse transmission is the major cause of latent period.

Contraction period (CP): It is the period between the point of contraction to the point of maximum contraction. The normal duration of contraction period is 0.04 second.

Relaxation period (RP): It is the period between the point of maximum contraction to the point of relaxation of muscle. The normal duration of RP is 0.05–0.06 second.

QUESTIONS AND ANSWERS

Q1. What is meant by twitch?

Ans. A rapid brief contraction followed by brief relaxation.

Q2. What are the different periods of simple muscle twitch?

Q3. How much is the duration of latent period, contraction period and relaxation period?

Q4. What are causes of latent period?

Ans. 2, 3 and 4—see text

Q5. What are the conditions when latent period is decreased or prolonged?

Ans. *Causes of decreased latent period are*:
  1. Increased temperature of surrounding of the muscle.
  2. Stimulation of nerve near to muscular end.
  3. Decreasing the load on the muscle.

  Causes of increased latent period are:
  1. Decreased temperature of surrounding medium.
  2. Stimulation of nerve near to vertebral end.
  3. Increasing the load on the muscle.

Q6. Mention the nerve and muscle properties which are elaborated by this experiment.

Ans. The properties of nerve demonstrated in this experiment are excitability and conductivity and properties of muscles are excitability, conductivity and contractility.

Q7. What is the purpose of suspending weight from lever?

Ans. It decreases the height of contraction and so that the graph may be obtained on the drum. It overcomes the inertia of lever.

Q8. How the point of stimulus is marked and what is its importance?

Ans. Read the method. Point of stimulus is used to measure the latent period. Moreover in some experiments, effects of some alterations are compared with normal simple muscle graph and here point of stimulation should be same.

Q9. How many milliseconds will have in a wave of tunic fork having frequency 100/sec?

Ans. 10 msec

Q10. What would happen if length of wire of writing lever is changed?

Ans. *Writing lever has three parts*: Metallic plate, wire and pointer. On increasing the length of wire magnification will be increased and vise versa.

Q11. What are events which occur on giving stimulus to the nerve?

Ans. *Various events occur as*:
   a. Impulse is conducted along nerve fibre.
   b. Neuro-transmitter ACh is released in the synaptic cleft.
   c. Binding of neurotransmitter with nicotinic receptor.
   d. Opening of sodium channel and influx of sodium.
   e. Development of motor end plate potential and opening of voltage gated sodium and potassium channels and generation of action potential.
   f. Propagation of action potential along the muscle membrane and transmitted to T tubule.
   g. Release of calcium from cisternae.
   h. Binding of Ca^{++} to troponin which causes lateral displacement of tropomyosin and exposure of active sites on the actin filament resulting in the binding of myosin head to the actin filament.
   i. Sliding of thin filament over thick filament.
   j. Muscle contraction.

Q12. What are the conditions in which height of contraction is increased/decreased?

Ans. *Height of contraction is increased in*:
   a. Increasing strength of stimulus.
   b. Increased initial length of muscle.
   c. Increased temperature of surrounding of muscle.
   d. Increased length of wire.
   e. Lowering of inertia of lever.

   Height of contraction is decreased in all opposite of abovementioned conditions.

Q13. What is the role of ATP molecules in muscle relaxation?

Ans. After the power stroke of myosin head, it remains engaged with actin binding site. And on binding of ATP to myosin head, it immediately disengages from actin molecules, so ATP molecules are required for contraction as well as for relaxation.

OBSERVATIONS: EXERCISE FOR STUDENTS

....

....

....

....

5

Effect of Temperature on Simple Muscle Twitch

Aim: To study the effect of temperature on simple muscle twitch.

Material and Instrument: Same as for recording simple muscle twitch except that Lucas chamber is used in place of myograph board, thermometer and cold and warm amphibian Ringer solutions.

Method

1. Arrange nerve muscle preparation; remember Lucas chamber is used in place of myograph board. Fill the chamber with amphibian Ringer solution at room temperature and record the simple muscle twitch using maximal stimulus; as explained in earlier practical of simple muscle twitch. Note the temperature of the Ringer solution.
2. Drain off the Ringer solution and replace it with fresh hot Ringer solution having temperature of about 40°C. Now without changing the strength of stimulus and using the same baseline and point of stimulus, record another simple muscle twitch.
3. Repeat the whole procedure using cold Ringer solution having temperature of about 10°C.
4. Take the time tracing in the usual manner.

OBSERVATION AND RESULTS

On exposing nerve muscle preparation to warm surrounding, duration of latent period, contraction period and relaxation period is decreased and the height of contraction is increased. Warm Ringer solution raises the temperature of the muscle, hence reducing its inertia and the delays on neuromuscular junction are minimized. This is due to increase in enzymatic and metabolic processes, decrease in viscosity of muscle and increase in velocity of nerve conduction and transmission.

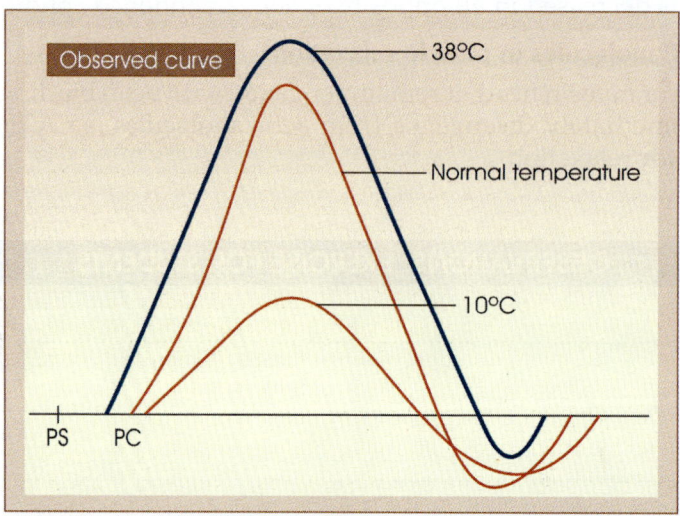

Fig. 5.1: Effect of temperature on simple muscle twitch

The effect of cold Ringer solution on muscle contractile response is exhibited as increase in latent period, contraction period and relaxation period and decrease in the amplitude of muscle contraction.

This is due to decrease in enzymatic and metabolic processes, increase in viscosity of muscle protein and decrease in velocity of nerve conduction and transmission.

PRECAUTIONS

1. For warm saline, the temperature must not go beyond 42°C because muscle proteins are denatured at higher temperature.
2. After taking normal simple muscle twitch record, effect of warm Ringer should be observed first and then record the effect of cold saline as with cold saline metabolic activity is depressed and recovery is delayed.
3. Every time ensure that point of stimulation should be same as that of normal recording.
4. For all recordings, strength of stimulus should be the same.
5. Wait for 2–3 minutes after pouring different temperature Ringer saline, then record the twitch.

QUESTIONS

Q1. What is the effect of high temperature on muscle twitch?

Q2. What is the effect of low temperature on muscle twitch?

Q3. What physiological changes occur at high and low temperature?

Ans. 1, 2 and 3—see text.

Q4. What is heat rigor?

Ans. Heat rigor is the development of permanent contraction of muscle if temperature of Ringer is increased beyond 45°C due to denaturation of muscle proteins.

Q5. Give the reason that effect of hot saline is demonstrated earlier than the effect of cold.

Ans. By cold saline, muscle is inactivated and it take much time to revive and sometime recovery is incomplete so effect of hot is seen earlier than the effect of cold is observed.

Q6. What is the effect of rise of temperature on velocity of contraction of muscle?

Ans. Rise of temperature causes increase in velocity of contraction because of decreased viscosity and increased force of contraction.

Q7. What is warm up and how does it provide benefit for performance of skeletal muscle?

Ans. A warm up is light aerobic exercise prior to the main activity. It includes mobilising exercises for the joints, some stretching exercises for the muscles and some easy rehearsal of the skills to follow.

The warm up will have benefits on the speed and strength of muscular contraction due to the increase in temperature of the muscles.

OBSERVATIONS: EXERCISE FOR STUDENTS

....

....

....

....

....

....

Velocity of Nerve Impulse

Aim: To find out the velocity of nerve impulse of sciatic nerve of frog.

Material and Instrument: Same as for recording simple muscle twitch.

RELATED THEORY

1. Conduction velocity of a nerve is defined as distance travelled by electrical impulse along a nerve fibre in a unit time. In frog, the value of nerve conduction of sciatic nerve is 40 meters/second. In amphibian experiments the conduction velocity is determined by stimulating nerve at two points, i.e. one at muscular end and another at vertebral end. Length of nerve fiber is measured and time taken by an impulse from one end of nerve to the other end of the nerve is taken as difference of latent periods of two simple muscle curves and nerve conduction is calculated as distance divided by time.

2. Various factors influence the nerve conduction like diameter and mylination of nerve fibre and temperature of the surrounding.

3. Nerve conduction in human being is done in patients of neurological disorders as a diagnostic tool in many clinical conditions where nerve conduction is decreased.

Method

1. Arrange nerve muscle preparation as done to record the simple muscle twitch using maximal stimulus muscle twitch.

2. Stimulate the sciatic nerve at the muscle end and take the recording as in the case of simple muscle twitch. Mark this graph as M graph.

3. On the same baseline keep the point of stimulus at the same position and stimulate the nerve by placing electrode at its vertebral end and take recording of simple muscle twitch.

4. Take the time tracing below the baseline by using tuning fork of frequency of 100 Hz. Now find the difference between latent periods of two simple muscle twitches which is the time taken by nerve impulse to travel from one end to the another end.

5. Measure the length of sciatic nerve and calculate the conduction velocity by using the following formula:

$$= \frac{\text{Distance travelled in centimeter}}{\text{Time taken by nerve impulse to travel from one end to the another end (sec)}}$$

6. Convert the results as metre per sec.

OBSERVATION AND RESULTS

1. On applying stimulus on muscle end of nerve latent period is shorter as compared to the vertebral end.

2. The difference of latent periods of two graphs is the time taken by a nerve impulse to travel from vertebral end to muscular end.

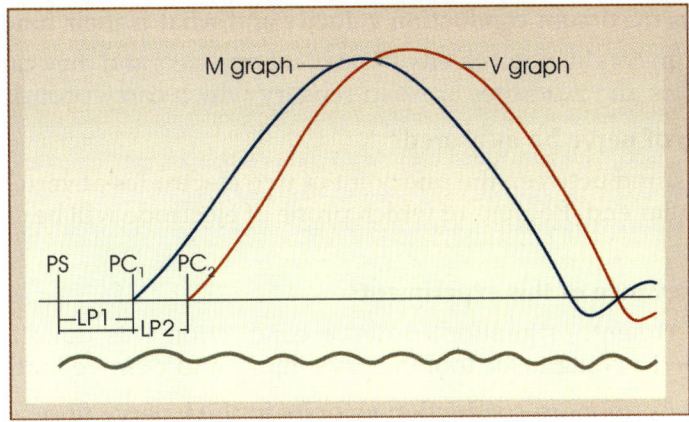

Fig. 6.1: Measurement of nerve conduction velocity

PRECAUTIONS

1. Point of stimulus and strength of stimulus should be the same.
2. While stimulating nerve at muscle and vertebral end the electrode should be on the extreme position.
3. Measure the difference of latent periods accurately.

QUESTIONS AND ANSWERS

Q1. Define the nerve impulse.

Ans. A wave of action potential which run along the nerve fibre is called nerve impulse.

Q2. Define the nerve conduction velocity.

Q3. How much is the nerve conduction of frog sciatic nerve?

Ans. Q2 and Q3: See text of related theory.

Q4. What are the factors on which impulse conduction along a nerve fibre depends?

Ans. *The various factors on which nerve conduction depends are:*
1. **Species difference:** The conduction velocity of nerve is different in different species. Frogs have lower conduction velocity as compared to the mammals.
2. **Types of fibers:** Mylinated fibers have fast nerve conduction as compared to non-mylinated fibres.
3. **Diameter of nerve fiber:** Nerve fibre having more diameter will have more nerve conduction than fibre having less diameter.
3. **Temperature:** Increase in the temperature of conducting media in which nerve is placed causes increase in nerve conduction.

Q5. How will you classify nerve fibre?

Ans.
a. Sensory and motor nerve fibre.
b. Medulated and non-medulated nerve fibre.
c. Erlanger and Gaser classification based on diameter and conduction velocity of fibres.

Fibre type		Diameter (μm)	Conduction velocity (metre/sec)	Function
	Aα	12–20	70–120	Proprioception and somatic motor
	Aβ	5–12	30–70	Touch and pressure
A	Aγ	3–6	15–30	Motor to muscle spindle
	Aδ	2–5	12–30	Pain, touch, and temperature
B fibre		< 3	3–15	Pre-ganglionic autonomic fibre
C fibre	I	0.4–1.2	0.5–2	Dorsal root pain touch temperature
	II	0.3–1.3	0.7–2.3	Post-ganglionic sympathetic fibre

Q6. Which type of fibre has maximum conduction velocity and what is their function?

Ans. Aα fibres have maximum conduction velocity (70–120 metres/sec) and they carry motor signals to extrafusal fibres of skeletal muscles and Aα fibres are also sensory which carry proprioception sensation.

Q7. How should the length of nerve be measured?

Ans. Length should be measured between the midpoint of two electrodes at vertebral end and midpoint of two electrodes at the muscular end. Because of which prone of electrode will be cathode or anode is not known to us.

Q8. What is the clinical relevance of this experiment?

Ans. Although in this experiment, estimation of nerve conduction was done in frog but in humans nerve conduction is performed as diagnostic tool in nerve injury and de-myelinating diseases.

Q9. Give physiological basis of more conduction velocity in thick nerve fibre as compared to thin fibre?

Ans. Thick fibres have less axoplasmic resistance as compared to thin fibre.

Q10. Enumerate the common clinical conditions in which nerve conduction is slower.

Ans.
a. Nerve injury
b. Diabetic neuropathy
c. Guillain-Barré syndrome
d. Alcoholic neuropathy
e. Toxic neuropathy.

OBSERVATIONS: EXERCISE FOR STUDENTS

7

Effects of
Two Successive Stimuli

Aim: To demonstrate the effects of two successive stimuli on skeletal muscle contraction.

Material and instrument: Same as for recording simple muscle twitch.

RELATED THEORY

1. Two successive stimuli (one after the other) are given at different intervals of time and the effect of second stimulus on muscle twitch is observed every time. The effect of second stimulus depends on time gap between first and second stimuli as it can be produced during latent period, contraction phase and relaxation phase of simple muscle twitch.

2. The refractory period in skeletal muscle is less than 0.005 second and it has two phases.

   a. Absolute refractory period: It is the period during which a second stimulus does not produce a response irrespective of the intensity of the stimulus.

   b. Relative refractory period: It is the time period during which if a second stimulus of stronger intensity is provided, it can produce a response. It corresponds with the second half of latent period.

3. Summation means a process of adding things together. Increase in the response of tissues on giving multiple stimuli as compared to the single stimuli is called summation. Summation is the property observed by nerve and muscle and other tissues.

4. In muscles, two types of summation is observed, i.e. summation of stimuli and summation of response.

5. Summation of stimuli: Single sub-minimal stimulus is not able to elicit any response but when multiple sub-minimal stimuli is given in quick succession, they give response due to summation of stimuli.

6. Summation of response: On applying two successive stimuli when response is of increased magnitude as compared to that of single stimulus, it is called summation of response. In this experiment, it is the summation of muscle contraction.

7. Beneficial effect: When two successive muscular activities are performed, the second muscular activity has better performance, it is called beneficial effect. (Actually, second activity is benefitted from the first muscular activity.) The second stimulus gets benefitted by the changes produced in the muscle due to the first stimulus.

The causes of this effect are:

a. Normally in a contraction phase, the Ca^{++} are released from the sarcoplasmic reticulum into the sarcoplasm and are rapidly transported back to sarcoplasmic reticulum during relaxation phase. But on applying second stimulus in quick succession, additional calcium ions are released and Ca^{++} of previous stimulus are not still transported back which causes availability of more Ca^{++} resulting in the prolonged active stage and increased force of contraction.

b. Increase in the temperature of muscle.

c. Decrease in the internal viscosity and resistance of the muscle.

d. Decrease in inertia of the recording system.

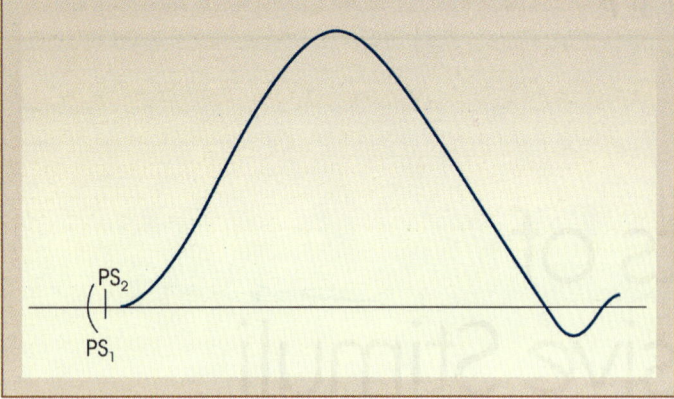

Fig. 7.1: Effect of second stimulus when induced during refractory period

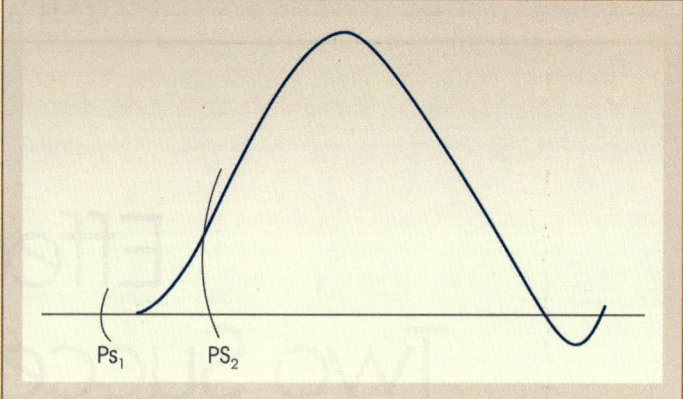

Fig. 7.2: Effect of second stimulus when induced during contraction phase

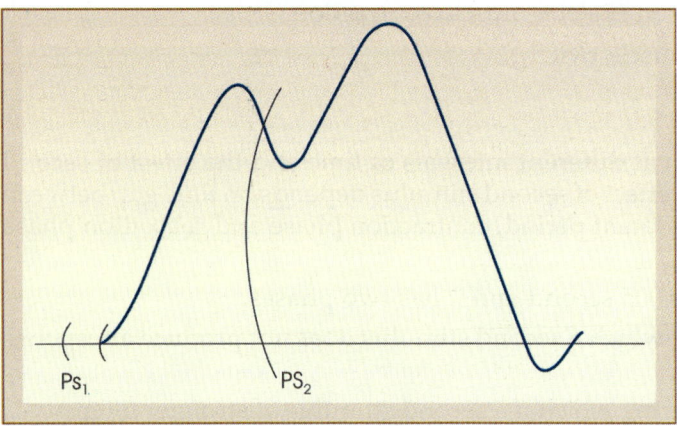

Fig. 7.3: Effect of second stimulus when induced during relaxation phase

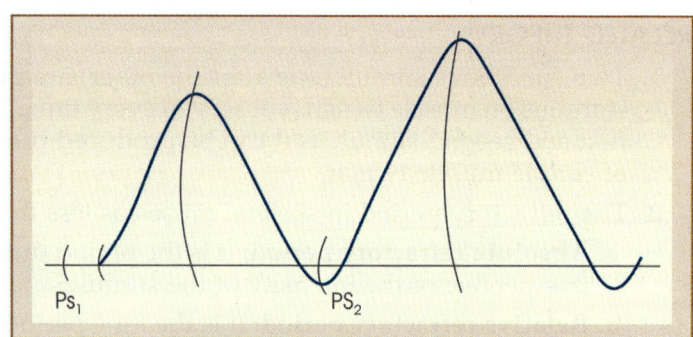

Fig. 7.4: Effect of second stimulus when induced after relaxation phase

METHOD

1. Arrange nerve muscle preparation and record the simple muscle twitch as explained in earlier practical of record of simple muscle curve.

2. The projecting strikers are separated slightly so that they strike the contact button in close succession. The distance between the strikers is so adjusted that a second stimulus should fall in the first half of the latent period of the simple muscle twitch of the first stimulus. The contraction is to be recorded using the same stimulus strength. The points of stimulation are to be marked.

3. The same procedure is repeated after progressively widening the distance between the strikers so as the second stimulus falls in the second half of the latent period, in the contraction period, in the relaxation period and lastly immediately after the relaxation period. Take the time tracing in the usual manner as explained in experiment of recording of simple muscle twitch.

OBSERVATION AND RESULTS

When two successive stimuli of maximal strength are induced to a skeletal muscle, the response to the second stimulus depends upon time gap when the second stimulus is given after the first stimulus.

1. If the second stimulus falls during the latent period of the muscle, the muscle is said to be completely refractory as there is no additional response. First half of latent period is absolute refractory period and second half of latent period is the relative refractory period.

2. If time of application of second stimulus falls during contraction, the height of contraction is increased.

3. If time of application of second stimulus falls during relaxation phase, second muscular response is observed.

4. When second stimulus falls after completion of relaxation phase of muscle twitch, a complete another muscle twitch having more height of contraction is obtained. The increase in the height of the second twitch is due to beneficial effect.

PRECAUTIONS

1. Maximal stimulus must be applied in this experiment.
2. Before recording the effect, check and mark the point of second stimulus.

QUESTIONS AND ANSWERS

Q1. What is refractory period?

Q2. How much is refractory period of skeletal muscle?

Q3. What is meant by summation of stimuli and summation of response?

Ans. 1,2,3 see the text of related theory.

Q4. In the graph, explain the response of second stimulus applied in different phases of muscle twitch.

Ans. See the text of observation and results.

Q5. What is beneficial effect and what are responsible factors for it?

Ans. See the text of related theory.

Q6. Which additional properties of skeletal muscles are elicited in this experiment as compared to SMT?

Ans. Refractory period and summation of response.

Q7. How will you ensure that second stimulus falls in the desired phase of muscle twitch?

Ans. After recording the simple muscle graph, open the two arms of striker, the arm which comes first in contact with electric contact block, mark it first and another second. Keep second arm in contact with electric contact block, the position of first arm will indicate the site of actual fall of second stimulus.

OBSERVATIONS: EXERCISE FOR STUDENTS

....

....

....

....

....

....

....

....

....

....

....

8

Genesis of Fatigue in the Isolated Nerve Muscle Preparation

Aim: To demonstrate the genesis of fatigue in the frog's nerve muscle preparation.

Material and instrument: Same as for recording simple muscle twitch.

RELATED THEORY

1. Fatigue is reduced or absence of response of the cell, tissue organ or body due to its excessive activity and can retain normal function after appropriate time gap (rest). Fatigue is the property of a skeletal muscle.
2. Initially, on repeated stimulation of nerve muscle preparation in quick succession, the progressive increase in force of contraction occurs due to the beneficial effect of the previous contraction.
3. Later on, the height of contraction is progressively decreased and latent period, contraction period and relaxation period is prolonged. Ultimately muscle stop giving response.
4. The causes of fatigue are depletion of acetylcholine, accumulation of metabolic waste products like lactic acid and decrease store of glycogen and creatine phosphate.
5. The synapse is the first site of fatigue in an intact animal. Neuromuscular junction is the site of fatigue in an isolated preparation. The fatigue is rapidly developed by increase of frequency of stimulation, increase in temperature or lack of O_2.

METHOD

1. Arrange nerve muscle preparation and record the simple muscle twitch as explained in earlier practical of recording of simple muscle twitch.
2. Record the first three simple muscle graphs and stop the kymograph and label the three curves.
3. Remove the writing lever from the drum and allow the kymograph to rotate and the muscle to contract.
4. Apply the writing lever to the drum and then record every 10th contraction till the muscle contractions cannot be recorded.
5. Take the time tracing below the simple muscle curves, close to the baseline.
6. Take record on another drum or on another place by directly stimulating the skeletal muscle. After gap of 10 minutes take record of SMT by stimulating the nerve.

OBSERVATIONS

1. When a muscle is repeatedly stimulated initially in the first few contractions, there is increase in amplitude due to beneficial effect and there is reduced latent period.
2. But when further stimulated, amplitude of contraction decreases along with increase in the latent period, contraction period and relaxation period. There is incomplete relaxation results in contraction remainder and finally the muscle does not respond to any further stimuli.
3. After the development of fatigue muscle shows contraction on giving direct stimulation to muscle which reflect that muscle is not fatigued.
4. After a gap of time, response of muscle is recovered even on stimulation of the nerve.

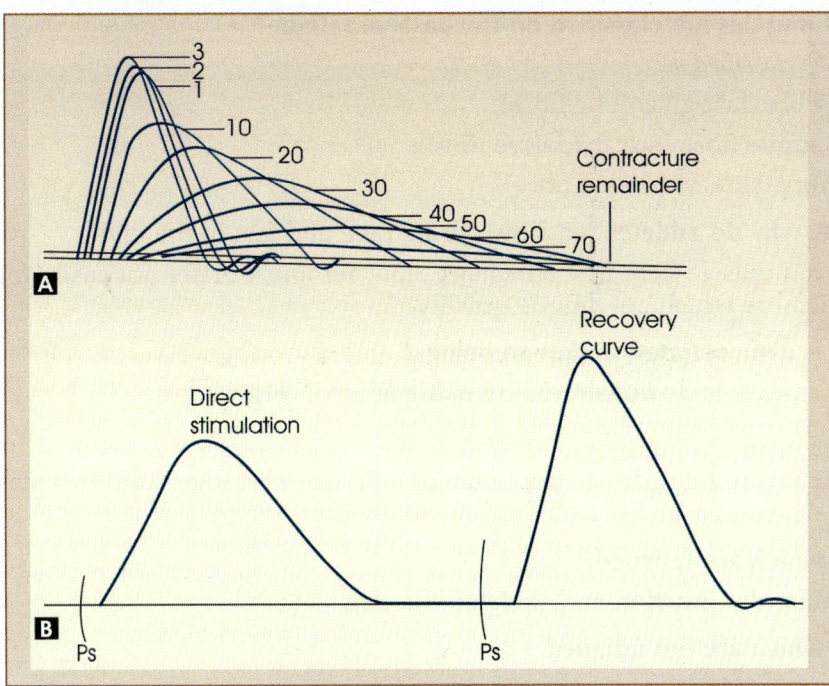

Fig. 8.1: Genesis of fatigue

QUESTIONS AND ANSWERS

Q1. What is fatigue?

Ans. Fatigue is defined as the inability of muscle to respond to a stimulus any further even after repeated stimulation.

Q2. What is the site of fatigue in this experiment?

Ans. Neuromuscular junction is the site of fatigue as muscle shows contraction on direct stimulation of muscle instead of nerve. Nerve is not the site of fatigue, can be demonstrated by the following method.

Make two nerve muscle preparations. Place one in muscle trough containing Ringer solution and another mount on myograph board and give continuous repeated stimulation till the fatigue is established. Now take fresh preparation place on myograph board in such a position that nerves of two preparations are crossed. On stimulation the nerve of fatigue preparation, the muscle of fresh preparation will show contraction that demonstrate that nerve is functioning and not fatigued.

Q3. What is the site of fatigue in intact muscles of human beings?

Ans. First sign of fatigue may be psychological as person can continue to work even if complaining of fatigue, if he compelled or motivated. Subsequently fatigue occurs due to exhaustion of fuel and accumulation of metabolites including lactic acids.

Q4. What is contraction remainder/physiological contracture and what is its cause?

Ans. When muscle is getting fatigued, it is not achieving completely relaxed state rather remain in partial contracted state which is known as *contraction remainder*. Since ATP molecules are required for detachment of myosin head from actin filament and for transporting Ca^{++} ions from the cytoplasm to back to sarcoplasmic reticulum during the relaxation phase. So decrease of ATP molecules and accumulation of metabolites are responsible for contraction remainder.

Q5. Which type of skeletal muscle fibres are easily fatigued?

Ans. The white muscle fibres are fast and easily fatigued.

Q6. How the skeletal muscles are classified on the basis of fatigue?

Ans. *Skeletal muscles are classified as:*

    a. Rapid fatigue fibre (fast glycolytic fibre).

    b. Intermediate fatigue fibre (fast oxidative fibre).

    c. Slow fatigue fibre (slow oxidative fibre).

Q7. In marathon race, why do athletes run slow during race and fast in the end?

Ans. The athlete uses red muscle fibre first which are slow aerobic, but are not easily fatigued. In the end, they use fast anaerobic fibre which get fatigue quickly.

Q8. How the fatigue is demonstrated in human beings?

Ans. In human being, fatigue is demonstrated by using Mosso's ergograph.

Q9. What is rigor?

Ans. The muscle is not able to relax due to depletion of ATP during fatigue and this state of partial contraction is called rigor.

Q10. Name the tissue which are fatigued.

Ans. Synapse, neuromuscular junction and skeletal muscles.

Q11. Name the tissue which are not fatigued.

Ans. Nerve and cardiac muscles.

OBSERVATIONS: EXERCISE FOR STUDENTS

Effect of Increasing the Strength of Stimulus

Aim: To study the effect of increasing strength of stimuli on skeletal muscle contraction.

Instruments and chemicals: Same as for the recording of simple muscle twitch.

RELATED THEORY

1. As already discussed in Chapters 1 and 2 that in labs, strength of stimuli is modified by changing the distance between the primary and secondary coil in Du Bois-Reymond induction coil. Depending on the degree of strength, stimulus can be sub-threshold, threshold, sub-maximal, maximal and supra-maximal.
2. Motor unit: A single nerve fibre supplying the number of muscle fibres constitute the motor unit.
3. On increasing the strength of stimulus, increased number of motor units are recruited and magnitude of response is heightened.

METHOD

1. Arrange the nerve muscle preparation as for recording a SMT except that the drum is not included and in its place an electromagnetic signal marker is included into the primary circuit in series.
2. The drum is placed in neutral gear and put in stationary position. The signal marker pointer is brought in conduct with the drum.
3. The primary key is kept closed and short circuiting key open. Move the secondary coil farthest away from the primary coil. Press tap-key briefly and then release it. The signal marker moves and marks the point of stimulus on the drum.
4. Rotate the drum manually so that the pointer moves about 1 cm on the drum. Then move the secondary coil near the primary coil by 1 cm at a time and press the tap-key and release it. At every point, test the response of the muscle to make and break shock separately.
5. Continue the experiment till further increase in the intensity of stimulus is not producing any increase in the height of the contraction.

PRECAUTIONS

1. At least 15 sec must elapse between make and break shocks to avoid beneficial effect.
2. Note the distance between primary and secondary coil after each make and break and label it simultaneously.

OBSERVATION AND RESULTS

1. On giving a stimulus of subminimal strength, there is no response.
2. When the strength of stimulus is increased to a threshold level, a response is produced.
3. Further progressive increase of strength of stimulus cause increase in the response of the muscle. The threshold of excitation of different motor neurons supplying a single skeletal muscle differs, therefore, with the increase in strength of stimulus, more and more motor units get recruited and thereby the height of contraction increases.
4. Response of break shock is higher than the make shock due to generation of stronger stimulus at break.
5. At specific strength of stimuli, all motor units are stimulated which is maximal stimulus.

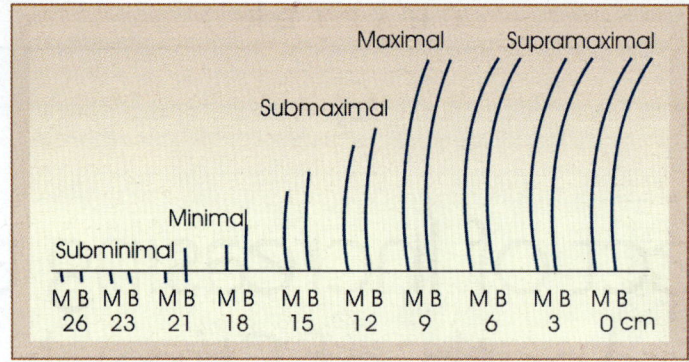

Fig. 9.1: Effect of increasing the strength of stimuli

6. Hereafter even if supra-maximal stimulus is applied no further increase in the response is observed because by then all the motor units have been activated.

QUESTIONS AND ANSWERS

Q1. **What are various types of stimuli depending on strength of stimuli?**

Q2. **What is meant by the term subthreshold, threshold, submaximal, maximal and supramaximal stimuli?**

Ans. 1 and 2: See Chapter 1 (Page 284).

Q3. **Explain the reason of generation of higher response at break shock than the make shock.**

Ans. Higher response at break is produced due to generation of stronger stimulus (induced current) due to rapid change in magnetic flux.

Q4. **What are the components of the motor unit?**

Ans. Alpha motor neuron, its axon and terminal branches and all muscle fibres supplied by it constitute the motor unit.

Q5. **What is the mechanism that cause increase in contraction on increasing the strength of stimulus?**

Ans. With the increase in the strength of stimuli, number of excited nerve fibres increases which ultimately causes contraction of more and more muscle fibres. In other words, with stronger stimulus, more motor units are recruited for muscular activity which causes increase in contraction.

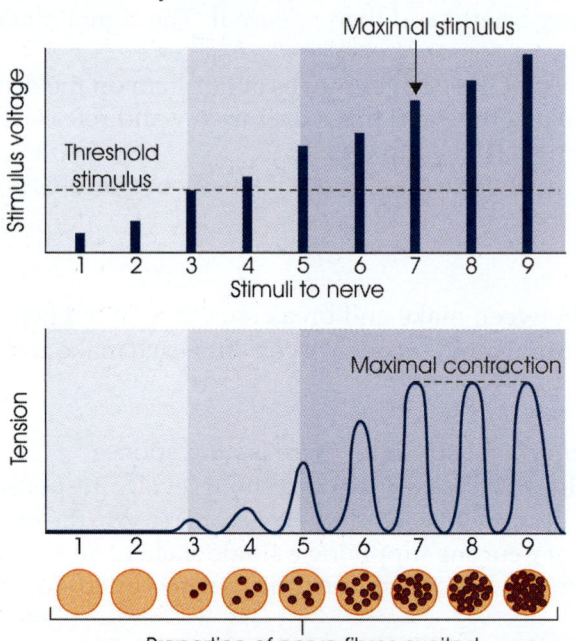

Fig. 9.2: Relation of strength of stimulation, recruitment of motor unit and height of contraction

Q6. What are various mechanisms for altering the force of contraction?

Ans.
1. By recruitment of motor units.
2. By altering the frequency of stimuli.
3. By changing initial length of skeletal muscle.

Q7. What is all or none law?

Ans. The strength by which a nerve or muscle fibre responds to a stimulus is independent of the strength of the stimulus. If that stimulus exceeds the threshold potential the nerve or muscle fibre will give a complete response otherwise there is no response.

Q8. Does motor units follow all-or-none law?

Ans. Yes, it follows all-or-none law.

Q9. Enumerate tissue or organ or physiological phenomenon which follows all-or-none law.

Ans. Skeletal muscle fibre, cardiac muscles as syncitium, nerve fibre, action potential and motor unit.

Q10. What is the physiological relevance of this experiment?

Ans. This experiment demonstrates the mechanism of applying different strength of muscular force for day-to-day life. For smaller muscular force, a few motor units and for large muscular force, many motor units are recruited.

OBSERVATIONS: EXERCISE FOR STUDENTS

....

....

....

....

....

....

....

....

....

....

....

....

....

....

....

....

10

Genesis of Tetanus

Aim: To demonstrate the effect of increasing frequency of stimuli on skeletal muscle contraction.

Instrument and chemicals: Same as for recording a simple muscle twitch, electromagnetic signal marker and vibrator variable interrupter.

RELATED THEORY

1. In previous chapters, effect of two successive stimuli have been studied and in the present section effects of multiple successive stimuli will be dealt. The effect of repeated multiple stimuli on the contractile response of a skeletal muscle depends on the number of stimuli (frequency of multiple stimuli). The response obtained will depend on whether next stimulus falls after the first twitch, in relaxation phase of first twitch, in the contraction phase or to second half of latent period of first twitch.

2. **Treppe or staircase phenomenon:** When multiple successive stimuli of lower frequency (5–10/sec) are given such that next stimuli appear at the completion of relaxation of previous response, the progressive increase of height of contraction is observed in subsequent contraction. This is called treppe/staircase phenomenon.

3. **Clonus:** When the frequency of multiple stimuli is such that next successive stimuli falls during mid relaxation phase of previous twitch then the succeeding contraction obtained will be superposed over the previous twitch due to incomplete summation of waves. This state is called clonus or sub-tetanus or incomplete tetanus. This occurs at a frequency of 20 vibration/sec. There is partial fusion of individual contractions due to incomplete relaxation and as a result curves do not touch baseline.

4. **Tetanus:** When the frequency of multiple successive stimuli is further increased so that each successive stimuli fall during contraction period of previous one. There is a smooth sustained contraction due to mechanical fusion of curves.

5. **Critical fusion frequency:** The minimum frequency of multiple stimuli, at which tetanus occurs is called critical fusion frequency. The critical fusion frequency usually depends on duration of contraction period and is inversely proportional to the contraction period. The conditions which increase the contraction period such as cold or fatigue will decrease the critical fusion frequency. At a frequency of 30 vib/sec complete fusion of contractions take place, thereby producing a smooth sustained contraction called tetanus.

METHOD

1. The nerve muscle preparation is arranged similar to that for recording a simple muscle twitch. Exclude the drum from the circuit and connect an electromagnetic signal marker and a variable interrupter into the primary circuit in series in the place of drum.

2. Adjust the induction coil so that it delivers a maximal stimulus.

3. Set the variable interrupter into operation adjusting the vibrating rod to give five stimuli per sec and start the drum at slow speed (12.5 mm/sec) and record 5–6 contractions on the drum.

4. Increase the frequency of stimuli progressively to 10 and 20 per sec and take a record of muscle response.

5. **Replace the variable interrupter from primary circuit with Neef's hammer and take the recording after adjusting the frequency of stimuli 30/sec, 40/sec and 50/sec or till the muscle tetanizes.**

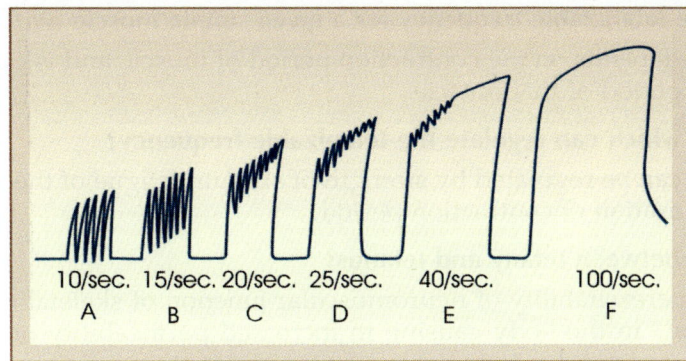

Fig.10.1: Genesis of tetanus

OBSERVATION AND RESULTS

1. When frequency of multiple stimuli is lower (5–10 vib/sec), successive stimuli falls at the completion of relaxation of previous twitch and each successive contraction has higher amplitude than the previous one (staircase phenomenon).
2. When frequency of multiple stimuli is more (15–20 vib/sec), successive stimuli falls in the relaxation phase of previous twitch. There is incomplete relaxation and baseline is not touched (incomplete tetanus/ clonus).
3. When frequency of multiple stimuli is further increased (30–50 vib/sec), successive stimuli falls in the contraction phase of previous twitch so that the individual responses fuse into one continuous contraction.

PRECAUTIONS

1. Exclude the drum from the primary circuit.
2. Avoid unnecessary stimulation.
3. Pour saline on preparation continuously to prevent drying.
4. Connect first variable interrupter and later Neef's hammer.

QUESTIONS AND ANSWERS

Q1. Define treppe, incomplete tetanus and tetanus.

Q2. What is the difference between incomplete and complete tetanus?

Ans. See text of related theory.

Q3. What is the beneficial effect?

Ans. On giving multiple successive stimuli just after relaxation of muscle each time, there is progressive increase in height of first 4–5 contractions. This is called beneficial effect as each contraction is benefitted from previous contraction and is the basis of staircase phenomenon. It occurs due to availability of more Ca^{++} from the previous contraction.

Q4. Justify that skeletal muscle is tetanised and cardiac muscle is not tetanised.

Ans. Skeletal muscle has refractory period of 5 to 10 ms which corresponds with the latent period and it can be excited during contraction period by successive stimuli and it shows sustained contraction. Heart muscles have long refractory period of 250 ms which correspond with contraction period and can be excited only after second half of diastole and hence cannot be tetanised.

Q5. Comment whether the summation of stimuli or summation of contraction is occurring in this experiment.

Ans. In this experiment, no summation of stimuli is taking place but summation of contraction is occurring. When a skeletal muscle is stimulated and a second stimulus is applied before the completion of relaxation, the second contraction having a greater tension develops and is fused to the first contraction.

Q6. What is tetanising frequency or fusion frequency?

Ans. See in text of related theory.

Q7. How will you calculate tetanizable frequency for a given simple muscle twitch?

Ans. Tetanizable frequency depends on the contraction period of muscle and is calculated by dividing the one second by contraction period of that muscle.

Q8. Enumerate the factors which can regulate the tetanizable frequency?

Ans. Tetanizable frequency can be regulated by strength of stimuli, fatigue of the muscle and temperature. All these factors modify duration of contraction period.

Q9. What is the difference between tetany and tetanus?

Ans. Tetany is a state of hyperexcitability of neuromuscular junction of skeletal muscles of extremities due to decrease in ionized Ca^{++} in the body causing in increased permeability of Na^+. Tetanus is a sustained contraction of skeletal muscles due to increased frequency of stimulation.

Q10. What is the difference between physiological tetanus and pathological tetanus?

Ans. Physiological tetanus is a sustained contraction of skeletal muscles due to increased frequency of stimulation. Pathological tetanus also shows sustained contraction of skeletal muscles which is caused by a toxin of bacteria *Clostridium tetani*.

Q11. What is the physiological relevance of this experiment?

Ans. *This experiment explains the following facts:*

    a. Incomplete tetanus type of contractions are occurring in maintaining the posture.

    b. For increasing the muscle force the CNS operates by two ways. One is recruitment of more motor units and another is by increasing the firing frequency which causes increase in muscle force.

    c. The three different conditions, pathological tetanus and physiological tetanus and tetany have almost similar mechanism of increasing the muscular contractions.

OBSERVATIONS: EXERCISE FOR STUDENTS

....

....

....

....

....

....

....

....

....

....

....

....

....

Effect of After Load and Free Load on Muscle Contraction and Calculation of Work Done

Aim: To demonstrate the effect of free load and after load on skeletal muscle contraction.

Material and instrument: Same as for recording simple muscle curve and weight of 10 gm, 20 gm, 30 gm, 40 gm, 50 gm, 60 gm.

RELATED THEORY

1. Two terms load and tension are used. Load is the force which is applied on the muscle by the weight of an object and tension is the force exerted by the contractile muscle on an object. Three types of muscle tension are active tension, passive tension and total tension.

2. Load can act in two situations—free load and after load. Free load is the force which is acting on muscle before the contraction has started. After load is the load applied on the muscle after the contraction has begun but not acting before contraction.

3. Frank-Starling law states that "within the physiological limits, the force of contractions is directly proportional to the initial length of muscle fibres. In free loaded condition, the initial length of muscle is increased and force of contraction is more.

4. The muscular activity can be calculated as work done during isotonic contraction.

5. Optimal load is that load at which work done is maximum. For load having magnitude less than optimal load, the initial length, force of contraction and work done is less. On increasing load more than optimal load, the work done is also less.

METHOD

The experiments can be done on rotating drum, but it is easy to perform on stationary drum.

After Loaded Condition

1. Arrange nerve muscle preparation and exclude the drum from the primary circuit. Record the simple muscle twitch as explained in the practical of effect of increasing strength of stimuli on skeletal muscle contraction.

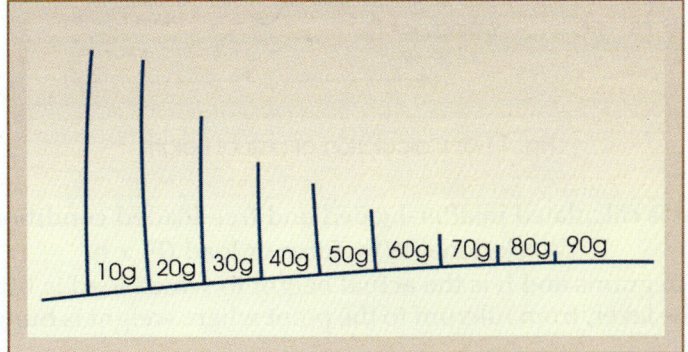

Fig. 11.1: After loaded condition

2. Adjust the screw of fulcrum in after load position so that it touches the vertical arm of the writing lever and hang weight of 10 gm and record simple muscle twitch.
3. Move the drum manually about 2 cm forward from recording and keep 20 gm of weight in place of now take recording.
4. Repeat the procedure by adding 10 gm of weight each time till the muscle is unable to lift the weight any more.

Free Load Condition

1. Arrange nerve muscle preparation and exclude the drum from the primary circuit. Record the simple muscle twitch as explained in the practical of effect of increasing strength of stimuli on skeletal muscle contraction.
2. For recording in free loaded condition, adjust the screw of fulcrum so that it does not touch the vertical arm of the writing lever and hang weight of 10 gm and record simple muscle twitch.
3. Move the drum manually about 2 cm forward from recording and keep 20 gm of weight in place of 10 gm, pointer will move downward and now take recording.
4. Repeat the procedure by adding 10 gm of weight each time till the muscle is unable to lift the weight any more.

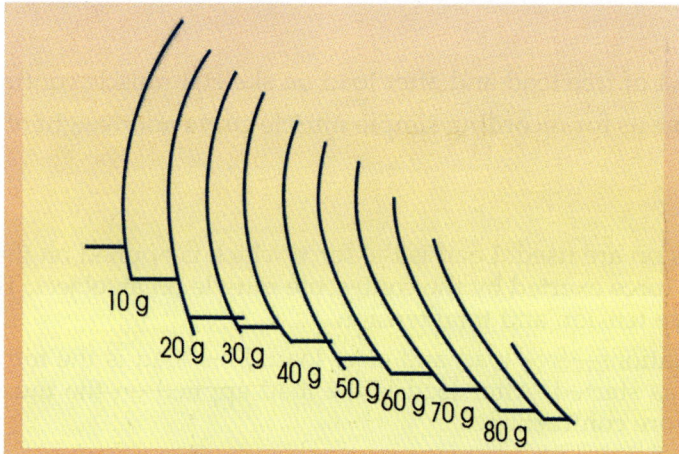

Fig. 11.2: Free loaded graph

Calculations of work done

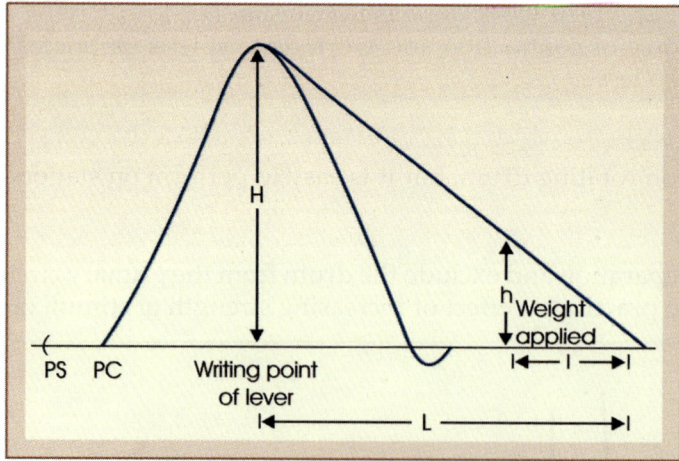

Fig. 11.3: Calculation of actual height

Work done for each weight is calculated in after-loaded and free-loaded condition of the muscle as follows:

$$\text{Work done (W) = force or load (F)} \times h$$

Where, F is the load lifted in grams and h is the actual height to which load is lifted (in cm) which is taken as $h = l/L \times H$, l is short arm of the lever, from fulcrum to the point where weight is hung and L is the long arm of the lever, from fulcrum to the stylus.

H is the height of contraction of curve for each weight. Multiply with 981 to express the result in ergs.

OBSERVATIONS

1. On progressive increase in the load, the amplitude of contraction decreases.
2. The contraction obtained for a given weight in pre-loaded or free-loaded condition is of higher amplitude than that obtained for the same weight in after load because in free load condition the initial length of the muscle is increased so there is increase in force of contraction. The Starling's law is applicable in this condition.

PRECAUTIONS

1. Label the each record simultaneously before changing the weight.
2. Strength of stimuli should be same for each recording.
3. If recording is done on moving drum, the point of stimulus should be kept same.

QUESTIONS AND ANSWERS

Q1. Define load and tension.

Q2. What is meant by free load and after load and optimum load?

Q3. What is Frank-Starling law?

Ans. 1, 2, and 3 see text of related theory.

Q4. What do you mean by active and passive tension?

Ans. Passive tension is the force exerted by the muscle on an object when muscle is resting state and active tension is the force acting on object during contraction of muscle.

Q5. Give examples of free-loaded and after-loaded condition of muscle.

Ans. **Examples of after-loaded conditions:** Lifting the weight from ground.
Examples of free load: Filling water from a tap by holding a bucket in the hand. Weightlifter allows the weight to stretch their muscle before they lift the weight.

Q6. What is the value of optimum load?

Ans. It is about 40% of the weight that is muscle is not able to lift.

Q7. What is the cause of more work done in free-loaded condition?

Ans. In free load, the force of contraction and work efficiency of muscle increase. In free load, the initial length of muscle increases to resting length which generates maximum force and by adding an elastic recoil force to the muscle during its contraction.

Q8. Enumerate various types of muscle lengths and define initial length.

Ans. Resting length, initial length, equilibrium length and optimum length. Initial length is the length of muscle just before it contracts and it is variable.

Q9. What are the shatters waves?

Ans. A few waves/oscillations are recorded after the completion of muscle twitch resulting from elasticity of muscles or jerking of lever on the stop screw due to its momentum are called shatters waves or physiological waves.

Q10. How will you ensure that simple muscle twitch have been recorded in free-loaded or after-loaded condition?

Ans. In after-load, the shatter waves appear mainly above the baseline but in free-load the waves appear below the baselines.

Q11. How much tension is developed during a complete tetanus?

Ans. During a complete tetanus, tension developed is about four times that developed by the individual twitch contraction.

Q12. What is the free and after load for cardiac muscle?

Ans. End diastolic volume is the free load and diastolic blood pressure is the after load for ventricle muscle.

Q13. Draw a flow chart of primary circuit in which drum is excluded.

Ans.

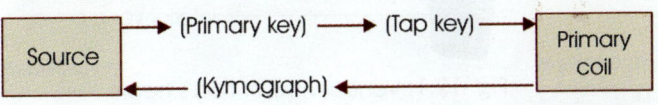

12

Recording of Normal Cardiogram

Aim: To record the normal beating of the heart of frog.

INSTRUMENTS AND CHEMICALS

Stunning rod, pithing needle, scissors, forceps, starling heart lever, thread, cotton, amphibian Ringer's solution, hook, myograph board with stand and kymograph with cylinder fitted with smoked paper.

Animal species: Frog.

RELATED THEORY

1. Frogs heart is composed of a sinus-venosus, right and left atrias (auricles), and a ventricle and truncus arteriosus. Sinus venosus is thin walled chamber which receives blood from three venae-cavae and transfer into the right atrium. The left atrium receives the blood from lungs by pulmonary vein. Both atria transfer the blood into ventricle.

2. The blood leaves the heart from the ventricle via a single truncus arteriosus which is short and branches further into two aortic arches and it loops left and right run dorsal to the heart to rejoin as a single aorta in the mid-dorsal region.

3. The excitation of the frog heart is myogenic as contraction of the heart originates within the muscle. In frog, the sinus venosus is an enlarged region between the vena cava and the right atrium and has pacemaker at the junction of sinus venosus and atrium in the form of white crescentic line. Cells of the pacemaker are termed leaky as sodium ions leak into the cells. Leaking of positive ions causes a slow depolarization to threshold, thus initiating an action potential that quickly spreads throughout the muscle producing muscular contraction.

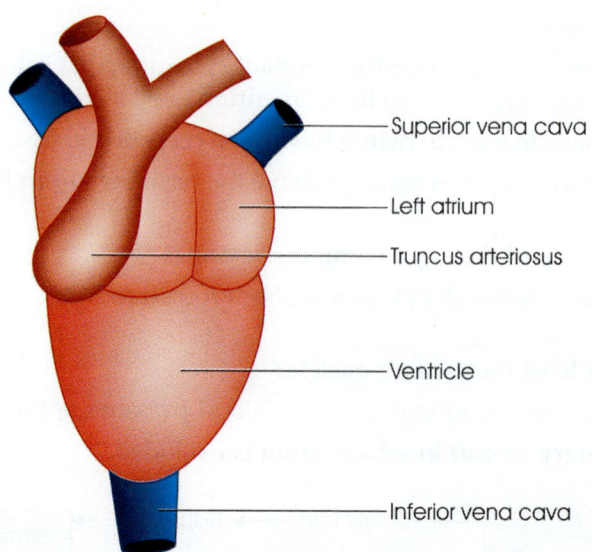

Superior vena cava

Left atrium

Truncus arteriosus

Ventricle

Inferior vena cava

Fig. 12.1: Ventral view of frog's heart

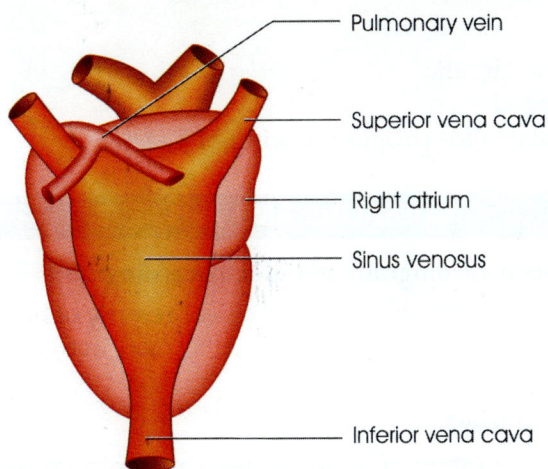

Fig. 12.2: Dorsal view of frog's heart

EXPOSURE OF THE HEART

1. Stun and pith a frog as done in nerve muscle preparation.
2. Place the frog on its dorsal surface as dissection is done on its ventral surface.
3. Give midline incision through skin of chest and abdomen. Now give bilateral horizontal incision through skin at the level of upper limb and middle of abdomen for proper exposure.
4. With the help of forceps, lift the xiphisternum and separate it from underlying tissue. Cut the intercostal cartilages and pectoral cartilage on both sides and remove the chest wall in one piece.
5. Heart will be seen as beating in the pericardial sac. Slit through the pericardium and remove it right up to base of the heart.
6. Examine the heart carefully and identify its various parts: One ventricle, two atria, truncus arteriosus, sinus venosus and superior and inferior venae cavae.
7. During systole, sinus venosus contracts first followed by the auricles, then single ventricle and lastly bulbous arteriosus.
8. Mount the frog on the myograph board. Place the preparation near the recording drum of kymograph.
9. Attach the starling heart lever on the vertical rod of the myograph stand at the height slightly above the heart. Gasp the apex of the ventricle using a blunt forcep and gently penetrate the point of the 'J'-shaped hook into the apex of the ventricle. Adjust the tension of thread with the help of supporting arm of liver to keep the recording liver horizontal in contact with the drum.
10. Move the drum in low speed of 2.5 mm/sec and take recording of contracting heart.

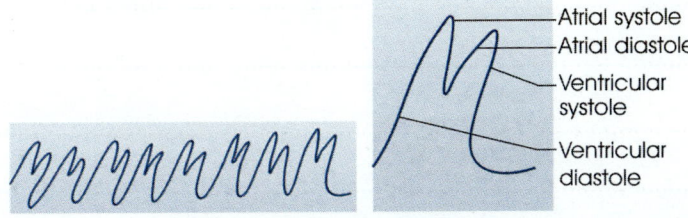

Fig. 12.3: Normal cardiogram

OBSERVATIONS

1. The rhythm of the heart is noted and the heart rate is calculated. Frogs heart rate remains in the range of 30 to 50 beats per minute depending on the physiological and environmental condition.
2. The down stroke is contraction and upstroke is the relaxation of heart.
3. In usual course, two waves of atrial and ventricle systole are recorded. Smaller down stroke is atrial systole and smaller upstroke is atrial diastole. Longer downstroke and upstroke is due to ventricle systole and diastole respectively.
4. Ventricular systole has more force of contraction than atria due to larger size of ventricular chamber.

PRECAUTIONS

1. Do not include the drum in the circuit.
2. Let the drum move at slow speed.
3. Pour the Ringer solution regularly for proper working of heart.

QUESTIONS AND ANSWERS

Q1. What is the difference between cardiogram and electrocardiogram?

Ans. Cardiogram is the graphical representation of mechanical activity of heart, i.e. systole and diastole, whereas electrocardiogram is graphical representation of electrical activity of heart, i.e. depolarization and repolarization.

Q2. How much is the heart rate of frog?

Ans. Frogs heart rate remains in the range of 30 to 50 beats per minute depending on the physiological and environmental condition.

Q3. What are the components of normal cardiogram?

Ans. Normally two waves of atrial systole and diastole and ventricle systole and diastole is seen, but waves of sinus venosus can also be recorded and three waves can be observed.

Q4. Name the tissue (part of heart) which act as pacemaker in the heart of frog.

Ans. The white crescentic line of sinus venosus is acting as pacemaker.

Q5. Name the properties of cardiac muscle which can be demonstrated in frog heart.

Ans. The properties such as excitability, automaticity, rhythmicity, conductivity, contractility, staircase phenomenon, refractoriness and all-or-none law are studied in frog heart.

Q6. What is the nerve supply of heart?

Ans. Sympathetic nerve supply is from cervicothoracic sympathetic chain.
Parasympathetic nerve supply is from vagus nerve.

Q7. What do you mean by vagal tone?

Ans. Both sympathetic and parasympathetic nerves innervate the heart but in basal conditions parasympathetic tone for heart is more than sympathetic tone which is called vagal tone.

OBSERVATIONS: EXERCISE FOR STUDENTS

....

....

....

....

....

....

....

....

....

13

Effect of Temperature on Frog's Heart

Aim: To demonstrate the effect of hot and cold saline on frog's heart.

INSTRUMENTS AND CHEMICALS

Same as in Chapter 12, thermometer, hot and cold saline.

METHOD

1. Expose the heart and take recording of normal cardiogram as done in Chapter 12. Take the time tracing with electromagnetic signal marker.
2. Pour warm Ringer solution having temperature 40°C on the heart with the help of dropper or cotton and record the effect for 5–7 contractions.
3. Stop the drum and pour normal saline and wait for some time so that normal rhythm is recovered.
4. Adjust the writing pointer again and ensure it touches the drum surface lightly.
5. Pour cold Ringer solution having temperature 10°C on the heart with the help of dropper or cotton and record the effect for 5–7 contractions.
6. 5-second time tracing below the graph is recorded.
7. Label the point position where hot and cold Ringer was applied. Calculate the heart rate at varied temperatures and note your results.

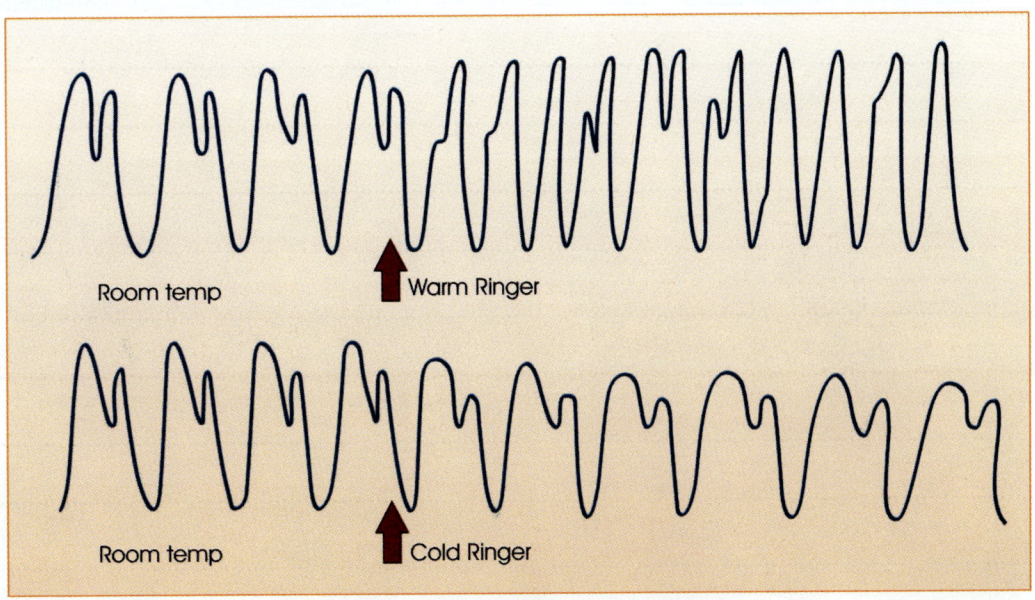

Fig. 13.1: Effect of hot and cold saline

OBSERVATIONS

1. On pouring of hot Ringer solution, pacemaker cells generate more cardiac impulses per unit time, thereby increasing the heart rate.
2. The increased metabolic activity in the cells of the atria and ventricle further increases the force of contraction.
3. The cold has the reversal effects due to decrease in the metabolic activity decreasing heart rate and force of contraction.

PRECAUTIONS

1. Same as in recording of normal cardiogram.
2. Do not use Ringer solution of more than 45°C.

QUESTIONS AND ANSWERS

Q1. What is the effect of warm saline on cardiogram of frog heart?

Ans. Warm saline acts on pacemaker cells in sinus-venosus and causes increase in heart rate and increase in force of contraction by directly acting on myocardium.

Q2. What is the effect of cold saline on cardiogram of frog heart?

Ans. Cold saline causes decrease in heart rate by influencing pacemaker cells and decrease in force of contraction by directly acting on myocardium.

Q3. What are the functional alteration caused by warm and cold saline?

Ans. Warm temperature increases the permeability of the cardiac muscle membrane to ions that controls heart rate resulting in acceleration of the self-excitation process. High temperature enhances the metabolic rate of ventricle muscles and causes increase in force of contraction. Cold produces opposite changes.

Q4. What is clinical relevance of this experiment?

Ans. This experiment demonstrates that alteration of temperature influences the activity of heart, e.g. exercise, fever and hypothermia.

Q5. Name conditions other than fever where heart rate and force of contraction are increased.

Ans. Anxiety, exercise, change in posture from lying down to standing, hypoxia, during inspiration and direct stimulation of sympathetic nerves.

OBSERVATIONS: EXERCISE FOR STUDENTS

....
....
....
....
....
....
....
....
....
....

14

Properties of Cardiac Muscle

Aim: To demonstrate the various properties of cardiac muscles.

INTRODUCTION

Cardiac muscle has various properties, i.e. automaticity, rhythmicity, excitability, conductivity, contractility, long refractory period, extrasystole and compensatory pause, all or none phenomenon, staircase phenomenon. Some of them were already demonstrated in previous chapters, extra systole and compensatory pause and stannius ligatures will be discussed in this chapter and the properties which are demonstrated on quiescent heart will be dealt in the next chapter.

EXTRASYSTOLE AND COMPENSATORY PAUSE

Instruments and chemicals: Same as in Chapter 12.

RELATED THEORY

1. Extra systole is the contraction of the heart prior to the time that normal contraction would have been expected. Normally the ventricle muscle contracts in response to impulse coming from pacemaker but if impulse come from some ectopic focus before the impulse reaches from the SA node the ventricle contracts in response to nonpacemaker stimuli.
2. Compensatory pause is the time gap during which the ventricle does not show any response to the impulse coming from SA node but remain silent due to refractory period of ventricle muscles.
3. Cardiac muscles have long refractory period. The normal refractory period of ventricle muscles is 250 msec and atrial muscles are 150 msec. So ventricle muscles do not respond to any stimulus during systole and early part of diastole.

METHOD

1. Expose the heart and take recording of normal cardiogram as done in previous chapters.
2. Apply wire electrodes 1 around auriculoventricular groove and other to the hooked pin passing through the apex of the heart.
3. Keep signal marker in the primary circuit.
4. Now stimulate the ventricles at different phases of the cardiac cycle, i.e. during systole and early and late diastole.

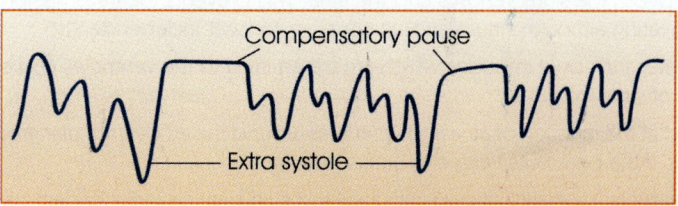

Fig. 14.1: Extra systole and compensatory pause

OBSERVATIONS

1. When artificial stimulus is given in systole and early part of diastole, the ventricle muscle does not respond due to refractory period.
2. When stimulus is given in late part of diastole, the ventricle muscle contracts and show extra systole.
3. Extra systole is followed by compensatory pause.

PRECAUTIONS

Same as in normal cardiogram.

QUESTIONS AND ANSWERS

Q1. What do you mean by extrasystole and compensatory pause?

Q2. What is the mechanism of compensatory pause?

Q3. Define refractory period.

Q4. How much is the refractory period of atrial and ventricle muscles?

Ans. 1, 2, 3 and 4 see text of related theory.

Q5. How much is the absolute and relative refractive period of ventricle muscles?

Ans. Absolute refractive period of ventricle is 200 msec and relative refractory period of ventricle is 50 msec.

Q6. Is there any benefit from the long refractory period of cardiac muscle?

Ans. Yes, the long refractory period of cardiac muscle prevents the cardiac muscle to get tetanized.

Q7. Enlist predisposing factor for extrasystole in human beings.

Ans. *The predisposing factors are*:
  - Caffeine, tobacco, alcohol and illicit drugs.
  - High blood pressure (hypertension).
  - Anxiety.
  - Heart disease, including congenital heart disease, coronary artery disease, heart attack, heart failure and a weakened heart muscle (cardiomyopathy).
  - Hyperthyroidism.

Q8. Can extra systole occur in persons without any cardiac disease?

Ans. Yes, they can be seen with certain predisposing factors and 2–4 extra systole/min are regarded as normal.

HEART BLOCK: STANNIUS LIGATURE

Instruments and chemicals: Same as in Chapter 12 and cotton thread.

RELATED THEORY

1. Heart block: When the impulse generated by the pacemaker is not transmitted to atrial or ventricular muscle, the heart is said to have heart block.
2. Stannius ligature: The transmission of an impulse can be blocked in frog heart by applying mechanical pressure by tying threads knots at various sites which is called stannius ligatures. These are of two types: 1st and 2nd stannius ligature
3. The 1st stannius ligature is tied between the sinus venosus and the atria. This prevents the transmission of an impulse from sinus venosus to atria. So atria and ventricle stop beating although sinus venosus continue to beat independently.

   After some time, the atrium generates their own impulses which are transmitted to the ventricles and atrium and ventricles start beating at a rate which is slower than the rate of sinus venosus.
4. Second stannius ligature is applied at the junction of atria and ventricles around the atrioventricular groove. By this ligature the impulse is not transmitted from atria to ventricles. Atria beat buts ventricles stops beating.

   After a short interval of time the ventricle generates its own impulses and start beating independent of atria at a much slower rate and this is referred to as idio-ventricular rhythm.

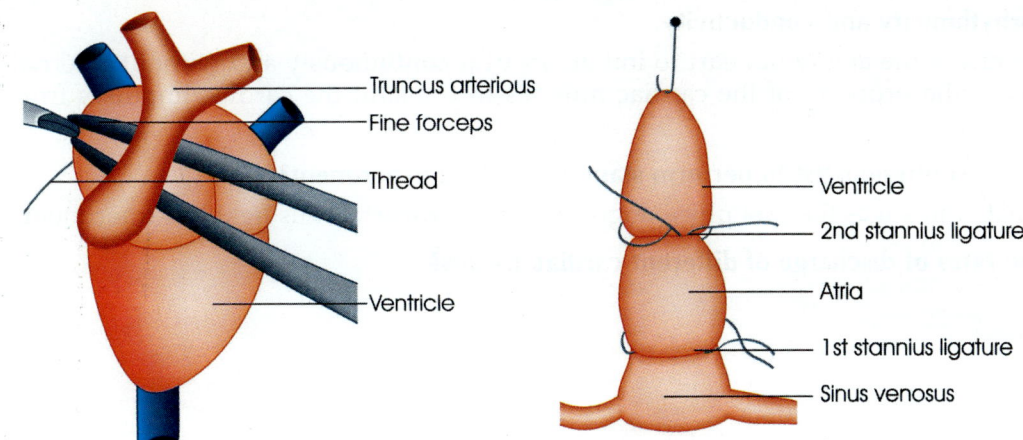

Fig. 14.2: Making a loop for 1st stannius ligature   Fig. 14.3: Site of stannius ligature

METHODS

1. Expose the heart as done previously.
2. Pass a thread with a help of fine forceps behind the truncus-arteriosus and make a loop posteriorly at white crescentic line.
3. Arrange the frog in the same way as in normal cardiogram and record the normal cardiogram on a slow moving drum.
4. Tie the knot to the loop of the thread passed around the white crescentric line. This is 1st stannius ligature. Heart will stop beating.
5. After a short interval of time, heart will start to beat again because of atrial rhythm.
6. Apply the 2nd stannius ligature at the auriculo-ventricular groove with thread.
7. Atrium continue to beat but ventricle stops beating again for some time and restart beating with very slow rate (idio-ventricular rhythm). Now auricles and ventricles have different rhythm.

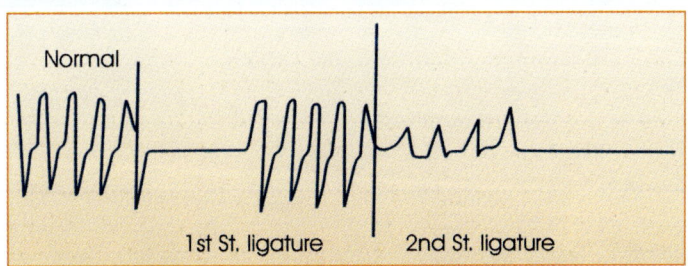

Fig. 14.4: 1st and 2nd stannius ligature

OBSERVATIONS

1. The conductivity of impulse from pacemaker to ventricular myocardium can be blocked at different levels.
2. Pacemaker, atrium and ventricular muscle have ability to generate impulses called self-excitation. But their rate of generation of impulses is different.
3. After applying 1st ligature heart stops beating and then restart with slow atrium rhythum.
4. After applying 2nd ligature atrium continue to beat but ventricle stop beating.

QUESTIONS AND ANSWERS

Q1. Define heart block.

Q2. What is stannius ligature?

Q3. What is idio-ventricular rhythm?

Ans. 1, 2 and 3 see text of related theory.

Q4. Name the properties which are demonstrated on applying the stannius ligature.

Ans. Conductivity and autorhythmicity.

Q5. Define autorhythmicity and conductivity.

Ans. Autorhythmicity is the ability of heart to initiate its beat continuously and without external stimulation. Conductivity is the property of the cardiac muscles to transmit the cardiac impulses from one part to another.

Q6. Who was the first physiologist to perform stannius ligature experiment?

Ans. Hermann F. Stannius was the first physiologist who performs stannius ligature experiment.

Q7. What are the rates of discharge of different cardiac tissues?

Ans.

Pacemaker tissue	Rate of discharge
SA node	60–100
AV node	40–60
Bundle of His	25–40
Purkinje fibre	25–40
Ventricle muscle	15–30

Q8. What are the types of heart block?

Ans. SA nodal heart block, AV nodal block and bundle branch block.

Q9. What is the significance of conducting stannius ligature experiment?

Ans. Stannius ligature experiment demonstrates the effects of heart block and property of automaticity and their hierarchy in the frog's heart.

OBSERVATIONS: EXERCISE FOR STUDENTS

....

....

....

....

....

....

....

....

....

....

....

....

....

15

Properties of
Cardiac Muscle II

Aim: To demonstrate the all or none phenomenon, staircase phenomenon, summation of subminimal stimuli in cardiac muscles.

INTRODUCTION

These properties are elicited on the quiescent heart and the pattern of giving stimulus is specific in each phenomenon.

> **Note:** The readers have to differentiate between the types of stimulus to elicit these properties.

Instruments and chemicals: Same as in Chapter 13.

ALL OR NONE PHENOMENON

Related Theory

1. **All-or-none phenomenon:** It expresses relation between response and stimulus. This law states that "the magnitude of response of a tissue to stimuli remains same irrespective of the strength of stimuli".
   If that stimulus exceeds the threshold potential, the nerve or muscle fibre will give a complete response; otherwise, there is no response.
2. This property is found in nerve, skeletal muscle and cardiac muscle.

Method

1. Expose the heart and apply 1st stannius ligature to make the heart silent.
2. Arrange the connection and apparatus as done in normal cardiogram.
3. Give sub-threshold stimulus to the ventricle and then increase the strength of the stimulus till a contraction appears and record it and label it as threshold stimulus.
4. Give progressive enhanced strength of the stimulus after each 30 seconds regularly and take records every time.

OBSERVATION

Height of the contraction remains the same in spite of enhancing the strength of the stimulus which means that there is no relation between strength of stimulus and height of contraction.

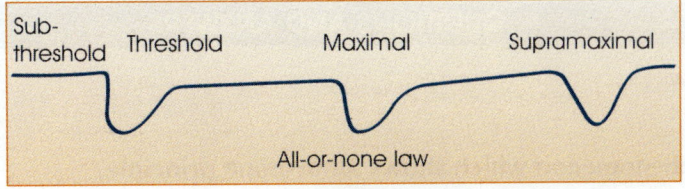

Fig. 15.1: All-or-none principle

Precautions: The stimulus should be given in quiescent heart.

STAIRCASE PHENOMENON

Related Theory

1. If a quiescent ventricle is stimulated repeatedly such that the interval between consecutive stimuli is less than 10 s, the first 4–5 contractions are of successive increased magnitude.
2. Progressive increase of force of contraction is due to the beneficial effect of previous contraction.

METHOD

1. Expose the heart and apply the 1st stannius ligature to make the heart silent.
2. Arrange the connection and apparatus as done in normal cardiogram.
3. Adjust the position of secondary coil for getting a single effective stimulus (supra-threshold stimulus)
4. Stimulate the ventricles repeatedly so that fresh contraction appears immediately after previous relaxation is over.

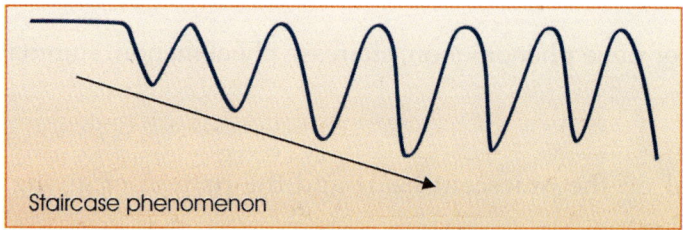

Staircase phenomenon

Fig. 15.2: Staircase phenomenon

OBSERVATION

On giving multiple suprathreshold stimulus to a quiescent heart there is a progressive increase in the height of a few initial contractions.

SUMMATION OF SUBLIMINAL STIMULI

When subthreshold stimuli is applied to the quiescent heart repeatedly at the interval of half to one second, the cardiac muscle shows contraction.

METHOD

1. Adjust the distance between the primary and the secondary coil to produce subminimal stimulus. Give one stimulus. This will not produce any response.
2. Now, give repeated sub-minimal stimuli in quick succession and finally the ventricle shows response.

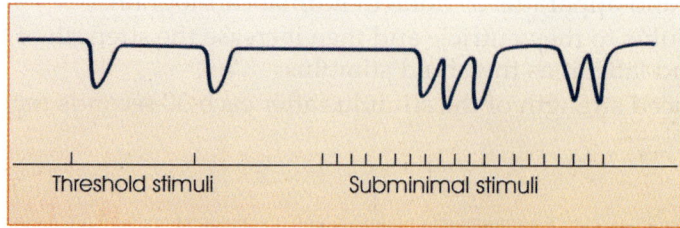

Threshold stimuli   Subminimal stimuli

Fig. 15.3: Summation of stimuli

QUESTIONS AND ANSWERS

Q1. Define all-or-none law.

Ans. See text.

Q2. Name the tissues or phenomenon which shows all-or-none principle.

Ans. Nerve, skeletal muscle, motor unit and cardiac muscle.

Q3. What is the cause for all-or-none law in cardiac muscle?

Ans. Cardiac muscle fibre acts as a functional syncytium due to low resistance gap junctions among the myocardial fibre.

Q4. What is the difference between skeletal muscles and cardiac muscles with respect to all-or-none law?

Ans. In skeletal muscles the all-or-none phenomena is applicable to single muscle fibre or single motor unit. In cardiac muscle it is applicable to syncytium.

Q5. Define staircase phenomenon and summation of stimuli.

Ans. See the above text.

Q6. What is the mechanism of staircase phenomenon?

Ans. Initial contractions are benefitted by each previous contraction. The amount of Ca^{++} ions released during each contraction is not completely pumped back into sarcoplasmic reticulum. First few contractions cause rise of temperature which decreases the viscosity of sarcoplasm and increases the metabolic activity.

Q7. What type of stimulus is given to elicit the all-or-none law, staircase phenomenon summation of stimuli?

Ans.

	All-or-none law	*Staircase phenomenon*	*Summation of stimuli*
Strength of stimulus	Different strength of stimulus is given	Suprathreshold stimulus is given	Subthreshold stimulus is given
Type of stimulus	Single stimulus of specific strength at one instance	Multiple stimuli	Multiple stimuli

OBSERVATIONS: EXERCISE FOR STUDENTS

....

....

....

....

....

....

....

....

....

....

....

....

....

....

16

Effects of Various Drugs on the Frog Heart Muscle

INSTRUMENTS AND CHEMICALS

Same as in Chapter 12 and drugs: Adrenaline, acetylcholine and atropine

RELATED THEORY

Adrenaline: Adrenaline is a sympatho-mimetic drug and has direct effect over the cardiac muscle cells. It acts on β_1 receptors and increases cardiac muscle cells permeability to Ca^{2+} and Na^+ ions. The Na^+ and Ca^{2+} influx increases in the pacemaker cells, thereby increasing the slope of the pacemaker potential and thus they reach the firing level and increase the heart rate. The increased influx of Ca^{2+} in the working cardiac muscle cells increases the force of contraction.

Acetylcholine (ACh): It acts on the pacemaker cells and increases their permeability to potassium ions and more of these potassium ions move out.

This causes hyper-polarization and decreases the slope of the pacemaker potential, thereby decreasing the heart rate. ACh increases the permeability of cardiac muscle cells to K^+ ions. The K^+ ions efflux outward shortening phase 2 of AP. This decreases the Ca^{2+} influx and decreases the force of contraction.

Atropine: It blocks the action of acetylcholine by adhering itself over the membrane receptors of cardiac muscle cells. The application of atropine on the heart after acetylcholine does not produce any effect but when applied before pouring acetylcholine, the atropine is blocking the inhibitory action of acetylcholine.

METHOD

1. Expose the heart and take recording of normal cardiogram as done in Chapter 12. Record the normal cardiogram with time tracing.

2. Stop the kymograph drum. A few drops of 1 in 10,000 solution of adrenaline is to be poured on the heart. There is increased heart rate and the force of contraction, record these tracings. The drum is stopped and fresh Ringer solution is poured. Record the normal cardiogram after the effect of adrenaline fades over.

3. Pour a few drops of 1 in 100,000 solution of acetylcholine over frog heart preparation. There is decreased heart rate and the force of contraction, record these tracing.

4. Then apply 0.5% atropine solution over frog heart preparation. The heart remains inhibited.

5. The drum is stopped and fresh Ringer is poured and it is washed.

6. Apply 0.5% atropine solution over frog heart preparation, then pour a few drops of 1 in 100,000 solution of acetylcholine over frog heart preparation and observed the effect of acetylcholine after applying atropine solution on the heart. The heart is not inhibited this time.

7. Remove the recording paper from drum and label the graph appropriately.

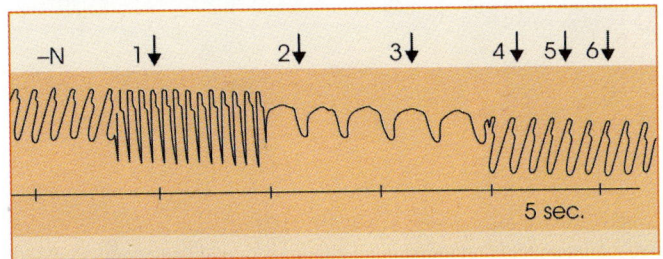

Fig. 16.1: Effect of drugs on heart of frog, N: Normal cardiogram; 1: Effect of adrenaline; 2: Effect of acetylcholine; 3: Effect of atropine; 4: Normal cardiogram; 5: Effect of atropine; 6: Effect of acetylcholine

OBSERVATIONS

1. Adreaniline increases heart rate as well as force of contraction.
2. Acetylcholine causes decrease of both heart rate and force of contraction.
3. Atropine blocks the action of acetylcholine.

QUESTIONS AND ANSWERS

Q1. What do you mean by the term chronotropic effect, ionotropic effect, bathmotropic and dromotropic effect?

Ans.
1. Chronotropic effect is related with change in the heart rate.
2. Inotropic effect is related with force of contraction.
3. Bathmotropic effect refers to modifying the degree of excitability specifically of the heart.
4. Dromotropic effect is related with the conduction speed.

Q2. Define the term Drug.

Ans. Drug is chemical substance that causes a change in an organism's physiology or psychology when consumed.

Q3. What are the effects of adrenaline, acetylcholine and atropine?

Ans. See the text.

OBSERVATIONS: EXERCISE FOR STUDENTS

....

....

....

....

....

....

....

....

....

....

Spotters 1
Amphibian Experiments

Q1. Identify the following spot and write its use in amphibian experiments.

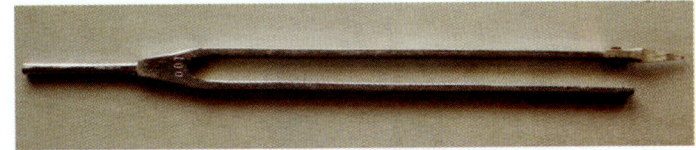

Ans. Tuning fork and used for recording time tracing in amphibian experiments.

Q2. Identify the following spot and write its use.

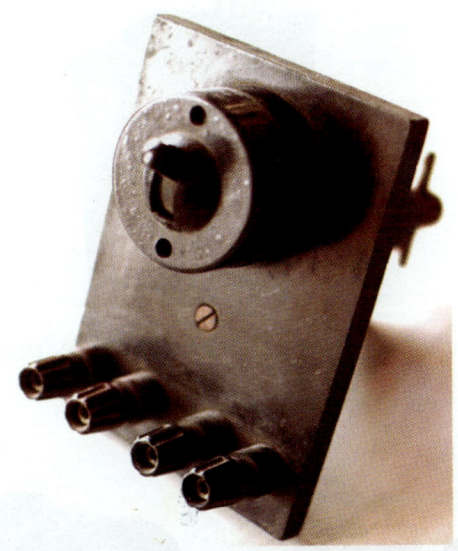

Ans. Short circuiting key and used for make and break of secondary circuit.

Q3. Identify the following spot and write its use.

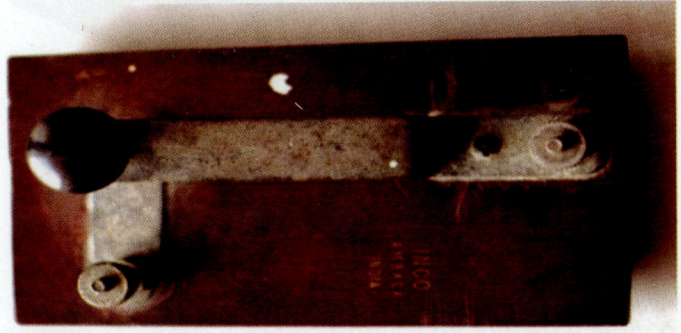

Ans. Tap key which is used to make and break of the circuit.

Q4. Identify the following spot and write its use.

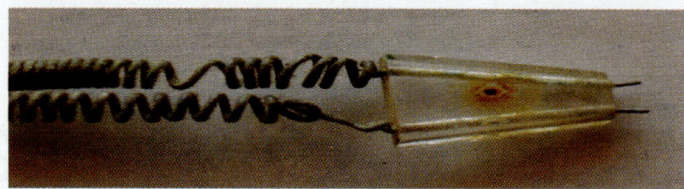

Ans. Stimulating electrode which is used for giving electrical stimulus to the tissues.

Q5. Identify the following spot and write its use.

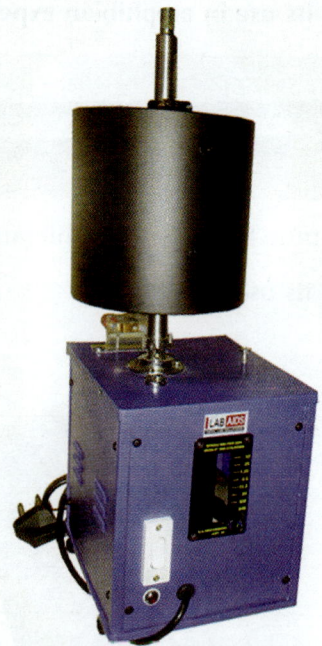

Ans. Kymograph and is used for recording the movement of tissue/organ on recording drum.

Q6. Identify the instrument shown below and write its use.

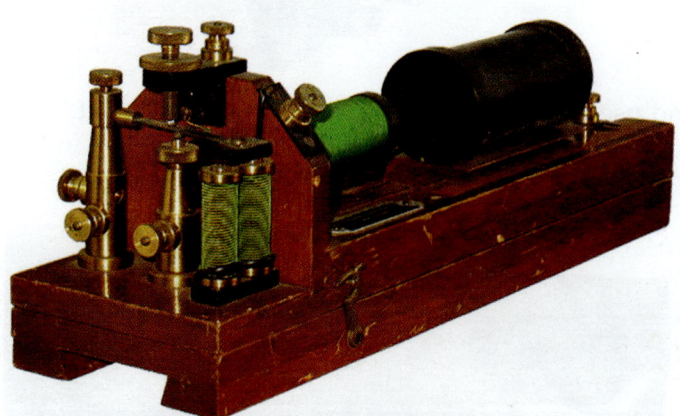

Ans. Du Bois-Reymond induction coil: It is used to convert the available low voltage, high ampere, direct (continuous current) into induced current of short duration. It is made up of primary and the secondary coils having insulated copper wire wound round a soft iron core. The primary coil terminals are connected to the DC source; and the secondary coil terminals are connected to the electrodes.

Q7a. Identify the following spot and write its use.

Q7b. Identify the following spot and write down the principle on which it works.

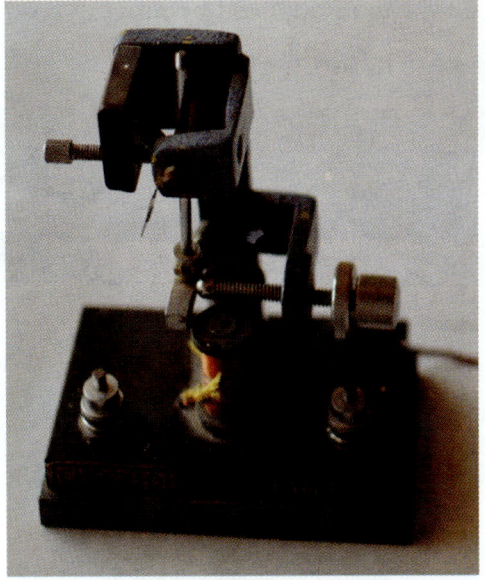

Ans. 7a. Vibrating variable interrupter and used to give multiple stimuli.

Ans. 7b. Vibrating variable interrupter and works on the principle of electric bell.

Q8. Identify the following spot and write its use.

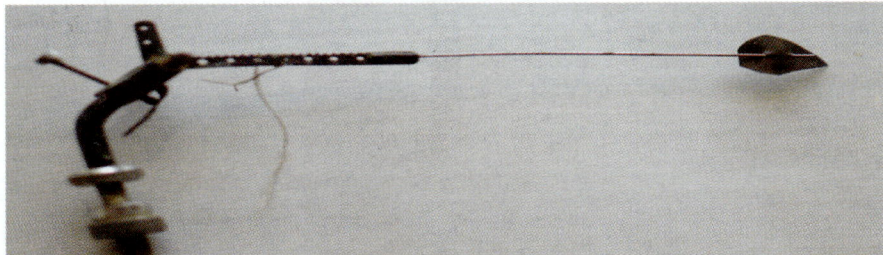

Ans. Isotonic muscle lever: It records as well as magnifies the muscle contraction on the drum of kymograph.

Q9. Identify the following spot and write its use.

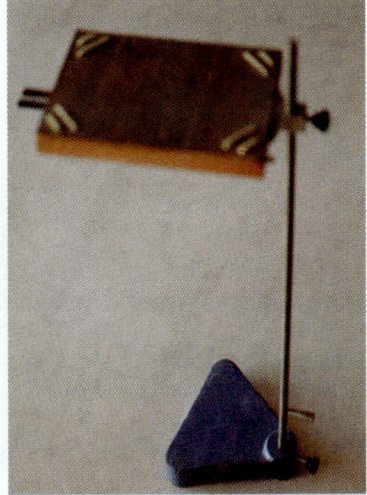

Ans. Myograph board and myograph stand.

Myograph board is a rectangular wooden board having clips on both the short sides. By one clip it is fixed with myograph stand and by another clip, writing liver is attached. The nerve muscle preparation and frog for other experiments is placed on the myograph board to get record on the drum of kymograph.

The position of myograph board can be adjusted by moving vertically along rod of myograph stand.

Q10. Identify the following spot and write its use.

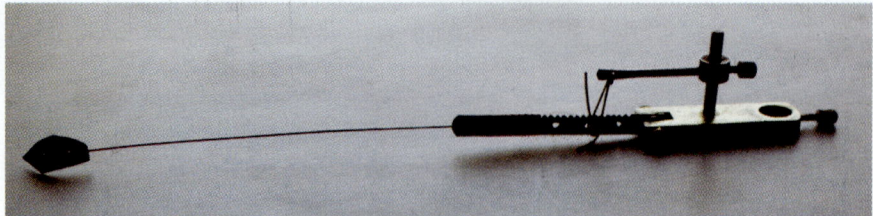

Ans. Starling heart lever and it is used for recording the contractions of heart.

Q11. Identify the spot shown below. What is its use?

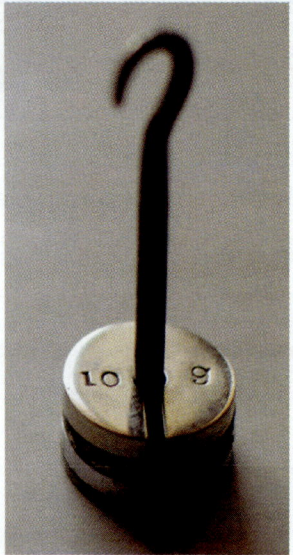

Ans. Weights which are used for lowering the inertia and for making appropriate size of recording graph.

Q12a. Identify the following picture.

Q12b. Write down the appliances of primary and secondary circuits.

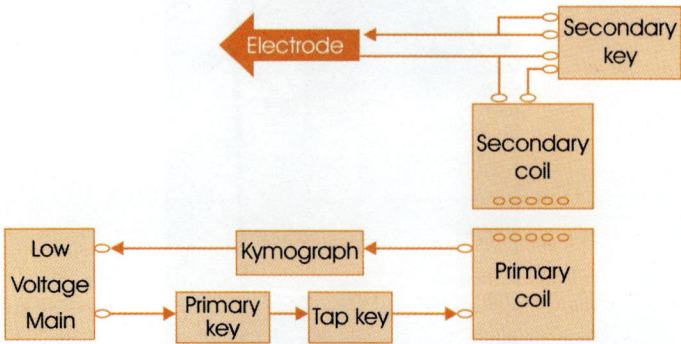

Ans. 12a. The above picture shows connections of primary and secondary circuits.

Ans. 12b. Appliances of primary circuit: Low voltage main, primary key, tapping key, primary coil of induction of coil.

Appliances of secondary circuit: Secondary coil, secondary keys and stimulating electrode.

Q13. What is the composition of amphibian Ringer solution?

Ans. The composition of amphibian Ringer solution:

Sodium chloride: 0.6%

Potassium chloride: 0.014%

Calcium chloride: 0.012%

Sodium bicarbonate: 0.02%

Sodium biophosphate: 0.001%

Q14. Identify the following spot and label the parts marked as 1, 2 and 3.

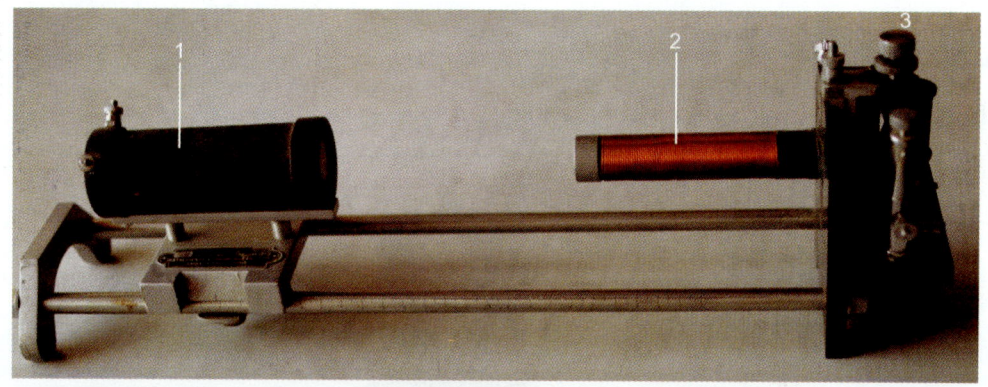

Ans. Du Bois-Reymond induction coil and parts are:

1. Primary coil

2. Secondary coil and

3. Terminal of primary coil.

Q15. Identify the following spot and label the parts marked as 1,2 and 3.

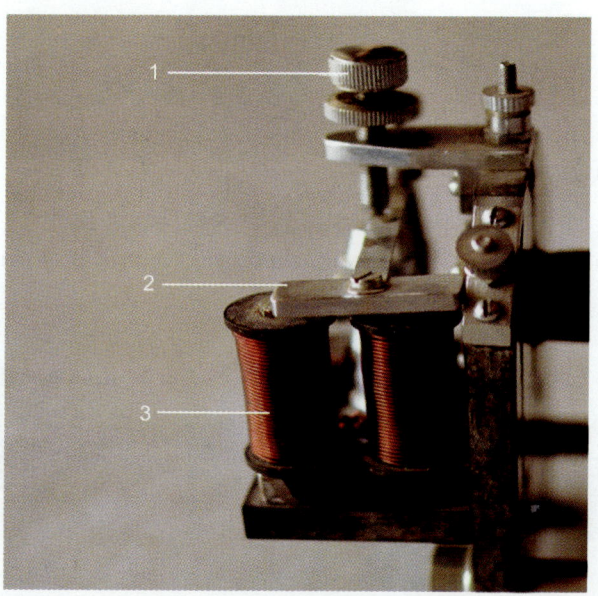

Ans.

1. Terminal of Neef's hammer

2. Neef's hammer, and

3. Electromagnet

Q16. Identify the following spot and label the parts marked as 1, 2, 3, 4 and 5.

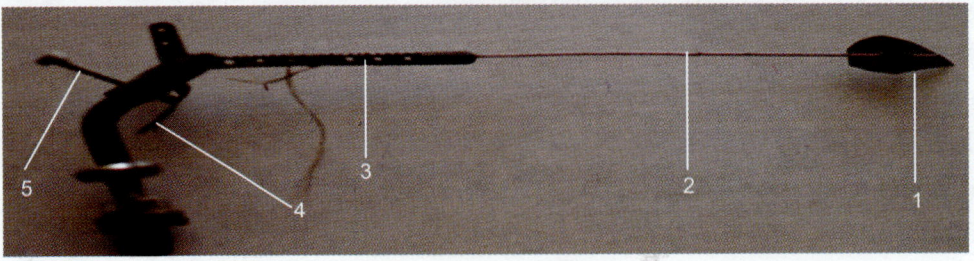

Ans. Isotonic muscle lever and its parts are:

1. Pointer   2. Wire

3. Metallic plate   4. Hook

5. After loaded screw

Q17. Label the following any 4 parts of a kymograph

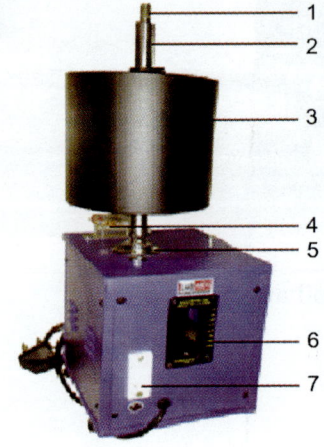

Ans.

1. Screw lift
2. Spindle
3. Drum
4. Electric contact block
5. Striker
6. Calibrated speed setting system and
7. On off switch.

Q18. Identify the following spot and label the parts marked as 1, 2, and 3, 4 and 5.

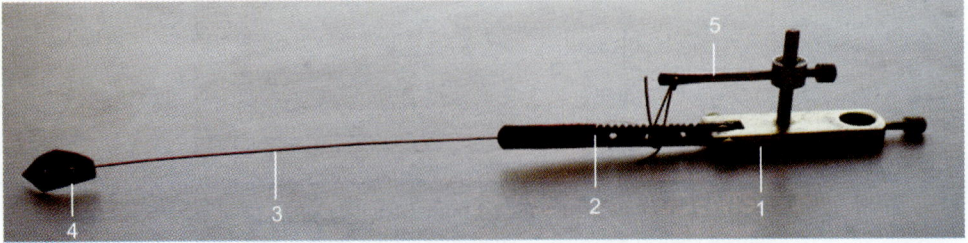

Ans.

1. Metallic frame
2. Metallic plate
3. Wire
4. Pointer
5. Supporting arm

Q19. Identify the graph below. Describe the phase of this graph.

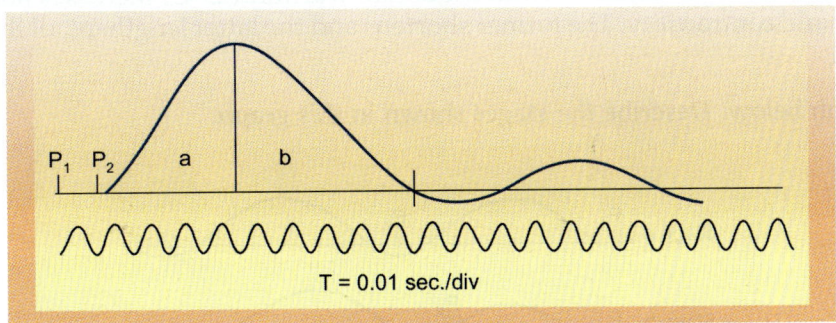

T = 0.01 sec./div

Ans. The graph is of simple muscle curve: P1: Point of stimulation, P2: Beginning of contraction

a. Latent period

b. Contraction phase

c. Relaxation phase.

Q20. Time tracing below the graph of simple muscle twitch has frequency of 100 vibs/sec. Calculate the time period of latent period contraction phase and relaxation phase in m sec.

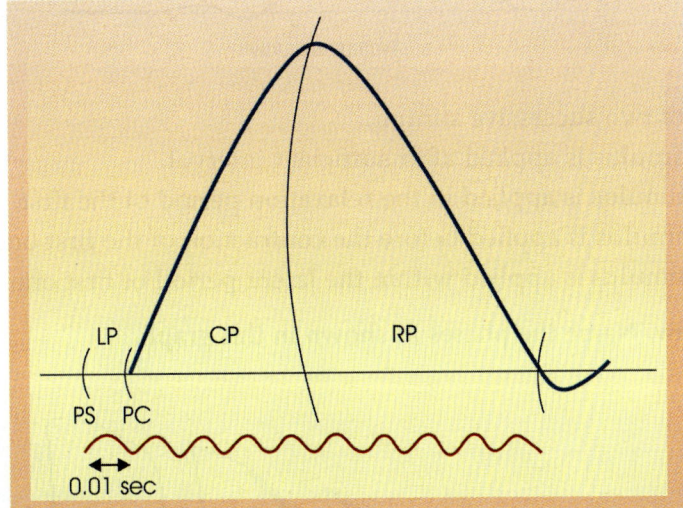

0.01 sec

Ans. Latent period = 0.01 sec/10 m sec. Contraction period = 0.04 sec/40 m sec. Relaxation period = 0.5 sec/50 m sec.

Q21. Identify the graph below and explain regarding the same.

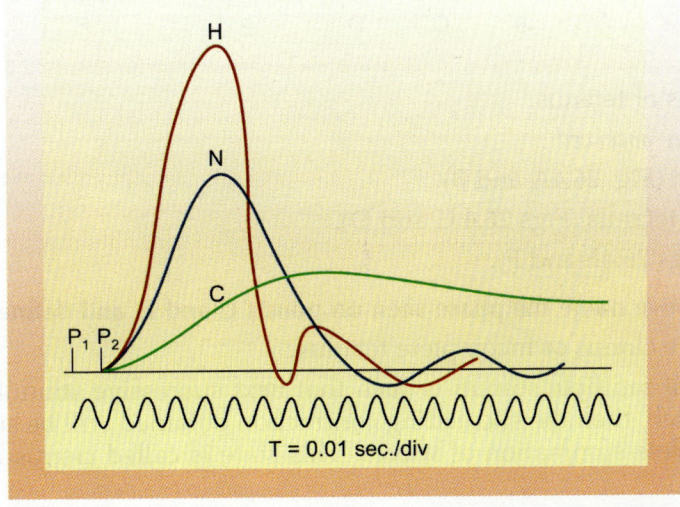

T = 0.01 sec./div

Ans. Effect of temperature on simple muscle twitch. P_1: Point of stimulation, P_2: Onset of contraction, H: Effect of heat, N: Normal curve, C: Effect of cold. Moderate warmth (25°C) increases and cold (5°C) depresses both excitability and contractility. The former shortens and the latter lengthens all the periods of the muscle curve.

Q22. Identify the graph below. Describe the stages shown in this graph.

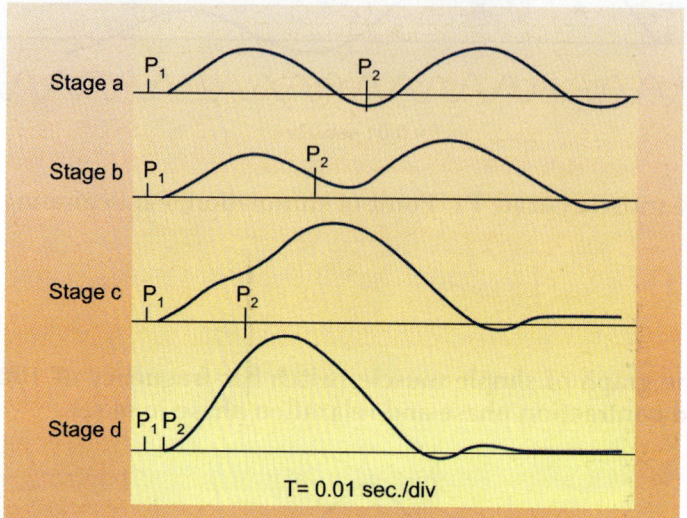

Ans. The graph is of effect of two successive stimuli.

Stage a: The second stimulus is applied after sufficient interval.

Stage b: The second stimulus is applied in the relaxation period of the first.

Stage c: The second stimulus is applied before the contraction of the first one is over.

Stage d: The second stimulus is applied within the latent period of first one.

Q23. Identify the graph below. Name the phases as shown in this graph.

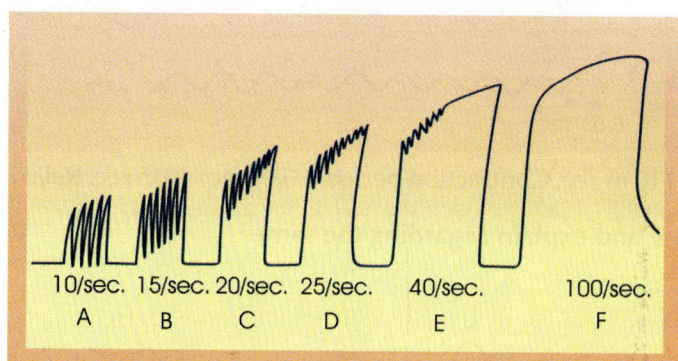

Ans. The graph is of genesis of tetanus.

Following phenomena are observed:

Staircase phenomenon (Fig. 26.4A and B).

Clonus or incomplete tetanus (Figs 26.4 C and D).

Complete Tetanus (Figs 26.4E and F).

Q24. In the graph shown above name the phase seen on points C and D and define this observation.

Ans. The points C and D are clonus or incomplete tetanus.

When the frequency of multiple stimuli is such that next successive stimuli falls during mid-relaxation phase of previous twitch, then the succeeding contraction obtained will be superposed over the previous twitch due to incomplete summation of waves. This state is called clonus or subtetanus or incomplete tetanus.

Q25. In the graph shown below name the phase seen on points E and F and define this observation.

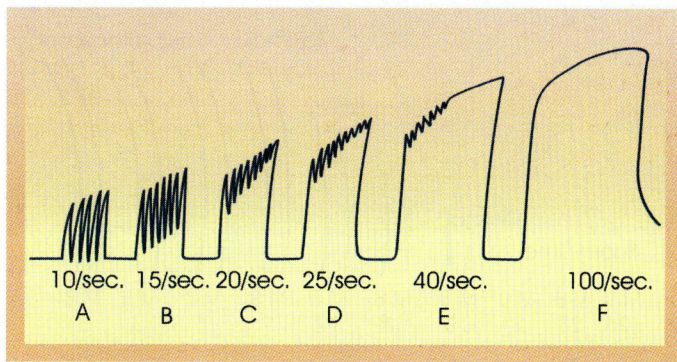

Ans. The points E and F are complete tetanus.

Tetanus: When the frequency is more, so that the stimuli fall within the latent period of the previous curve, the record traces a clear steady line, which rise first abruptly and then gradually, till maximum contraction takes place. This is called tetanus.

Q26. Identify the graph below and explain regarding the same.

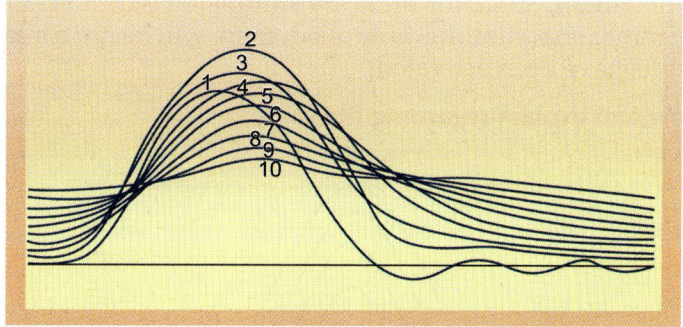

Ans. The graph above is of genesis of fatigue in skeletal muscle. The diagram indicates successive stage of the curve (beginning from 1). 2 and 3 are higher than the 1 due to beneficial effect of contraction. 10 shows the maximum development of the contracture. When repeatedly stimulated, the muscle loses its irritability, becomes gradually less excitable and ultimately ceases to respond. This phenomenon is called fatigue.

Q27. Identify the graph below and explain regarding the same.

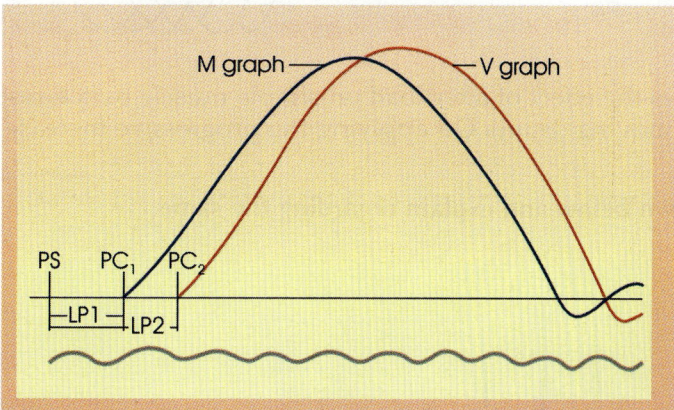

Ans. The above graph shows estimation of nerve conduction of the sciatic nerve of frog.
1. The nerve conduction is estimated by giving stimulus at vertebral end and muscular end of the nerve.
2. On applying stimulus on muscle end of nerve, latent period is shorter as compared to the vertebral end
3. The difference of latent periods of two graphs is the time taken by a nerve impulse to travel from vertebral end to muscular end.

Q28. Identify the graph below and explain regarding the same.

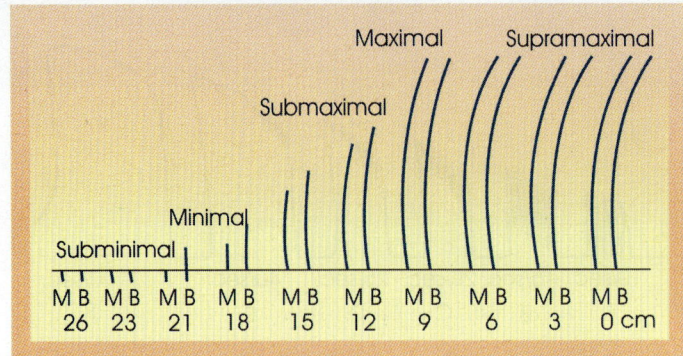

Ans.

1. On giving a stimulus of subminimal strength there is no response.
2. When the strength of stimulus increased to a threshold level a response is produced.
3. Further progressive increase of strength of stimulus causes increase in the response of the muscle. The threshold of excitation of different motor neurons supplying a single skeletal muscle differs, therefore, with the increase in strength of stimulus, more and more motor units get recruited and thereby the height of contraction increases.
4. At specific strength of stimuli, all motor units are stimulated which is maximal stimulus.
5. Hereafter even if supramaximal stimulus is applied, there will be no increase in the response because by then all the motor units have been activated.

Q29. Identify the graph below and explain regarding the same.

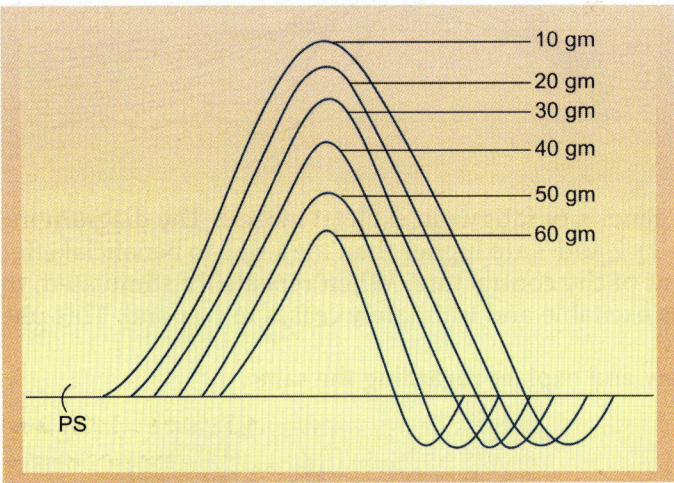

Ans. The above graph shows the effect of after load on simple muscle twitch response with increasing weight (recording is done on moving drum). On applying the progressive increase of the load, the amplitude of contraction decreases.

Q30. Identify the graph shown below and explain regarding the same.

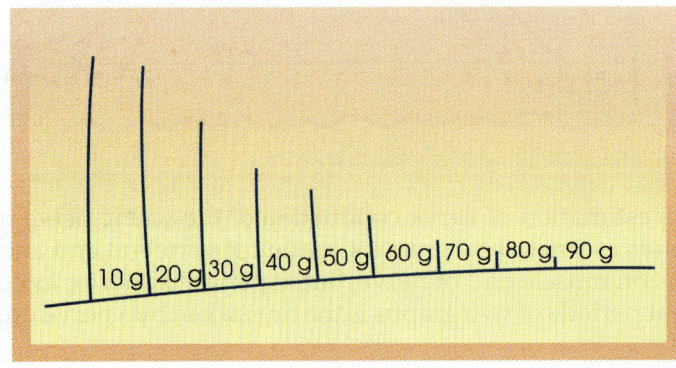

Ans. The above graph shows effect of after load on simple muscle twitch with increasing weight (recording is done on stationary drum). On applying the progressive increase of the load, the amplitude of contraction decreases.

Q31. Identify the graph below and explain regarding the same.

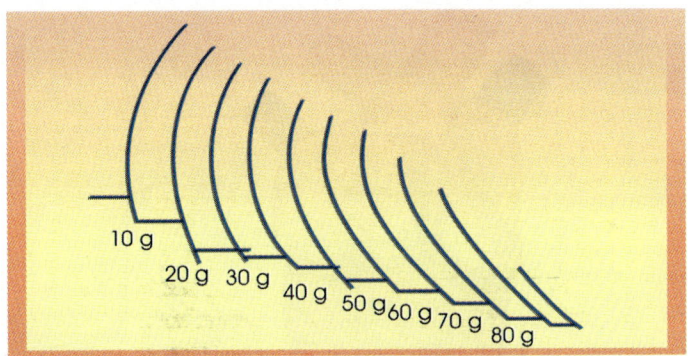

Ans.

1. The above graph shows effect of free load on simple muscle twitch response and on progressive increase in the load, the amplitude of contraction decreases.
2. The contraction obtained for a given weight in pre-loaded or free-loaded condition is of higher amplitude than that obtained for the same weight in after load because in free load condition the initial length of the muscle is increased so there is increase in force of contraction. The Starling's law is applicable in this condition.

Q32. Identify the spot shown below and explain regarding the same.

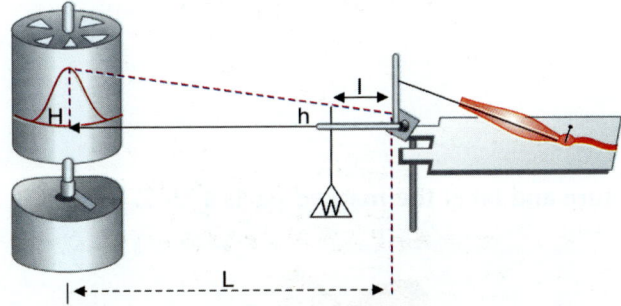

Ans. Experiment setup to calculate the work done by a single muscle twitch.
Thus the calculation for actual height will be $h = H \div (L/l)$ or $(H \times l)/L$. If w is the weight in grams lifted then work done $W = F \times h = w \times h$

Q33. Identify the spot shown below and explain regarding the same.

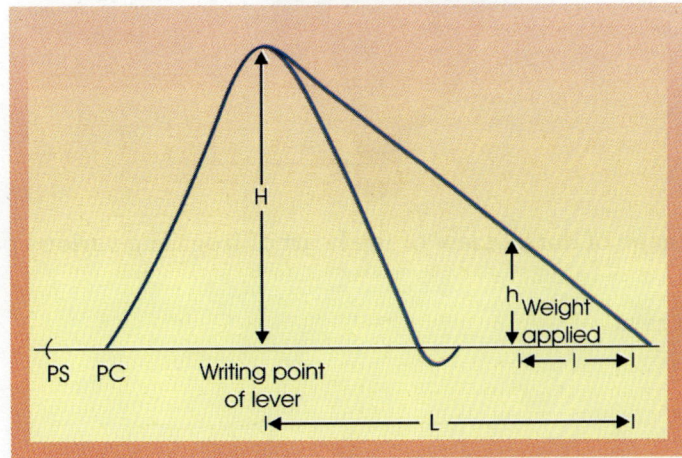

Ans. The graph of SMT showing the measurements for calculations of actual height. Thus the calculation for actual height will be h = H ÷ (L/l) or (H × l)/L . If w is the weight in grams lifted then work done W = F × h = w × h

Q34. Identify the following picture and label the marked parts 1 to 5.

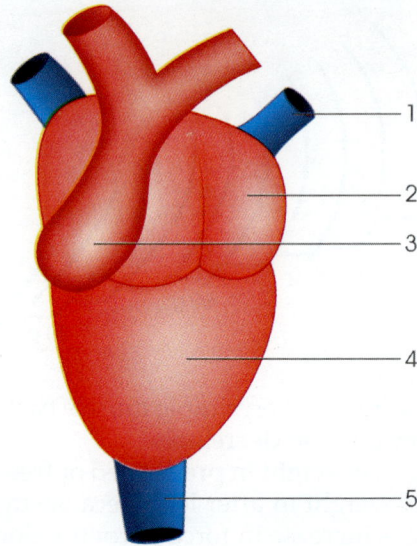

Ans. The above picture is image of ventral view of the heart of frog. The various parts from above downwards are:

1. Left superior vena cava
2. Left atrium
3. Truncus arteriosus
4. Ventricle
5. Inferior vena cava.

Q35. Identify the following picture and label the marked parts 1 to 5.

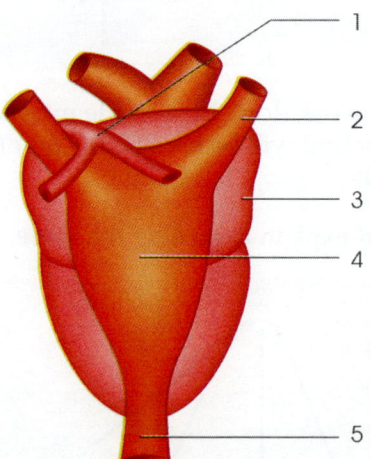

Ans. The above picture is image of dorsal view of the heart of frog. The various parts are:

1. Pulmonary vein
2. Right superior vena cava
3. Right atrium
4. Sinus venosus and
5. Inferior vena cava

Q36. Identify the following graph and explain it.

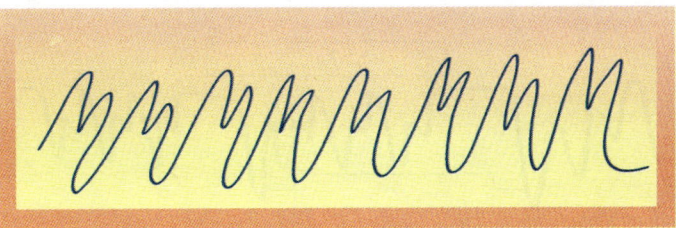

Ans. The above graph is of normal cardiogram which shows smaller downstroke of atrial contraction, smaller upstroke of atrial relaxation, larger downstroke of ventrical contraction and larger upstroke of ventrical relaxation.

Q37. Identify the following graph and label the following 1 to 4.

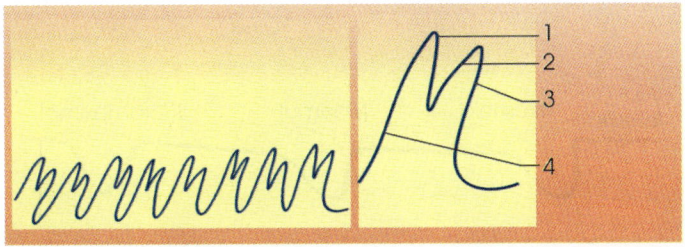

Ans. The above graph is of normal cardiogram and 1—atrial contraction, 2—atrial relaxation, 3—ventrical contraction, 4—ventrical relaxation.

Q38. Identify the following graph. What changes do you observe?

Q39. Identify the following graph. Explain the mechanisms of changes with hot and cold saline.

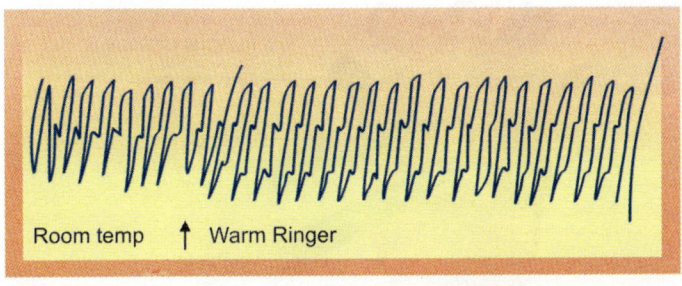

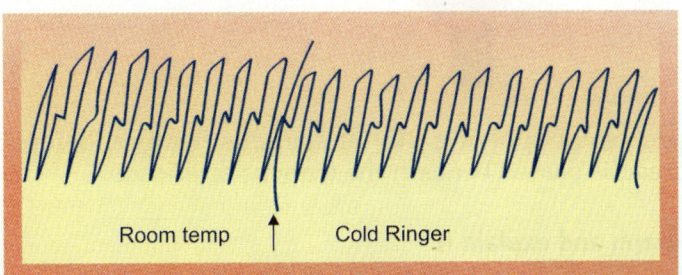

Ans. 38. Above two graphs show the effect of temperature on frog heart. With warm Ringer solution, heart rate and force of contraction increases with cold saline reverse changes occur.

Ans. 39. Above two graphs show the effect of temperature on frog heart.

Metabolic activity of the pacemaker cells increases on poring of hot Ringer solution as it generates more cardiac impulses per unit time, thereby increasing the heart rate. The increased metabolic activity in the cells of the atria and ventricle further increases the force of contraction. The cold has the reversal effects due to decrease in the metabolic activity decreasing rate and force of contraction.

Q40. Identify the following graph and explain it.

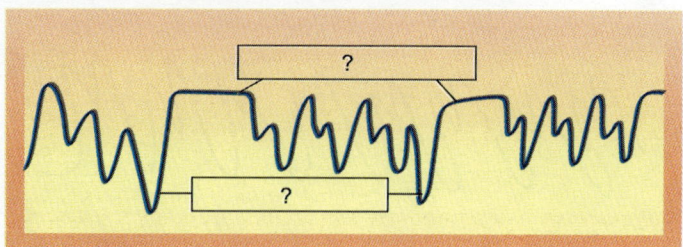

Ans. The above graph demonstrates the extrasystole and compensatory pause. When artificial stimulus is given in late part of diastole the ventricle muscle contracts and show extrasystole which is followed by compensatory pause.

Q41. Identify the following graph and explain it.

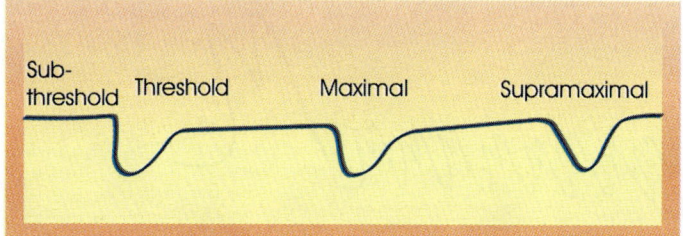

Ans. The above graph demonstrates the phenomenon of all-and-none law. Stimuli of different strengths have been applied to quiescent heart but the magnitude of the response remains same.

Q42. Identify the following spot.

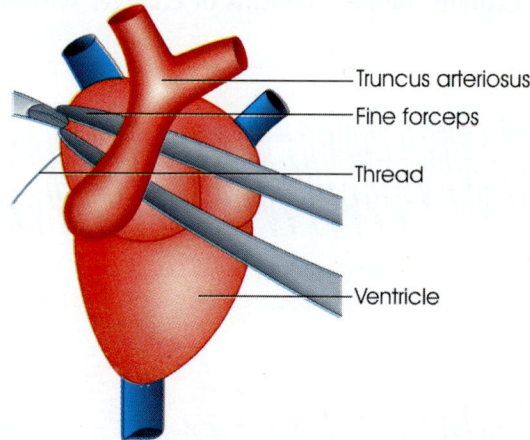

Ans. This spot shows the process of applying the 1st stannius ligature. Before making knot of 1st stannius ligature, the loop of thread is passed beneath the truncus arteriosus.

Q43. Identify the following graph and explain it.

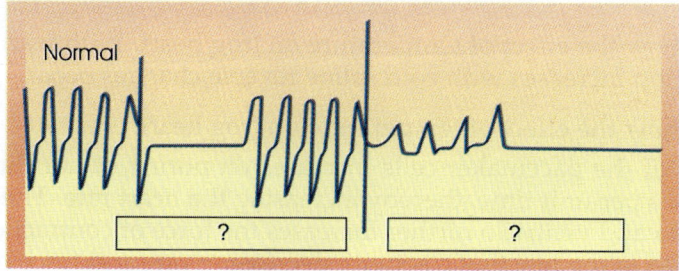

Ans. This spot shows the effect of 1st and 2nd stannius ligature. After applying knot of 1st stannius ligature, heart stops beating and after some gap it begins beating with lower rate with rhythm of atrium. After applying knot of 2nd stannius ligature, heart stop beating but atria continue to beat without contractions of ventricle.

Q44. Identify the graph shown below and explain it.

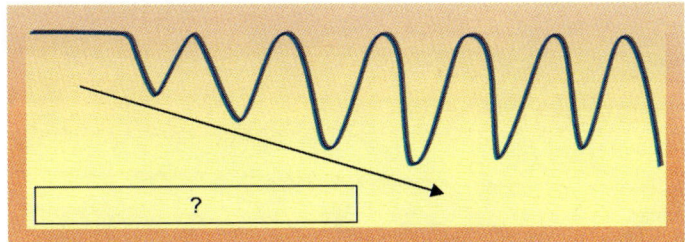

Ans. Staircase phenomenon: If a quiescent ventricle is stimulated repeatedly such that the interval between consecutive stimuli is less than 10 s, the first 4–5 contractions are of successive increased magnitude. This is called staircase phenomenon. Successive increased in the force of contraction of the ventricle is due to beneficial effect (more amount of calcium is made available with each successive contraction) producing staircase effect.

Q45. Identify the following graph and explain it.

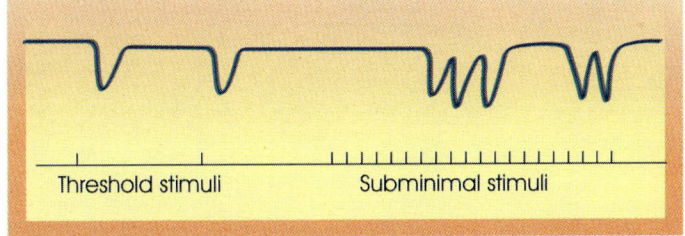

Ans. The above graph shows summation of subminimal stimuli.

Q46. Identify the following graph and explain it.

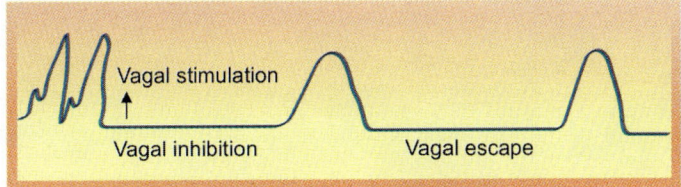

Ans. When there is excessive vagal stimulation, the heart stops beating. After a short time (few seconds), the ventricles again begin to beat at a lower frequency. This phenomenon is called vagal escape. It may be due to generation of an idio-ventricular rhythm.

Q47. Identify and explain the following graph.

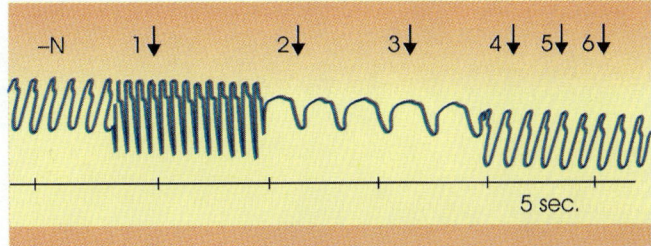

Ans. This graph shows the effect of drugs on heart of frog, N: Normal cardiogram; 1: Effect of adrenaline; 2: Effect of acetylcholine; 3: Effect of atropine; 4: Normal cardiogram; 5: Effect of atropine; 6: Effect of acetylcholine.

Appendices

Appendix 1

Photometry and Spectrophotometry*

Photometry: When monochromatic light (light wave of a specific wavelength) is passed through a coloured solution, certain wavelengths are selectively absorbed. This is called **absorbance (A).** The light that is not absorbed is transmitted through the solution. This is called **transmittance (T).** The colour of the solution is because of this transmitted light.

If the concentration of the substance in solution is increased, absorbance increases in a linear fashion and transmittance decreases. This means that absorbance is directly proportional to the concentration of the substance in the solution and is inversely proportional to the transmittance.

When absorbance (A) is plotted versus the wavelength (λ) it is called the absorption spectrum of the compound. The wavelength at which maximum absorption takes place is called the absorption maximum (λ_{max}).

When a monochromatic light with an original intensity (I_o) passes through a solution that can absorb a certain wavelength, the intensity of transmitted light (I_t) will be less than I_o.

Some of incident light energy could be reflected or absorbed by the cell containing the solution. (To eliminate these factors, a **blank** solution is used.)

Therefore, absorbance is defined as:

$$\text{Absorbance (A)} = \log \frac{1}{T} = \log \frac{I_o}{I_t}$$

And transmittance (T) is:

$$T = \frac{I_t}{I_o}$$

The ratio of I_t/I_o is described as percentage,

So, $\%T = I_t/I_o \times 100\%$

As the concentration of a compound increases, less light is transmitted. %T varies inversely and logarithmically with the concentration, therefore it is convenient to use absorbance (A) (as optical density) which is directly proportional to the concentration.

Thus, Photometry is Governed by Two Laws

Beer's law: Amount of light transmitted by a substance in solution decreases exponentially with an increase in the concentration of the substance. In other words, the amount of light absorbed by a coloured substance is proportional to the concentration of the substance.

A α concentration C

Therefore, A = kC

(Where k is the proportionality constant).

Lambert's law: The amount of light absorbed by a coloured solution is proportional to the pathlength (l), of the solution through which the light passes.

$$A \alpha l$$
$$A = kl$$

*by Dr Jyoti John, Addtional Professor, Department of Biochemistry, All India Institute of Medical Sciences, Nagpur, Mh.

If we combine these two laws, we get:

A = kCl

(Where k = the proportionality constant also known as the **molar absorption coefficient.** It is specific for a given substance at a given wavelength. It is the absorbance shown by a one molar (1M) solution of a substance with a light path of 1 cm.)

If we have a standard solution, we can calculate the concentration of a substance as follows:

A = kCl

(The light path (l), is usually 1 cm, and kept constant in photometric instruments)

Thus, A = k C

$A_T = k\ C_T$ (where C_T = concentration of unknown substance to be tested)

$A_S = k\ C_S$ (C_S = concentration of standard)

and

$$\frac{A_T}{A_S} = \frac{kC_T}{kC_s}$$

Therefore

$$C_T = \frac{A_T \times C_S}{A_S}$$

Blank solution: This contains all the reagents but will not have the substance to be analyzed. The blank test tube helps to set the 'zero' reading.

Standard: This solution represents a **known** concentration of the substance whose concentration is to be estimated. The concentration of the substance in the test sample can be calculated by comparing its absorbance with the absorbance of a known concentration of a standard solution. (A series of standards of known concentration can be prepared, to plot a standard curve.)

INSTRUMENTS BASED ON PHOTOMETRY

Colorimeter

Colorimeters are based on the basic principles of photometry, but only coloured solutions (that absorb light in the visible range) can be used. In the lab, colourless compounds can be converted into coloured compounds using certain chemical reactions. The amount of colour generated is proportional to the amount of the compound to be measured.

In a colorimeter, light from a lamp (for example, a tungsten lamp) is passed through a filter (in order to obtain light of a particular wavelength). In simple instruments coloured glass filters are used but prisms or diffraction gratings are used in sophisticated ones.

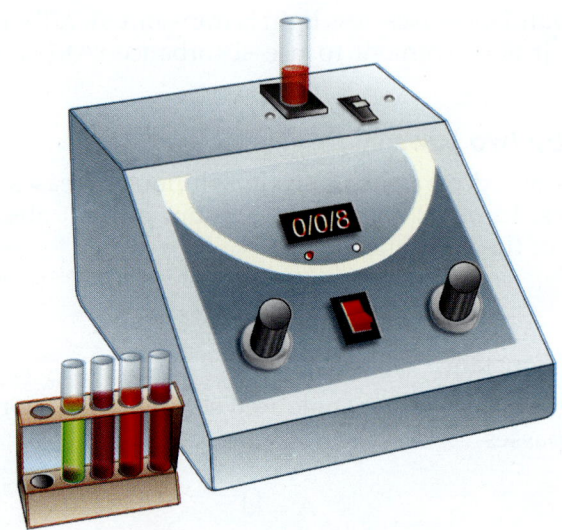

Fig. A1.1: Photocolorimeter

The monochromatic light is then passed through the solution. The solution is placed inside a cuvette. Glass Cuvettes are used in colorimetry for the visible range while quartz or fused silica cuvettes are used for readings to be taken in the UV range.

The transmitted light falls on the photosensitive surface of a photo cell (containing selenium) generating a current. The current generated is proportional to the light intensity. The photo cell is connected to a galvanometer which is calibrated to read either percentage transmittance or absorbance or both.

SPECTROPHOTOMETER

A spectrophotometer works on the same principle as a colorimeter but it is more sensitive than colorimeter. Also, it can operate in the infrared range, visible range (380–750 nm) and the ultraviolet range (200–380 nm) of the electromagnetic spectrum. Instead of glass cuvettes, quartz cuvettes are used in the UV light range. The wavelength selection is done by using a prism or diffraction gratings and consequently it is possible to select narrower bandwidths making it more sensitive than a colorimeter. In spectrophotometer it is not necessary that the compounds to be estimated be coloured. This is because light in the ultraviolet and infrared range is also emitted and hence these compounds can be measured if they show significant absorption at these wavelengths.

Acknowledgement: This topic has been written by Dr Jyoti John, Additional Professor, AIIMS Nagpur.

Appendix 2
Artificial Respiration or Resuscitation

Indication: In any condition where respiration fails but heart continues to beat, application of artificial respiration is indicated.

Principle: The purpose of giving artificial respiration is as follows:

1. By maintaining the vitality of the nerve centres, as well as that of the heart, the circulation is maintained. Artificial respiration also helps to maintain circulation. It is expected that after sometime, the respiratory centres will start functioning spontaneously.
2. During artificial respiration, the alternate inflation and deflation of lungs reflexly stimulate the respiratory centres, and thus help them to take up their own spontaneous rhythm.

METHODS OF ARTIFICIAL RESPIRATION

Manual Methods

Schafer's Method (Fig. A2.1)

The subject is laid in prone position and a small pillow is placed underneath the chest and epigastrium. The head is turned to one side. The operator kneels down by the side of the subject facing towards his head. Two hands are placed on the two sides of the lower part of the chest and then the operator slowly puts his body weight leaning forwards and pressing upon the loins of the subject. Intra-abdominal pressure rises, the diaphragm is pushed up and air is forced out of the lungs. After this the operator releases the pressure and comes back to his original erect position. The abdominal pressure falls, diaphragm descends and air is drawn in. These movements are repeated about twelve times a minute (roughly the normal rate of respiration). By this means it is possible to have a total pulmonary ventilation of 6,500 ml per minute, and this amount is sufficient for complete aeration of blood. The advantage of this method is that the patient being in the prone position, mucus or saliva comes out of the mouth and cannot obstruct his airways.

A = Laying casualty's face downwards with head turned to one side, arms bent and forehead resting on his hands with neck extended and kneeling to one side of casualty's hips facing his head; and placing hands flat on the small of casualty's back just above the top of pelvic bones, thumbs almost touched each other in the midline,

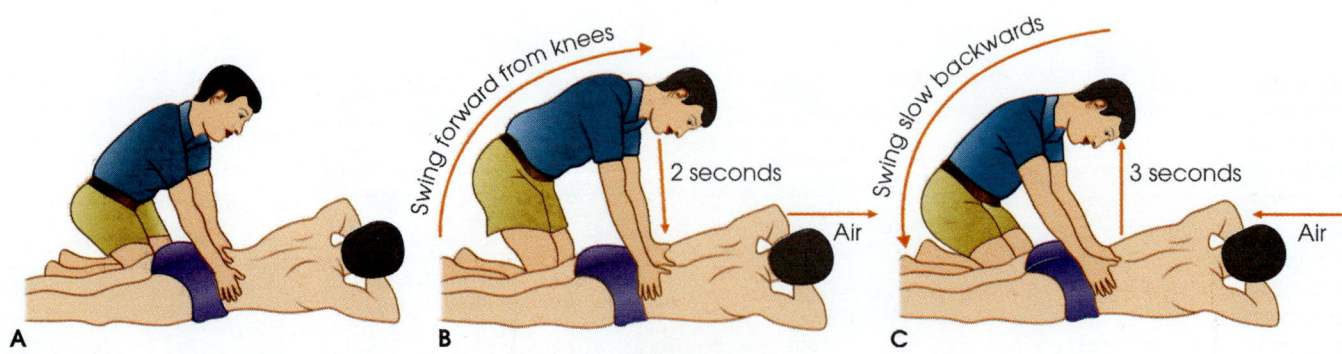

Fig. A2.1: Schafer's manual method for artificial respiration

fingers being spread over the loins and pointing towards the ground. B = Sitting on heels and swinging body slowly forward from knees being kept arms straight and hands in place all the time only applying gentle pressure by the body weight. Forcing air out of the lungs (expiration) to be maintained this position for two seconds counting 'one, two'. C = Relaxing the pressure by swinging quietly and gradually backwards on to heels allowing inspiration and counting three, four, five, in three seconds before swinging forwards again to first movement being kept arms straight and hands in place all the time. Until the last few years, Schafer's prone pressure method of artificially inflating the lungs was most widely practised. But nowadays either back-pressure-armlift method of Holger-Nielsen's method or the mouth-to-mouth method is practiced preferably.

Sylvester's Method

The subject is placed in supine position. The operator stands or kneels at the head end and holds the two arms of the subject. The operator then raises the subjects hands above his head and then folds the hands back upon the chest, compressing the chest wall at the same time. Such movements alternately increase and decrease the thoracic cavity, thus drawing in and pushing out air from the lungs. This method is most commonly used in the operation theatre or in other accidents. The tongue should be kept pulled out and the mucus from the mouth cavity should be wiped out from time to time. The rate is same as in Schafer's method. In drowning cases, the water in the lungs must, at first, be driven out, by holding the subject upside down or revolving the subject by holding his legs. After this the subject should be given artificial ventilation. Respiratory level and volume during the artificial method has been presented in Fig. A2.2C.

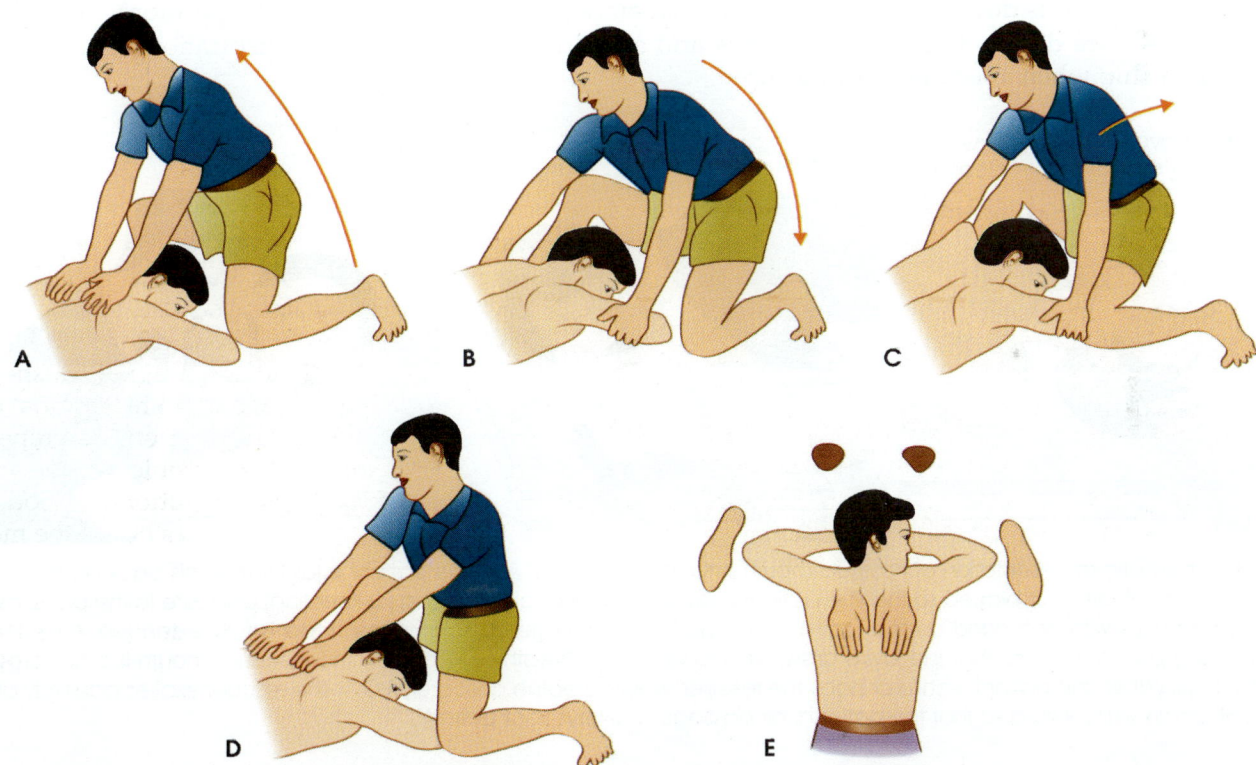

Fig. A2.2: Back-pressure-arm-lift method or Holger-Nielsen's manual method for artificial respiration. A = Rocking forward quietly with arms straight and applying light pressure to back by weight of the upper part of body only counting for two seconds, 'one, two' (expiration) B = Rocking back with arms straight releasing pressure gradually and sliding hands to elbows of casualty counting 'three' for one second. C = Raising and pulling casualty's arms until tension being felt for two seconds counting 'four', 'five' causing inspiration. D = Placing hands over casualty's shoulder blading with thumbs being touched in the midline and arms straight. Then lying casualty's arms down and placing hands on his back as in Figure A for one second counting 'six'. E = Position of casualty's and operator—laying casualty with face downwards and turning to one side arms bent and forehead rested on his hands being nose and mouth unobstructed and neck extended; and kneeling at this head being placed one knee near casualty's head and one foot alongside his elbow and hands being placed over casualty's shoulder blades with thumbs touching in the midline and fingers spreading out and being kept arms straight. [If arms being injured placing them by the sides of body doing the complete procedure but inserting hands under casualty's shoulders and raising them for inspiration. If arms and chest both injured to arm to be raised and lowered by inserting hands under casuality's shoulders.].

Holger-Nielsen Method (Fig. A2.2)

The subject is placed in the prone position with the arms abducted at the shoulders and elbows remaining flexed. The face is turned to one side and rests on the hands. The mouth is cleaned after wiping out mucus, fluid, etc. from it. The operator kneels down in front of the subject facing towards the head. Two hands are placed on the two sides of the back of the chest with the thumbs and fingers spread apart. Then the operator puts his body weight leaning forwards upon the subject's back. This compresses the chest and helps in expiration. The subject's arms forwards by holding them above the elbows. This helps in natural inspiration. This process is repeated about 10–12 times a minute. The respiratory level and volume during this artificial method have been presented in Fig. A2.2B.

Mouth-to-Mouth Method (Fig. A2.3)

The subject is laid in the supine position with extended head. The operator sits by the side of the subject's head. The operator holds the lower jaw of the subject by one thumb and index-finger and clamps the nostrils with the other thumb and index finger. The operator then keeps his mouth over the subject's mouth and exhales forcibly which causes inflation of the lungs and thorax. The operator then takes off his mouth and the process is repeated 10–20 times per minute. It is positive pressure breathing. The respiratory level and volume during this artificial method have been presented in Fig. A2.4.

EVE's Rocking Method

The patient is tied on a stretcher. The head and feet are alternately tilted through an angle of 45°. Eight or nine movements are carried out per minute, 7 seconds for each movement—4 seconds head down and 3 seconds feet down. When the head is down, the diaphragm, so that air is pushed out of the lungs (expiration).

When the feet are down, diaphragm descends and air is drawn into the lungs (inspiration). This method is useful aboard ship when a hammock can be used.

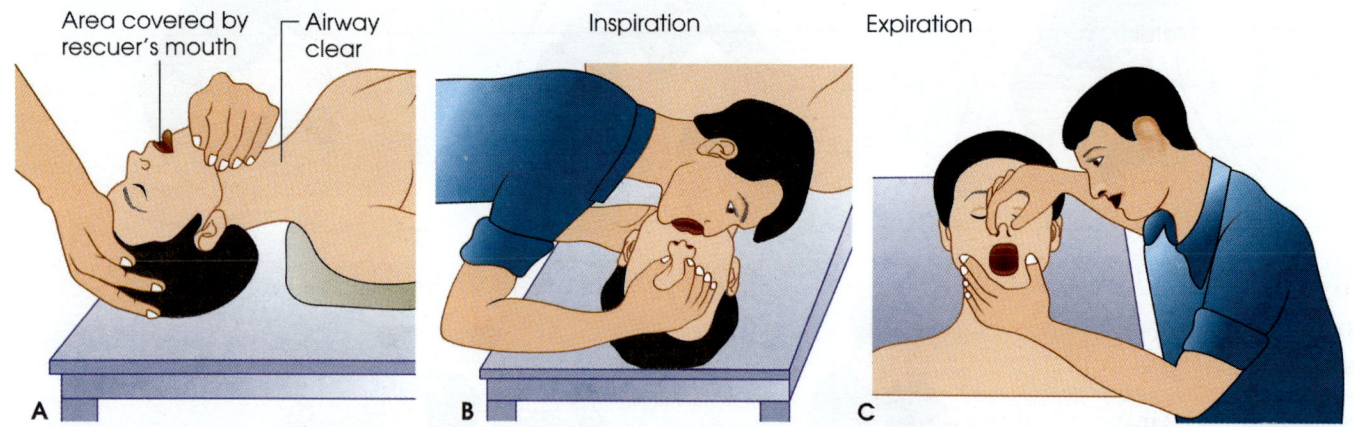

Fig. A2.3: Schematic representation of moth-to-mouth artificial ventilation. A = The patient is laid flat on his back on the patient's shoulders some soft article is placed so that the patient's head falls well back. Standing (or kneeling) opposite to the patient's head the rescuer presses with one hand on the crown of the patient's head gently so that the head is fully extended. Other hand is placed on the patient's jaw so that the jaw is drawn well forward. B = Breathing in deeply the rescuer's mouth is placed over the patient's lungs. [When the patient is child or baby the rescuer should breathe delicately.] C = The rescuer expires passively and the jaw is kept drawn well forward so that the patient's air passage is always kept patent

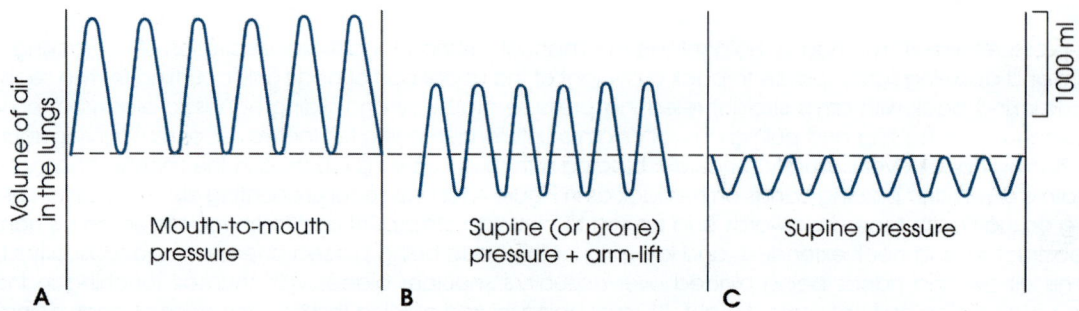

Fig. A2.4: Graphical representation of pressure of amount of gas during some artificial ventilation showing cessation of respiration in the dotted line

Instrumental Method

Instead of a human operator, machineries are used. The advantage is that it can be carried on for good length of time, whereas the human operator is likely to be fatigued. The machines generally work on two principles:

1. Negative-pressure breathing by alternately compressing and relaxing the chest wall and
2. Positive-pressure breathing by introducing air or oxygen directly into the lungs—intermittently or continuously. Some of the methods working on the first principle are mentioned below.

Drinker's Method (Fig. A2.5)

In this method the patient is placed in an airtight chamber, the head remaining outside. By mechanically driven pumps, the pressure in the chamber is alternately lowered and raised. When the pressure is lowered the chest swells up and air is drawn into the lungs. When the pressure is raised chest becomes compressed and air is pushed out. In this way, artificial ventilation may be continued for any length of time. These methods are very useful in cases where prolonged artificial respiration is necessary, such as in morphine poisoning, in paralysis of the respiratory muscles, as in poliomyelitis, pneumothorax, etc. [The so-called iron lungs is an instrument working on this principle.]

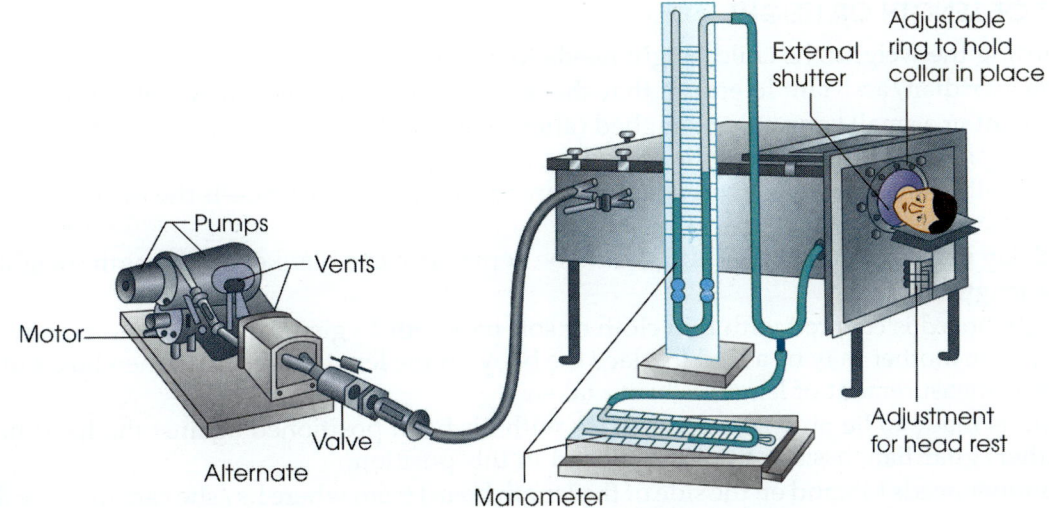

Fig. A2.5: Drinker's respiration (so-called iron lungs)

Resuscitator (Figs A2.6A and B)

This apparatus forces air through the mask that fits over the patient's face; into the lungs of the patient during the positive pressure cycle and then either allows air to flow out the lungs during the remainder of the cycle or pulls the air out by negative pressure. Resuscitator commonly has safety valve which prevents the positive pressure from rising normally about +14 mm Hg and the negative pressure from falling below –9 mm Hg.

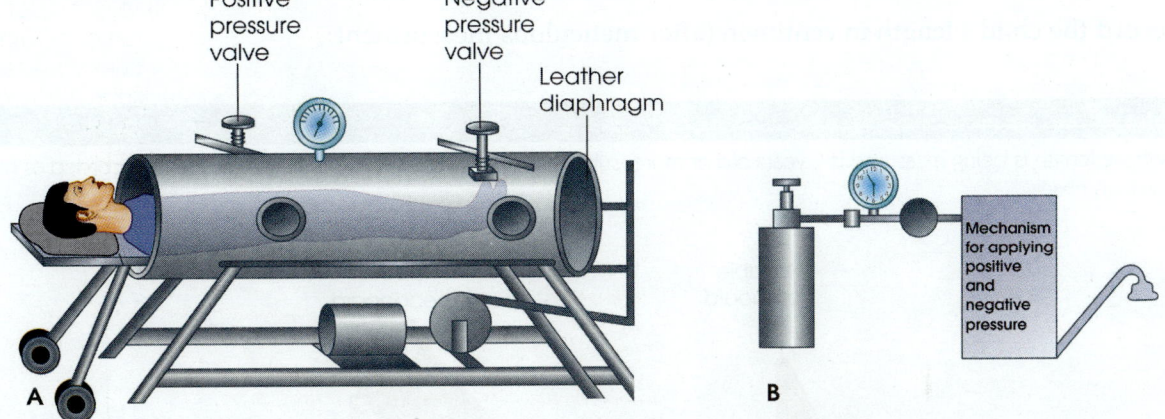

Fig. A2.6A and B: (A) Tank respirator; (B) Resuscitator

Exercise for Students

Practice and discuss the methods of artificial respiration.

Appendix 3
Anthropometric Measurement

MEASUREMENT OF LENGTH OR HEIGHT

1. After recording the weight; the child height needs to be measured.
2. Instruct the guardian/assistant to ensure that shocks, shoes and hair ornaments of child are removed.
3. In case of infant or a small baby being weighed (after removal of clothes) ensure a dry diaper can be asked to be worn as to prevent getting wet while recording length.
4. parents/or mothers help can be taken after explaining them the procedure if the child is anxius/crying so that child can be comforted.
5. In case of delay in measurement the child should be kept warm in a blanket until length/height is measured.
6. Measuring length of child:
   a. The length board is covered with thin cloth or soft paper for hygiene and for avoiding any discomfort to the baby. The mother may be asked to place the baby on the length board and then holds the baby's head in place as measurement of length is being taken.
   b. The child is made to lie on board on his back with his head positioned against the fixed headboard and the mother/guardian/assistant holds the head in this position.
   c. The examiner needs to stand on the side of the length board from where he/she can visualise the measuring tape and move the footboard.
   d. Ensure the child lies straight without moving his position along the board. Do not let shoulders touch the board, and the spine must not be in arched position. If required, hold down the child's legs with one hand and the footboard must be moved with the other hand. Ensure legs remain straight, otherwise apply gentle pressure to the knees to straighten the legs.

   > **Note:** The knees of newborns cannot be totally straightened hence apply minimum pressure, otherwise the fragile bones of newborn may be injured.

   e. Record the child's length in centimen (after meticulous measurment).

Key Notes

If the child whose length is being measured is 2 years old or more, subtract 0.7 cm from the length and the result is recorded as height in the monitoring growth chart.

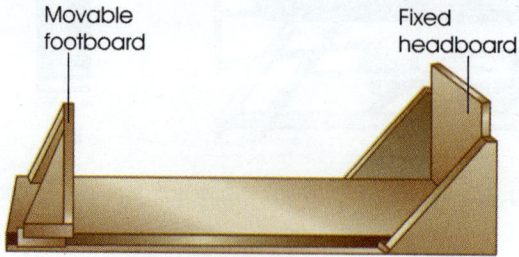

Movable footboard   Fixed headboard

Fig. A3.1: Length board

Standing Height Measurement

1. Seek assistance of mother/guardian to help the child to stand on the baseboard with feet positioned slightly apart. Ensure that the back of the head, shoulder blades, buttocks, calves, and heels touch the vertical board.
2. The mother/guardian/assistant can be asked to hold the child's knees and ankles gently, in order to keep the legs straight and feet flat, with heels and calves being touching the vertical board.
3. The heads need to be kept head in position, and as examiner one can hold the bridge between thumb and forefinger over the child's chin and use other hand to pull down the headboard so that it rests firmly on top of the head and compress the hair.
4. Record the child's height in centimeters to the last completed 0.1 cm. Remember: If the child whose height is being measured is less than 2 years old, add 0.7 cm to the height and record the result as length.

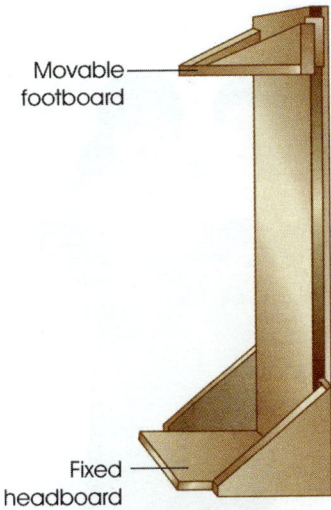

Movable footboard

Fixed headboard

Fig. A3.2: Height board

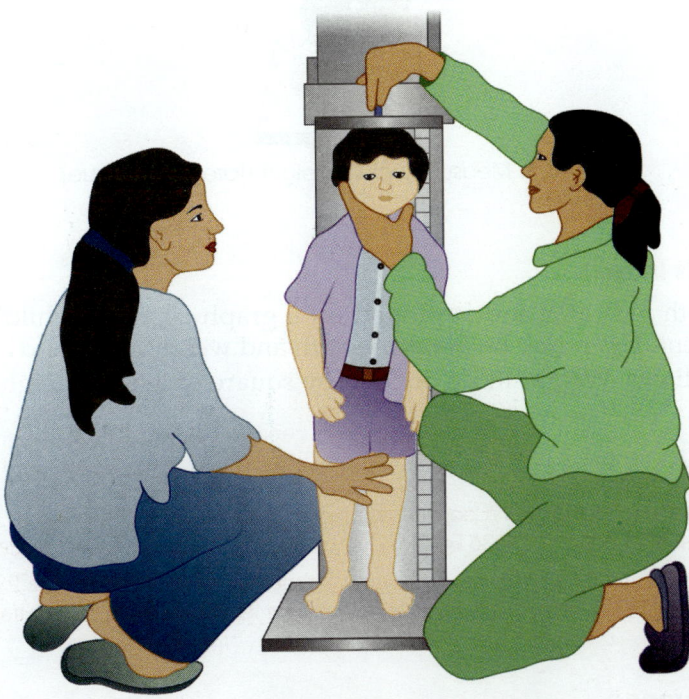

Fig. A3.3: Measuring standard height

Note: Stadiometer can be used to measure height in children above two years, when child is above to stand independently.

Measurement of Weight

Note: As per World Health Organization recommendation the weight should be recorded in children using a scale having solidly built and durability, it should be electronic (digital reading), should measure up to 150 kg, measures to a precision of 0.1 kg (100 g) and permits "Tared weighing" (the scale can be reset to zero (tared) with the individual just weighed still on it).

Thus, a mother can stand on the scale, be weighed, and the scale tared:

1. The child who can stand alone is to be weighed standing on a weighing scale. Otherwise, the mother is to be weighed alone; then the mother and child are to be weighed together and the mother's weight needs to be subtracted from joint weight (mother and child) to determine the child's weight.

Note: The child's clothes need to be removed for accurate measurement. Infants also are to be weighed naked; but they should be kept wrapped in a blanket to keep them warmed until weighing is completed. Older children/or in case of social inhibition it is advisable to have minimal clothing.

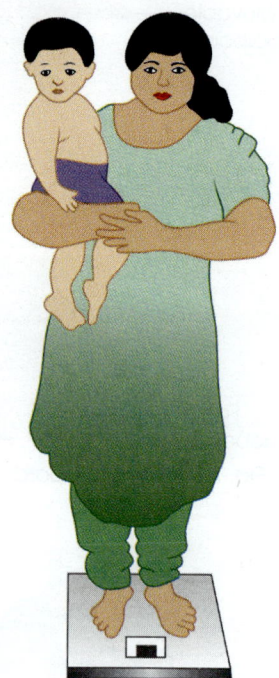

Fig. A3.4: Measuring child weight (Tared technique)

Determine BMI (Body Mass Index)

1. BMI is an useful growth indicator and is plotted on a graph against a child's age for monitoring body's growth and development depending on height/length and weight of a child.
2. BMI is calculated as follows: Weight in kg divided by square of length/height in metres and expressed as kg/m^2.

Note:

A. If the measurements of child have been recorded in pounds and inches, they must be converted to metric units before calculating BMI: 1 inch = 2.54 cm or 0.0254 m, and 1 pound = 0.4536 kg. BMI is to be rounded to one decimal place.

B. The length measurement for a child less than 2 years old and a height measurment for a child age 2 years or older is employed for BMI calculation. It is necessary, the convert height to length (by ading 0.7 cm) or length to height (by subtracting 0.7 cm) before calculating the child's BMI.

Measuring Head Circumference

The measuring tape recommended for babies and toddler is the non-stretch Teflon measuring tape and is used for measuring head circumference of the babies.

1. Approximate the measuring tape above the ears and in position midway btween the eyebrows and the hairline and to the occipital prominence at the back of the head. This is a standard guideline but one may come across with varied head shape in children and is advisable to measure the largest circumference possible.
2. Pull the measuring tape and align its end to confirm.
3. Take note of the reading of the measurement from the appropriately marked place on measuring tape.
4. The measurement must be taken to the nearest millimeter.

Bibliography

1. De Onis M, Onyango AW, Borghi E, Siyam A, Nishida C, Siekmann J. Development of WHO growth reference for school-aged children and adolescents. Bull world health Organ. 2007;85:660–667.
2. HARRIS, S. R. 2013. Congenital idiopathic microcephaly in an infant: Congruence of head size with developmental motor delay. Dev Neurorehabil, 16,129–32.
3. WHO Multicenter Growth Reference Study Group, author. WHO Child Growth Standards based on length/height, weight for age. Acta Paediatr. 2006; 450 (Suppl): 76–85.

Appendix 4
Interpretation of Growth Chart

Learning Objectives

The students after learning the practical should be able to:

1. Learn the intricate details of method to use the growth charts plotting and interpretation.
2. To identify normal growth for a given child, as well as growth problems or trends that suggest that a child is at risk of a problem.

Aim and objective: Interpretation of Growth Chart

INTRODUCTION

Growth is defined as progressive increase in the size of a child or parts of a child. It is different from development wherein there is a continuous on-going accession of various skills (abilities) such as neck holding, language learning, social and adaptive capabilities to interact with other people. Growth and development go hand-in-hand, but at different rates.

Background

Assessment of growth is done with the help of various growth indicators and due consideration is given to the child's age while interpreting the anthropometric measurements. Following growth parameters are commonly used for growth assessment.

1. Length/height-for-age
2. Weight-for-age
3. Weight-for-length/height
4. BMI (body mass index)-for-age
5. Head circumference.

This module describes how to interpret these growth indicators for a child:

Growth Charts

The growth charts used in this course were derived from the WHO Multicentric Growth Reference Study[1] and IAP growth charts revised in 2015.

The WHO growth charts demonstrate how healthy children should grow at a global level. This is because the study samples drawn from these six countries (including India) were believed to have an environment conducive for optimum growth. The standards describe the growth of children living in six countries (including India) in environments believed to support optimal growth. Breastfeeding was one of the many criteria defined for optimal growth. The WHO growth charts use the growth of breastfed infants as the norm for growth. This is in agreement with national guidelines that recommend breastfeeding as the optimal infant feeding method. The WHO growth charts should be used with all children up to aged 5 years, regardless of type of feeding.

The IAP growth charts are a national reference that represent how Indian children and teens grew primarily during the 1970s, 1980s and 1990s. The IAP recommends using the references from ages 5 through 18 years so health care providers can track weight, stature/height, and body mass index (BMI) from childhood through age 18 years. The WHO and IAP growth charts are provided for both sexes and by convention, are pink for girls and blue for boys.

Measurement and charting: The specific charts used will depend on the child's age, which determines whether the child will stand for measurement of height or lie down for measurement of length. The measurements will be plotted on growth charts in the Boy's Growth Record or the Girl's Growth Record so that trends can be observed over time and any growth problems identified. It is important to use the Growth Record for the correct sex since boys and girls grow to different sizes.

Method Protocol

1. Obtain accurate measurements: When weighing and measuring children, follow procedures that yield accurate measurements and use equipment that is well maintained.
2. Select the appropriate growth chart, based on the age and sex of the child being weighed and measured.
3. Record data after selecting the appropriate chart and entering the patient's name and record number, if appropriate, complete the data entry table.
4. Plot measurements on the appropriate WHO or IAP growth chart, plot the measurements recorded in the data entry table for the current visit.
   A. Find the child's age on the horizontal axis. When plotting weight-for-length, find the length on the horizontal axis. Use a straight edge or right-angle ruler to draw a vertical line up from that point.

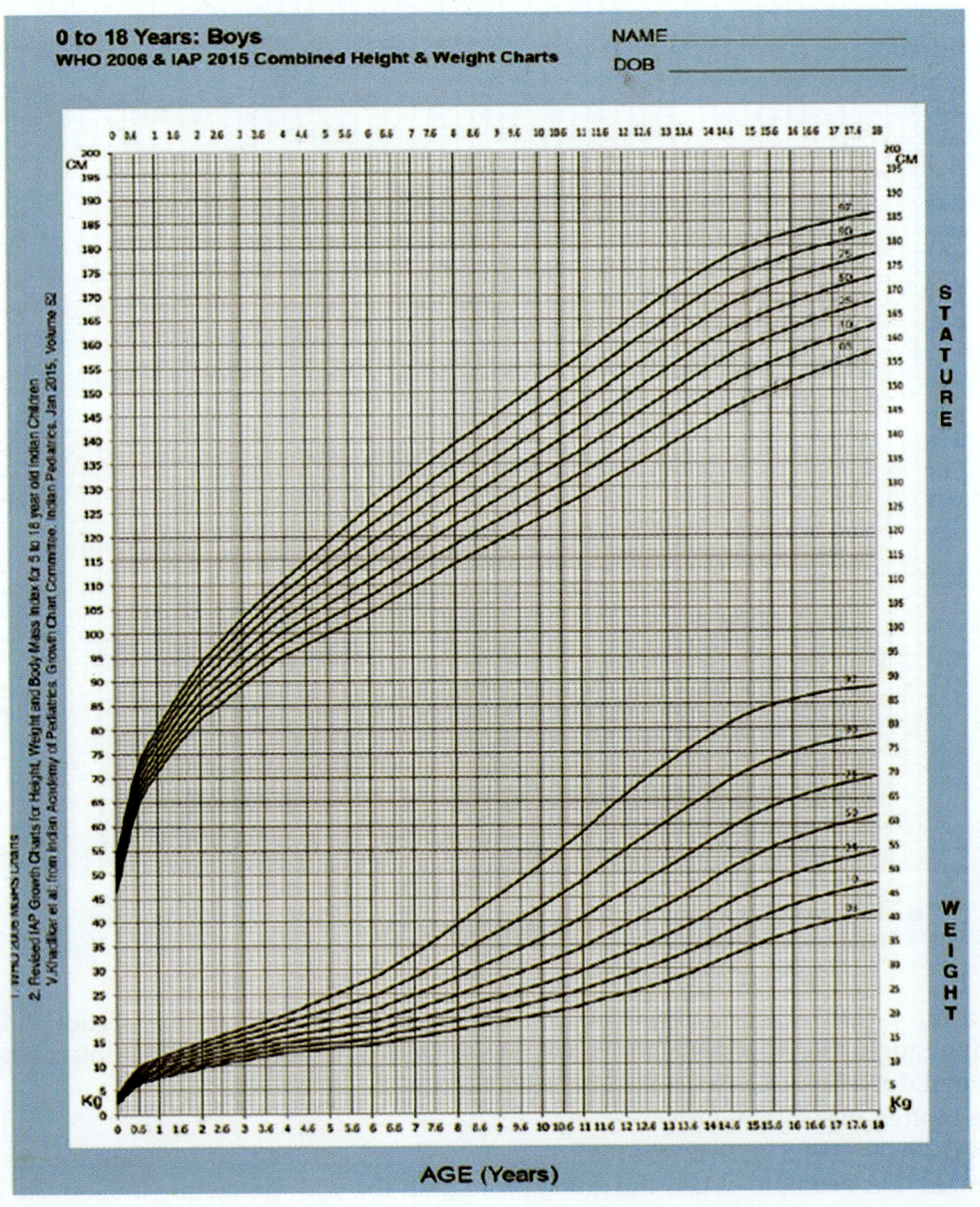

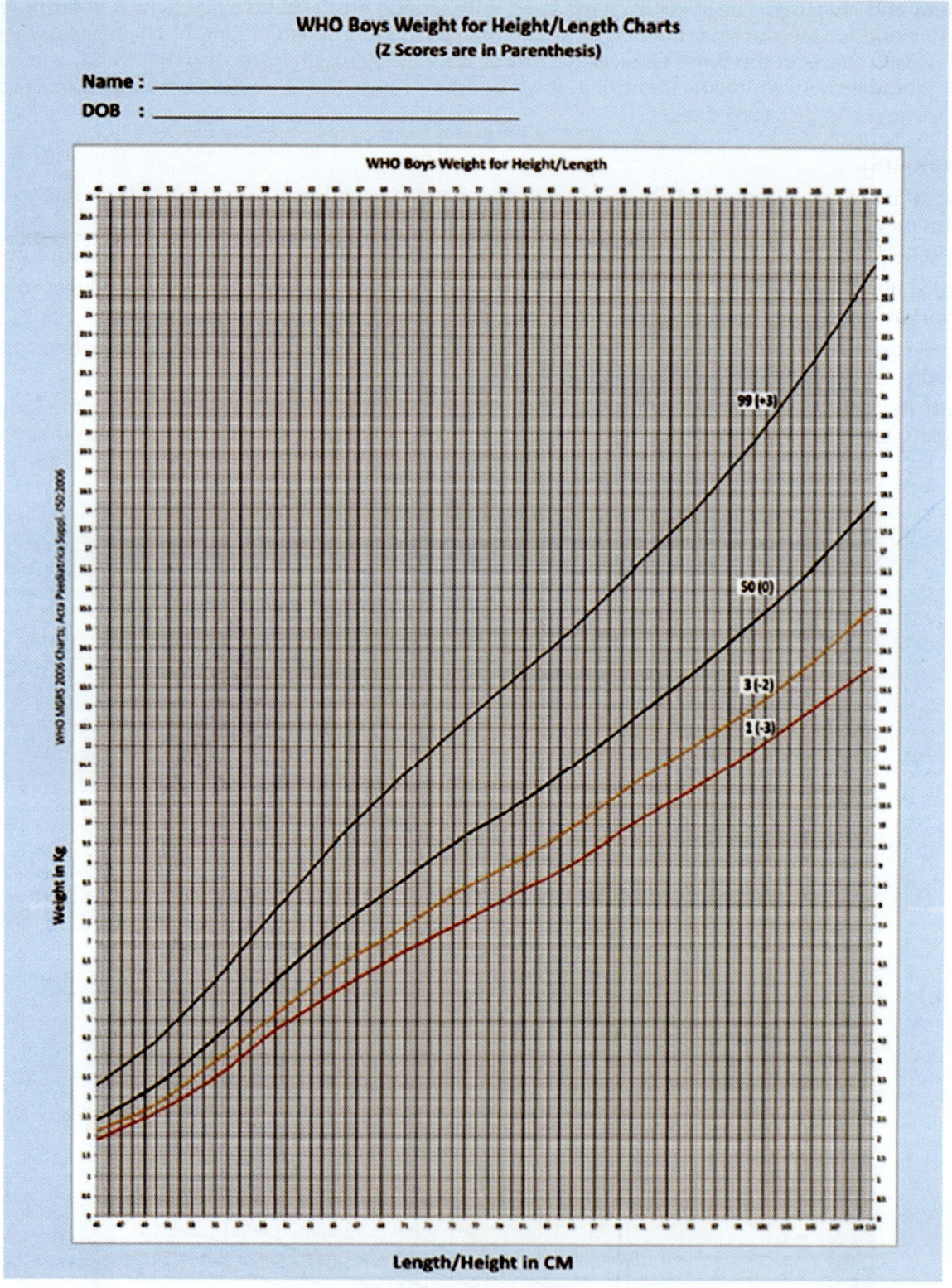

WHO Boys Weight for Height/Length Charts
(Z Scores are in Parenthesis)

Name : _____

DOB : _____

WHO Boys Weight for Height/Length

Weight in Kg

WHO MGRS 2006 Charts; Acta Paediatrica Suppl. 450 2006

99 (+3)

50 (0)

3 (-2)

1 (-3)

Length/Height in CM

B. Find the appropriate measurement (weight, length, stature, or BMI) on the vertical axis. Use a straight edge or right-angle ruler to draw a horizontal line across from that point until it intersects the vertical line.

C. Make a small dot where the two lines intersect.

5. Interpret the plotted measurements:

A. The curved lines on the growth chart show selected percentiles that indicate the rank of the child's measurement. For example, when the dot is plotted on the 95th percentile line on the IAP BMI-for-age growth chart, it means that 5 of 100 children (5%) of the same age and sex in the reference population have a higher BMI-for-age.

B. The WHO growth standard charts use the 3rd and the 97th percentiles as the outer most percentile cutoff values indicating abnormal growth.

The IAP growth reference charts similarly use the 3rd and the 97th percentiles as the outermost percentile cutoff values indicating abnormal growth.

C. Interpret the plotted measurements based on the percentile ranking on the WHO or the IAP growth charts and the percentile cutoff value corresponding to the nutrition indicator shown in the table below.

D. If the percentile rank indicates a nutrition-related health concern, additional monitoring and assessment are recommended.

E. Determine the percentile rank. Determine if the percentile rank suggests that the anthropometric index is indicative of nutritional risk based on the percentile cutoff value.

Compare today's percentile rank with the rank from previous visits to identify any major shifts in the child's growth pattern and the need for further assessment.

When transitioning from the WHO growth charts to the IAP growth charts at aged 5 years, a change in growth classification may occur. During this transition, caution should be used in interpreting any changes in classification.

Anthropometric index	Percentile cut-off values	Nutritional status indicator
WHO and IAP growth charts 3rd and 97th percentiles		
Length-for-age	<3rd percentile >97th percentile	Short stature/stunting Tall for age
Weight-for-age	<3rd percentile	Acute malnutrition
Weight-for-length (height)	<3rd percentile	Wasting-chronic malnutrition
Head circumference	<3rd percentile >97th percentile	Microcephaly Macrocephaly
IAP growth charts 3rd and 97th percentile cut-offs		
BMI-for-age	≥27th percentile (equivalent to 90th percentile of adult chart)	Obesity
BMI-for-age	≥23rd (equivalent to 71st percentile of adult charts)	Overweight
BMI-for-age	<3rd	Underweight

Bibliography

1. American Academy of Pediatrics. Pediatric Nutrition Handbook. 6th ed. Elk Grove Village, IL: American Academy of Pediatrics. 2009;559–564.

2. Vaman Khadilkar, Sangeeta Yadav, KK Agrawal, Suchit Tamboli, Monidipa Banerjee, *Alice Cherian, Jagdish P Goyal, Anuradha Khadilkar, V Kumaravel, V Mohan, D Narayanappa, I Ray and Vijay Yewale. Guidelines: Revised IAP Growth Charts for Height, Weight and Body Mass Index for 5- to 18-year-old Indian Children

3. World Health Organization. Physical Status: The Use and Interpretation of Anthropometry. Geneva: World Health Organization, 1995. WHO Technical Report Series 854.

4. World Health Organization. Training Course on Child Growth Assessment. Geneva, WHO, 2008.

5. World Health Organization. WHO Child Growth Standards: Length/Height-for-Age, Weight-for-Age, Weight-for-Length, Weight-for-Height and Body Mass Index-for-Age: Methods and Development. Geneva: World Health Organization; 2006.

*The WHO and CDC growth charts are available at http://www.cdc.gov/growthcharts/who_charts.htm and http://www.cdc.gov/growthcharts/clinical_charts.htm

Acknowledgements: This chapter has been authored by Dr Abhishek Madhura, Assistant Professor, Paediatric, Government Medical College, Nagpur.